Smart Innovation, Systems and Technologies

Volume 291

The Smart Innovation, Systems and Technologies book series encompasses the topics of knowledge, intelligence, innovation and sustainability. The aim of the series is to make available a platform for the publication of books on all aspects of single and multi-disciplinary research on these themes in order to make the latest results available in a readily-accessible form. Volumes on interdisciplinary research combining two or more of these areas is particularly sought.

The series covers systems and paradigms that employ knowledge and intelligence in a broad sense. Its scope is systems having embedded knowledge and intelligence, which may be applied to the solution of world problems in industry, the environment and the community. It also focusses on the knowledge-transfer methodologies and innovation strategies employed to make this happen effectively. The combination of intelligent systems tools and a broad range of applications introduces a need for a synergy of disciplines from science, technology, business and the humanities. The series will include conference proceedings, edited collections, monographs, handbooks, reference books, and other relevant types of book in areas of science and technology where smart systems and technologies can offer innovative solutions.

High quality content is an essential feature for all book proposals accepted for the series. It is expected that editors of all accepted volumes will ensure that contributions are subjected to an appropriate level of reviewing process and adhere to KES quality principles.

Indexed by SCOPUS, EI Compendex, INSPEC, WTI Frankfurt eG, zbMATH, Japanese Science and Technology Agency (JST), SCImago, DBLP.

All books published in the series are submitted for consideration in Web of Science.

More information about this series at https://link.springer.com/bookseries/8767

Md Atiqur Rahman Ahad · Sozo Inoue ·
Daniel Roggen · Kaori Fujinami
Editors

Sensor- and Video-Based Activity and Behavior Computing

Proceedings of 3rd International Conference on Activity and Behavior Computing (ABC 2021)

Springer

Editors
Md Atiqur Rahman Ahad
University of East London
London, UK

Sozo Inoue
Kyushu Institute of Technology
Fukuoka, Japan

Daniel Roggen
Sussex University
Brighton, UK

Kaori Fujinami
Tokyo University of Agriculture
and Technology
Koganei, Tokyo, Japan

ISSN 2190-3018 ISSN 2190-3026 (electronic)
Smart Innovation, Systems and Technologies
ISBN 978-981-19-0360-1 ISBN 978-981-19-0361-8 (eBook)
https://doi.org/10.1007/978-981-19-0361-8

This Springer imprint is published by the registered company Springer Nature Singapore Pte Ltd.
The registered company address is: 152 Beach Road, #21-01/04 Gateway East, Singapore 189721, Singapore

Organizing Committee

General Chairs

Sozo Inoue, Kyushu Institute of Technology, Kitakyushu, Japan
Md Atiqur Rahman Ahad, University of Dhaka, Dhaka, Bangladesh; Osaka University, Osaka, Japan

Program Chairs

Daniel Roggen, University of Sussex, Sussex, UK
Kaori Fujinami, Tokyo University of Agriculture and Technology, Tokyo, Japan

Preface

Focusing on the vision-based and sensor-based recognition and analysis of human activity and behavior, this book gathers selected papers presented at the 3rd International Conference on Activity and Behavior Computing (ABC 2021), https://abc-research.github.io/, on October 22–23, 2021. The respective chapters cover action recognition, action understanding, behavior analysis, and related areas. The 3rd Activity and Behavior Computing conference aims to be a venue to discuss some of the facets of computing systems, which are able to sense, recognize, and eventually understand human activities, behaviors, and the context within which they occur. This in turn enables a wide range of applications in a large variety of disciplines.

We received 21 submissions. After rigorous review by related top experts (number of reviewers per paper: minimum two to maximum five) and review rebuttal process, nine papers were accepted and included in this book. The process is summarized as follows: "The program chairs along with the general chairs had a rigorous meeting to decide the fate of the papers at the first round. After the rebuttals, another meeting was arranged and the final decisions are made. Even after the final decision, the program committee did a few stages of minor editing for some papers to enrich the quality of the chapters. The resulting selection of papers reflects the broad interests of this nascent community and is important to take stock of the state of the art and continued research challenges in the field." A reviewer had to answer several questions, and hence, the review process was rigorous, e.g., contribution to ABC, decision, what category best fits this paper?, originality, revision requirements, and your level of expertise on this subject.

Human–robot interaction is continuously evolving in industrial context for the betterment of services as well as ease and safety of human lives. Nowadays, we can see increasing collaborative works between humans and robots in almost every industry, from automobile manufacturing to food packaging. Despite the fact that the collaboration is making the overall industrial processes optimized and flexible, activity recognition during these processes is becoming more complex. Furthermore, to improve the interactions between human and robot, it is necessary for the robots to have a better understanding of human behavior and activities.

In recent years, there have been many works on identifying complex human activities and more research focusing on identifying human activities in human–robot collaboration (HRC) scenario. Research in this area can result in building a better system. So, with a goal of recognizing human activities in HRC context, in Bento Packaging Activity Recognition Challenge, we shared a dataset collected in a HRC context. For the dataset collection, we created an environment of Lunch-box (widely known as "Bento" in Japan) packaging on a moving conveyor belt performed by human subjects. The challenge participants were asked to predict the activities of these human subjects during the packaging. Apart from the regular nine papers, seven selected papers for this challenge are included along with the summary of the challenge.

We gladly thank the authors for their contributions and the reviewers for their time to review rigorously. We are thankful to other members and advisors of this conference. There are two keynote speakers who delivered the talks. We are thankful to them:

- Björn W. Schuller, Fellow IEEE (Imperial College London, UK, and University of Augsburg, Germany)—for his talk on "Multimodal Sentiment Analysis: Explore the No Pain, Big Gain Shortcut"; and
- Koichi Kise (Osaka Prefecture University, Japan)—for his talk on "Reading of Reading for Actuating: Augmenting Human Learning by Experiential Supplements".

We are thankful to the 11 panel speakers on the "The Future of Activity and Behavior Computing" and the session chairs for their valuable time. We thank the volunteers and the participants for their efforts to make it a wonderful event.

Finally, this book presents some of the latest researches in the field of activity and behavior computing. We hope that it will serve as a reference for researchers and practitioners in academia and industry related to human activity and behavior computing. We look forward to meet you all in the upcoming International Conference on Activity and Behavior Computing (ABC) in the coming years! Stay safe and stay strong.

Osaka, Japan — Md Atiqur Rahman Ahad
Fukuoka, Japan — Sozo Inoue
Brighton, UK — Daniel Roggen
Tokyo, Japan — Kaori Fujinami

About This Book

Focusing on the vision-based and sensor-based recognition and analysis of human activity and behavior, this book gathers selected papers presented at the 3rd International Conference on Activity and Behavior Computing (ABC 2021), https://abc-research.github.io/, on October 22–23, 2021. The respective chapters cover action recognition, action understanding, behavior analysis, and related areas. Human–robot interaction is continuously evolving in industrial context for the betterment of services as well as ease and safety of human lives. Human–robot collaboration (HRC) is an important area for the future. Hence, with a goal of recognizing human activities in HRC context, a new challenge is thrown in this event called "Bento Packaging Activity Recognition Challenge," where a dataset collected in a HRC context is introduced. For the dataset collection, an environment of Lunch-box (widely known as "Bento" in Japan) packaging on a moving conveyor belt performed by human subjects is created. The challenge participants were asked to predict the activities of these human subjects during the packaging. Selected challenge papers are included in this book. The book addresses various challenges and aspects of human activity recognition in both the sensor-based and vision-based domains, making it a unique guide to the field.

Highlighting Points

- Presents some of the latest researches in the field of activity and behavior computing;
- Gathers extended versions of selected papers presented at 3rd ABC 2021 on October 22–23, 2021;
- Serves as a reference for researchers and practitioners in academia and industry.

Contents

About the Editors

Md Atiqur Rahman Ahad Senior Member of IEEE, Senior Member of OPTICA (formerly the OSA), is a Professor at University of Dhaka (DU), and a Specially Appointed Associate Professor at Osaka University. He studied at the University of Dhaka, University of New South Wales, and Kyushu Institute of Technology. He authored/edited 10+ books, e.g., *IoT-Sensor Based Activity Recognition*; *Motion History Images for Action Recognition and Understanding*; *Computer Vision and Action Recognition.* He published ~200 journals, conference papers, book chapters, ~130 keynote/invited talks, ~40 Awards/Recognitions. He is an Editorial Board Member of *Scientific Reports*, Nature; Associate Editor of *Frontiers in Computer Science*; Editor of *International Journal of Affective Engineering*; Editor-in-Chief: *IJCVSP*; Guest-Editor of *Pattern Recognition Letters*, Elsevier; *JMUI*, Springer; *JHE*; *IJICIC*; Member: ACM, IAPR.

Sozo Inoue Ph.D., is Professor in Kyushu Institute of Technology, Japan. His research interests include human activity recognition with smart phones, and healthcare application of Web/pervasive/ubiquitous systems. Currently he is working on verification studies in real field applications, and collecting and providing a large-scale open dataset for activity recognition, such as a mobile accelerator dataset with about 35,000 activity data from more than 200 subjects, nurses' sensor data combined with 100 patients' sensor data and medical records, and 34 households' light sensor data set for 4 months combined with smart meter data. Inoue has a Ph.D. of Engineering from Kyushu University in 2003. After completion of his degree, he was appointed as Assistant Professor in the Faculty of Information Science and Electrical Engineering at the Kyushu University, Japan. He then moved to the Research Department at the Kyushu University Library in 2006. Since 2009, he is appointed as Associate Professor in the Faculty of Engineering at Kyushu Institute of Technology, Japan, and moved to Graduate School of Life Science and Systems Engineering at Kyushu Institute of Technology in 2018. Meanwhile, he was Guest Professor in Kyushu University, Visiting Professor at Karlsruhe Institute of Technology, Germany, in 2014, Special Researcher at Institute of Systems, Information Technologies and Nanotechnologies (ISIT) during 2015–2016, and Guest Professor at University of

Los Andes in Colombia in 2019. He is Technical Advisor of Team AIBOD Co. Ltd. since 2017, and Guest Researcher at RIKEN Center for Advanced Intelligence Project (AIP) since 2017. He is Member of the IEEE Computer Society, the ACM, the Information Processing Society of Japan (IPSJ), the Institute of Electronics, Information and Communication Engineers (IEICE), the Japan Society for Fuzzy Theory and Intelligent Informatics, the Japan Association for Medical Informatics (JAMI), and the Database Society of Japan (DBSJ).

Daniel Roggen Ph.D., received the master's and Ph.D. degrees from the École Polytechnique Fédérale de Lausanne, Switzerland, in 2001 and 2005, respectively. He is currently Associate Professor with the Sensor Technology Research Centre, University of Sussex, where he leads the Wearable Technologies Laboratory and directs the Sensor Technology Research Centre. His research focuses on wearable and mobile computing, activity and context recognition, and intelligent embedded systems. He has established a number of recognized data sets for human activity recognition from wearable sensors, in particular the OPPORTUNITY dataset. He is Member of Task Force on Intelligent Cyber-Physical Systems of the IEEE Computational Intelligence Society.

Kaori Fujinami Ph.D., received his B.S. and M.S. degrees in electrical engineering and his Ph.D. in computer science from Waseda University, Japan, in 1993, 1995, and 2005, respectively. From 1995 to 2003, he worked for Nippon Telegraph and Telephone Corporation (NTT) and NTT Comware Corporation as Software Engineer and Researcher. From 2005 to 2006, he was visiting Lecturer at Waseda University. From 2007 to 2017, he was Associate Professor at the Department of Computer and Information Sciences at Tokyo University of Agriculture and Technology (TUAT). In 2018, he became Professor at TUAT. His research interests are machine learning, activity recognition, human–computer interaction, and ubiquitous computing. He is Member of IPSJ, IEICE, and IEEE.

Toward the Analysis of Office Workers' Mental Indicators Based on Wearable, Work Activity, and Weather Data

Yusuke Nishimura, Tahera Hossain, Akane Sano, Shota Isomura, Yutaka Arakawa, and Sozo Inoue

Abstract In recent years, many organizations have prioritized efforts to detect and treat mental health issues. In particular, office workers are affected by many stressors, and physical and mental exhaustion, which is also a social problem. To improve the psychological situation in the workplace, we need to clarify the cause. In this paper, we conducted a 14-day experiment to collect wristband sensor data as well as behavioral and psychological questionnaire data from about 100 office workers. We developed machine learning models to predict psychological indexes using the data. In addition, we analyzed the correlation between behavior (work content and work environment) and psychological state of office workers to reveal the relationship between their work content, work environment, and behavior. As a result, we showed that multiple psychological indicators of office workers can be predicted with more than 80% accuracy using wearable sensors, behavioral data, and weather data. Furthermore, we found that in the working environment, the time spent in "web conferencing", "working at home (living room)", and "break time (work time)' had a significant effect on the psychological state of office workers.

Y. Nishimura (✉) · T. Hossain · S. Inoue
Kyushu Institute of Technology, Fukuoka, Japan
e-mail: nishimura@sozolab.jp

T. Hossain
e-mail: tahera@sozolab.jp

S. Inoue
e-mail: sozo@sozolab.jp

A. Sano
Rice University, Houston, TX, USA
e-mail: akane.sano@rice.edu

S. Isomura
NTT Data Institute of Management Consulting, Inc., Tokyo, Japan
e-mail: isomuras@nttdata-strategy.com

Y. Arakawa
Kyushu University, Fukuoka, Japan
e-mail: arakawa@ait.kyushu-u.ac.jp

M. A. R. Ahad et al. (eds.), *Sensor- and Video-Based Activity and Behavior Computing*, Smart Innovation, Systems and Technologies 291,
https://doi.org/10.1007/978-981-19-0361-8_1

1 Introduction

In recent years, research on mental health and well-being has attracted a lot of attention as a way to improve the quality of one's personal and professional life [1, 2]. Smart sensing, machine learning, and data analytics have been rapidly utilized to get new insights into human health, lifestyle, personality, and other human characteristics and behaviors.

It has been studied that many physical and mental disorders appear in a variety of physiological and behavioral manifestations before being diagnosed [3, 4]. If everyday health and well-being can be monitored using ubiquitous sensors, this assessment could help users reflect on their behaviors to prevent severe mental and physical disorders and help clinicians monitor users' conditions and diagnose disorder. In our daily life, work occupies a major part of individuals' days. It is necessary for employees and individuals to design a workplace that impacts them positively in order to enjoy a certain quality of life. Workplace stress, anxiety, and depression are harmful to human health and productivity, with major financial consequences. The number of companies that employ stress assessments to ensure a high-quality work environment has risen by 12% in 2021 compared to 2012 [5]. In addition, the number of companies that use the assessment results has also increased.

There are several reasons why companies should work to improve their employees' mental health. The first reason is the employee retention rate. The past research has shown that work environments with low levels of job satisfaction have higher turnover rates than those with high levels [6, 7]. The second reason is the maintenance of employee health. When people are under high negative psychological stress in the workplace, they are increasing the risk of physical illness as well as mental illness [8]. Well-being is also expected to have a significant impact on work productivity, and a high-well-being level group of individuals tends to perform better than a low-well-being level group of individuals [6, 7]. The majority of these studies rely on self-reported assessments and sensor data acquired passively from smartphones and other wearable devices.

In this research, we collected real-world 2-week data from $N = 100$ office workers engaged in intellectual work to discover knowledge about the impact of their behavior on the psychological measures. The dataset collected in this study consisted of three main types. (1) daily activity data using a Fitbit smartwatch which the subjects continuously wore during the experiment, (2) psychological data from questionnaires. Subjects self-reported their psychological states using their smartphones three times a day, (3) behavioral data self-reported on the smartphone application to record their work activity and environment-related information throughout the experiment. The behavioral data include the type of work tasks as well as the detailed situation when and how the work tasks were performed, such as "with whom", "the type of the work", and "the place where the work was performed". Also, this experiment was conducted while remote work was introduced. Therefore, the data were collected under the condition of working both in the office and at home.

We analyzed the collected data in two ways: (1) We developed prediction models for six psychological indicators of office workers each night and the following morning, and (2) we analyzed the contribution of features and SHAP (SHapley Additive exPlanations) value in the prediction models to analyze the correlation between behavioral data and psychological data. Our results showed that multiple psychological indicators of office workers can be predicted with an accuracy of 80% or more using wearable sensors, behavioral data, and weather data. Furthermore, we found work-related factors that affected the psychological indicators of office workers. For example, among behavioral data, the time spent on "eating", "working alone", "hobbies", "resting", and "traveling" had high effects on the psychological situation. In addition, "with whom the work was done" and "whether the work was standardized" were found to have high effects.

The main contributions of this paper are:

- The real-world office worker multimodal dataset, where the dataset contains objective physiological and behavioral sensor data, and work activities and work environment information with different psychological state information. The dataset depicts the status of real office workers states performing their everyday work under real-life stressors.
- Prediction of different mental states of office workers.
- Correlation analysis between behavior and psychological state of office workers to reveal the factors in the workplace that affect their psychological state.

We expect this dataset and analyses will contribute to design work behavior and environment and eventually improve the performance of employees, the turnover rate, and the solution of the shortage of human resources in the workplace. The remaining part of the paper proceeds as follows. First, Sect. 2, begins by reviewing the related literature on estimating stress, mood, and mental health. Section 3 explains data collection and explanation of data attributes. Section 4 describes the feature extraction of multimodal data, preprocessing, and model building process. Section 5 presents results about prediction models and correlation analysis among different psychological indexes and the behavior of office workers. In Sect. 6, results are discussed and the conclusions drawn are presented with some future work points in Sect. 7.

2 Related Research

Mood, health, and stress are three widely investigated well-being labels. In recent years, research on estimating stress, mood, and mental health indicators using sensor data has become popular [9–11]. Koldijk et al. [12] used a multimodal set of sensor data including computer logs, facial expressions, and posture data using webcam and Kinect, and to detect stress with 90% accuracy. Alberdi et al. [13] predicted stress and workload from ecological data and behavioral data of office workers under real stress factors in smart office environments.

Sano et al. [14] used smartphones, wearable sensors, and survey data to predict student performance, stress, and mental state with a precision of 67–92%. In another study, Li et al. [1] aim to create a deep learning framework that can predict human well-being from raw sensor signals to assist individualized long-term health monitoring and early-warning systems. The proposed framework was tested over a period of 6391 days utilizing wearable sensor data and well-being labels obtained from college students. Robles et al. [15] used log data from smartphones, wearable sensors, and social apps to develop a framework that can predict stress. Studies by Amamori and others estimated survey items related to HRQOL (Health-Related Quality of Life) using sensor data from wristband terminals and positional data from smartphones [16].

On the other hand, many researchers are working to discover workers' physical and mental discomfort experienced as a result of their day-to-day activities, workload, and work environment, which may lead to decreased work performance. Improving employee wellness services for managing these issues is critical, but understanding who requires attention is a prerequisite step toward proactive care. In this regard, Feng et al. [17] examined the impact of irregular work hours on health and showed the significant negative impact on health. According to the findings, night shift nurses were more sedentary and showed lower levels of life satisfaction than day shift nurses. There are many other studies on the psychological analysis of workers. Lee et al. [18] used intelligent worker physiological sensor data to predict the state of concentration at work. Fukuda et al. [19] used wristband wearable sensors to collect sleep data and estimated mood indicators from questionnaire surveys. The classification accuracy was 60–73%, which indicated the contribution of psychological prediction in sleep. In another worker stress study, the accuracy of psychological indicators has reached 71% [20], where, they used smartphones accelerometer sensor data to monitor behavior of subjects with their stress level from self-assessment questionnaire data.

Alexandros et al. [21] used data collected from banded wearable devices and smartphones to predict the mood of workers in an office environment. In this study, they used five levels of prediction for eight different types of moods, and the results were 70.6% for personalized prediction and 62.1% for generalized prediction using the Bagged Ensembles of Decision Trees. Mirjafari et al. [22] differentiated "*Higher*" and "*Lower*" job performers in the workplace. They used mobile sensing, wearable, and beacon data to train a gradient boosting classifier that can classify workers as higher or lower performers. The majority of these studies have relied on self-reported assessments as well as sensor data acquired passively from smartphones and other wearable devices. Table 1 shows the summary information about prior studies that predicted wellness and psychological state using sensor module and other data.

It has been shown that in many early researches passively collected sensor data, biometric sensor data, images, self-reported data, and acceleration data often aim to improve stress and mood recognition of office workers and students [25, 26], but few studies have used the type of person's behavior as an explanatory variable [13, 15, 16, 21, 22, 27]. There are also many studies that estimate mood and stress, but few studies have estimated fatigue, productivity, work engagement, and work

Table 1 A summary of previous studies for predicting wellness and psychological state

Research target	Participants (N)	Sensors/Module	Data used
Understanding how daily behaviors and social networks influence self-reported stress, mood, and other health or well-being-related factors [23]	University students, $N = 201$	Wrist-based sensors electronic diaries (e-diaries)	Questionnaires data acceleration and ambient light data
Differentiating higher and lower job performers in the workplace [22]	Working professionals, $N = 554$	Smartphones (i.e., Android and iOS), wearables (i.e., Garmin vivosmart) and Bluetooth beacon	Mobile sensing and daily survey data
Forecasting personalized mood, health, and stress [1]	College students, $N = 239$	Wearable sensor and self-report assessments	Skin temperature, skin conductance, and acceleration; self-reported mood, health, and stress scored
Multimodal analysis of physical activity, sleep, and work shift in nurses with wearable sensor data [17]	Nurses in a large hospital, $N = 113$	Fitbit, self-reported assessments of affect and life satisfaction	Sleep pattern data from Fitbit, demographic data
Detecting affective flow states of knowledge workers using physiological sensors [18]	Industrial research lab professionals, $N = 12$	Physiological sensors, webcam-based techniques for measuring a worker's pulse, respiration, affect, or alertness	Sensors and webcam data collected in a controlled lab setting
Using smart offices to predict occupational stress [13]	Office workers, $N = 25$	Mobi (TMSI) sensors with self-adhesive electrodes for ECG and skin conductance level (SCL)	Heart rate (HR), heart rate variability (HRV), SCL, self-reported stress and mental workload scores
Forecasting depressed mood based on self-reported histories via recurrent neural networks [24]	Random participants using the application from apps store, $N = 2382$	Smartphone application called "Utsureko" for collecting data from users	Self-reported historical data of mood, behavior log and sleeping log
Forecasting stress, mood, and health from daytime physiology in office workers and students [25]	Employees at a high-tech company in Japan and college students, $N = 240$	Skin conductance, skin temperature, and acceleration from a wrist sensor	Self-reported data and wrist sensor data

(continued)

Table 1 (continued)

Research target	Participants (N)	Sensors/Module	Data used
Understanding a relationship between stress and individual's work role [26]	Volunteers working in a research division of a large corporation, $N = 40$	Physiological data were collected from a heart rate monitor worn around the chest and a Fitbit	Cardiovascular data, multiple daily self-reports of momentary affect, and filled out a one-time assessment of the global perceived stress data
Mood recognition at work using smartphones and wearable sensors [21]	Recruited 4 users (researchers) to take part in this study which was conducted in an office environment, $N = 4$	Toshiba Silmee wristband sensor and smartphone app "HealthyOffice" to collect self-reporting data	Heart rate, pulse rate, skin temperature, 3-axial acceleration, and self-reported data

self-evaluation, etc., which are important for the performance of office workers by the same explanatory variable. Although several studies have been conducted to estimate psychological indicators based on data from working, there are few cases where people working for companies are tested as subjects, and it was difficult to collect data in actual workplaces. There are few studies that have focused on the analysis of the work environment during work behavior, and there have been few analyses that take into account where workers work, the people they work with, and the work environment.

Based on the above, this paper aims to analyze the psychological state of office workers to reveal the relationship between their psychological states and their work content, work environment, and behavior by using sensor data, self-reported time-series work task/environment data, and psychological index data together. The data collected in this research depict the behaviors of real office workers performing their natural office work under real-life stressors. We believe that this will contribute to the development of tools for improving the occupational health of office workers. This study will be also expected to help find knowledge to improve working methods by revealing the relationship between psychological indicators and behavior.

3 Data Overview

This experiment was led by NTT Data Management Institute and conducted to collect data from several companies that cooperated with the project. Sixty-three male and 37 female workers with an average age of 42.1 years participated in a 14-days data collection experiment in January 2021. The data collected in this experiment included sensor data, self-reported work task/environment data, weather data, and psychological index data obtained from questionnaires.

3.1 Sensor Data

The sensor data were collected using a wristband sensor, Fitbit [28]. Fitbit data included data on calorie consumption, heart rate, sleep characteristics, metabolic equivalent, step count, floor count, and activity characteristics. Heart rate was measured every 5 s, and all other Fitbit data were measured every minute.

3.2 Work Task/Environment Data

In order to collect behavioral data and questionnaire data, we used a nursing care behavior recording application fonlog [29] developed by Inoue and others for office workers. Behavioral data were collected by labeling the participants' behavior of what kind and what time they were doing. Participants provided an average of 9.1 behavioral labels per day. Table 2 shows the questionnaire items related to work. The types of behavioral labels are as follows: face-to-face meetings, meals, single work, hobby/break, housework/child-rearing, rest (during business hours), travel, web meetings, collaboration (with the communication), telephone (meetings), and non-business work. In particular, activities in the work were recorded not only by entering the type but also details of the task and the environment in which the task was performed also recorded.

3.3 Psychological Measures

In the questionnaire on psychological conditions, six indicators were used to evaluate the results.

- Depression and Anxiety Mood Scale (DAMS) [30]
  DAMS questions to evaluate each strength in 7 stages with respect to positive mood, depressive mood, and anxiety mood (9 questions). Therefore, each score is a value between 0 and 6. Each of the DAMS scores has been shown to be highly suitable for the study of cognitive-behavioral models that include both depression and anxiety, as they can sensitively capture changes in mood. Positive mood is the average of degree of "vivid", "happy", and "fun". Depressive mood is average of the degree of "gloomy", "Unpleasant", and "Sinking". Anxiety mood is average of the degree of "worried", "anxious", and "concerned".
- Subjective Pain [31]
  Subjective pain is a questionnaire that evaluates the type and degree of fatigue an individual is aware of. There are five questions each about sleepiness, discomfort, and lethargy, and each item is rated on a five-point scale, and the average of these scores is used as the score. Each score is a value between 0 and 4 (15 questions).

Table 2 Types of records and their values related to task description and work environment

Activities	Records	Values
Work tasks	Task description	Planning task
		Development task
		Sales task
		Management task
		Field task
		Office task
	Scope of the work	Core task
		Non-core task
	Novelty of the work	Standardized task
		Non-standardized task
	Position in the work	Managers
		Operators and participants
		Collaborators
		Managers and operators
Work environment	Work environment	Home (place for work)
		Home (living)
		Home (other)
		Workspace (outside)
		Store and outside
		Work place
	Task situation	Alone
		With others (no interaction)
		With others (colleagues)
		With others (family)
	Work environment assessment	Very comfortable
		Comfortable
		Neither
		Uncomfortable
		Extremely uncomfortable

- Recovery Experience [32]
  Recovery experience is a questionnaire to evaluate how an individual recovers from work in leisure time. The average score for each question is the average score for each question in the seven-step evaluation for "psychological distance to work", "relaxed", "learned new things", and "decided what to do by myself". Each score is a value between 0 and 6 (4 questions).
- Work Engagement [8]
  Work engagement questions assess how enthusiastic an individual is about their work. One question each on "vitality", "enthusiasm" and "immersion" in work

and the average of the seven steps is used as the work engagement score Each score is a value between 0 and 6 (3 questions).

- Productivity [33]
  Health and labor performance questions designed by the World Health Organization. The score is the self-assessment of the overall performance of the day. Each score is a value between 0 and 6.
- Evaluation of the Work
  Questions for participants to self-evaluate their work for the day. The score is based on a five-point scale for the following questions. Each score is a value between 0 and 4 (7 questions). (1) "I was able to concentrate on my work", (2) "I was able to work efficiently", (3) "I was able to work on schedule", (4) "I was able to communicate well with the people involved", (5) "I was able to communicate efficiently with the people involved", (6) "I was able to come up with new ideas", (7) "I was able to achieve results".

4 Methods

In this section, we describe the analysis methodology, starting with the feature extraction and preprocessing of sensor data, behavioral data, and questionnaire data separately, followed by a modeling approach.

4.1 Preprocessing and Feature Extraction

4.1.1 Sensor Data

The wristband device recorded calories burned, sleep characteristics, metabolic equivalents, the number of steps, the number of floors, and activity characteristics every minute, and heart rate every 10 s. All of these data were aggregated for each day for each participant. We used the mean, variance, and median values for each sensor over the course of a day as features. However, since the time of day for sleep was limited, data from 0:00 to 8:00 were aggregated. In the sleep data, the sleep state was expressed in three levels (awake, deep sleep, and light sleep state) so the sleep time for each sleep stage was aggregated.

4.1.2 Behavioral Data

Behavioral data are the types and functions of work tasks labels described in Sect. 3. The data were aggregated on a daily basis for each participant, and the value indicated the duration of the action in minutes. If the action was not performed, the value 0 (minutes) was entered.

4.1.3 Weather and Other Data

For the explanatory variables, in addition to the sensor data and behavioral data collected in the experiment, we added weather data, day of the week, and participant information for prediction models. Weather information is important not only because it directly affects people's psychology, but also because it affects when participants exercise and study [34]. Weather data were collected from the Japan Meteorological Agency's website based on the participant's residential area. The data were aggregated for each day, and the features below were computed: Average temperature, maximum temperature, minimum temperature, precipitation, sunshine duration, average wind speed, maximum wind speed, average pressure, and cloud cover. The participant information included age and gender.

4.1.4 Questionnaire Data

Each psychological index was scored for each questionnaire. The scoring method for each psychological indicator is shown in Sect. 3.3. The scores were computed in different ways for each psychological indicator and were continuous values. We considered the two classes of data, which were the lower 40% and the upper 40%, because we designed binary classification of each psychological trend which was either high or low. The data in the intermediate 20% bins were deleted. This labeling method was based on [34]. Figure 1 shows the histogram of the psychological indices of "DAMS" and "Subjective Pain" collected from the morning questionnaire, and Fig. 2 shows the histogram of the psychological indices of "DAMS", "Subjective Pain", "Recovery Experience", and "Recovery Experience" collected from the weekday evening questionnaire. The blue dotted lines on the histogram represent the 40th percentile and the red dotted lines represent the 60th percentile. Therefore, the values below the blue dotted line are the lower label and the values above the red dotted line were the upper label. The histogram without the blue dotted line shows the same value for the 40th percentile and the 60th percentile. For those indicators, the mental score $\geq$ 60 percentile was used as the upper label and the others as the lower label.

4.2 Model Development

For model development, we use the same day's all explanatory data when we detect the evening questionnaire and we use the previous day's explanatory data when we detect the morning questionnaire. LightGBM (Light Gradient Boosting Machine) was employed as the classification model. LightGBM is a tree-based learning framework for gradient boosting. It has been created to be distributed and efficient, with a faster training speed and greater efficiency. This learning model use Gradient Boosting Decision Tree (GBDT), which is a model using Gradient-based One-Side Sam-

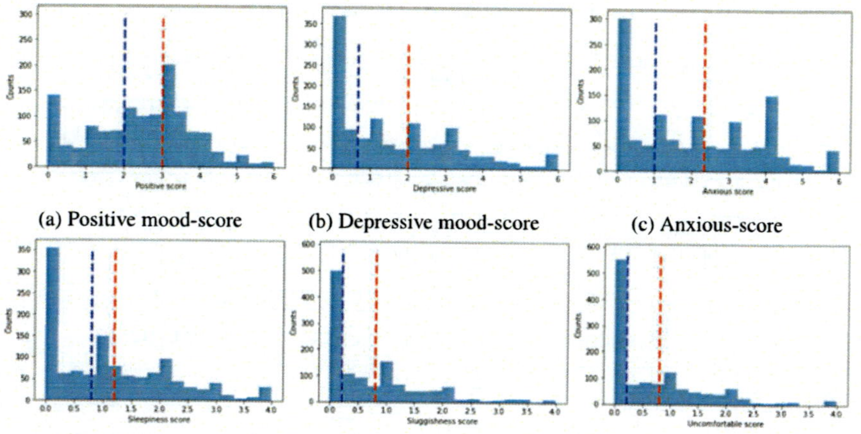

(a) Positive mood-score (b) Depressive mood-score (c) Anxious-score

(d) Sleepiness-score (e) Sluggishness-score (f) Uncounfortable-score

Fig. 1 Histograms show the distributions of scores on psychological indicators from the morning questionnaire. The blue dotted line indicates the 40th percentile of each psychological score, and the red dotted line indicates the 60th percentile of each psychological score (y-axis: data counts, x-axis: score for each indicator)

pling (GOSS) and Exclusive Feature Bundling (EFB) in comparison with the conventional GBDT model [35]. This mechanism enables accurate estimation of small amount of data and it is a suitable algorithm for handling sparse data. Hyperparameters for each classification model were set using grid search. The model was evaluated by fivefold cross-validation. The dataset was randomly divided into five parts, four of which were used as training data and one as validation data. We repeated the process five times and evaluated the average of the five times.

4.3 Gini Index

We can analyze how much the feature selection contributes to the classification of the target using the Gini index. First, to calculate the Gini index, we calculate the Gini impurity. The Gini impurity is expressed by the following Eq. 1, and is a measure of how poorly a target is classified. $G(k)$: Impurity at a given node k, n: Number of target labels, $p(i)$: frequency of target label i at some node k

$$G(k) = \sum_{i=1}^{n} p(i) \times (1 - p(i)) \tag{1}$$

The Gini importance is calculated based on the Gini impurity. This index shows "how much the Gini impurity can be reduced by dividing by a certain feature".

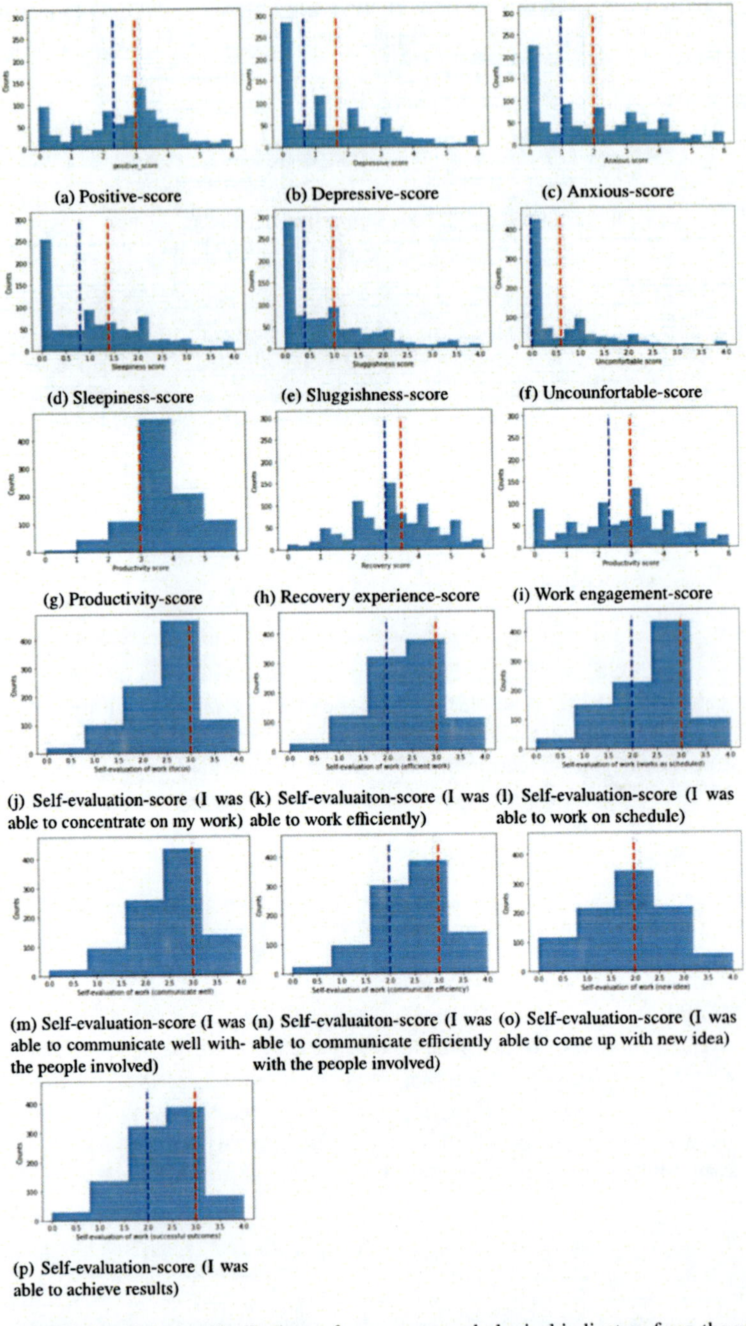

(a) Positive-score (b) Depressive-score (c) Anxious-score

(d) Sleepiness-score (e) Sluggishness-score (f) Uncounfortable-score

(g) Productivity-score (h) Recovery experience-score (i) Work engagement-score

(j) Self-evaluation-score (I was able to concentrate on my work) (k) Self-evaluaiton-score (I was able to work efficiently) (l) Self-evaluation-score (I was able to work on schedule)

(m) Self-evaluation-score (I was able to communicate well with- the people involved) (n) Self-evaluaiton-score (I was able to communicate efficiently with the people involved) (o) Self-evaluation-score (I was able to come up with new idea)

(p) Self-evaluation-score (I was able to achieve results)

Fig. 2 Histograms show the distributions of scores on psychological indicators from the weekday evening questionnaire. The blue dotted line indicates the 40th percentile of each psychological score, and the red dotted line indicates the 60th percentile of each psychological score (y-axis: data counts, x-axis: score for each indicator)

The importance of a feature j is defined by Eq. 2 below. $F(j)$: The set of nodes into which a feature j is to be split, N_{parent}: Samples counts at a node i, $N_{\text{leftchild}}$, $N_{\text{rightchild}}$: Samples counts on the left (right) side among the child nodes of a node N_{parent}: Gini impurity at a given node i, $G_{\text{leftchild}}$, $G_{\text{rightchild}}$: Gini impurity at the left (right)-hand side of the child nodes of a node i.

$$
\begin{aligned}
I(k) = \sum_{i=1}^{n \in F(j)} &(N_{\text{parent}}(i) \times G_{\text{parent}}(i)) - (N_{\text{leftchild}}(i) \times G_{\text{leftchild}}(i) \\
&+ N_{\text{rightchild}}(i) \times G_{\text{rightchild}}(i))
\end{aligned}
\quad (2)
$$

In this study, we used Gini importance as the feature importance. Gini importance is a feature importance used in decision tree models and is the weighted sum of the reduction in impurity of a node averaged over the entire decision tree. It is a measure of how much the impurity of a node is improved by using that feature.

4.4 SHAP Value Analysis and Comparison

It is important to interpret how the machine learning model makes its decisions in mental health prediction because it allows us to understand how each feature affects the participant's mental health. To interpret the model, several studies have begun to use SHAP (SHapley Additive exPlanations) [36, 37]. SHAP values are the contribution of each feature as determined by cooperative game theory [38]. The importance of a feature can be defined as the increase in the prediction error of the model after permuting the values of the feature. Thus, a feature can be considered important if its error increases after permuting it. If changing its value does not change the error, it is unimportant because the model is ignoring the feature in its decision. This method allows us to quantify the contribution of a feature, and its consistency in the classification prediction task has been demonstrated [39]. We analyzed the relationship between the explanatory and target variables by interpreting the model predicting the psychological indicators using their SHAP values. The SHAP values give an idea of the additivity of the features to the explanatory variables. It shows how much each feature positively or negatively affects the model. Specifically, we examined the relationship between office workers' behavior and their psychological state, as well as workplace factors that influence their mental health. Furthermore, we analyze work-related factors that affect the psychological indicators of office workers. For example, in terms of behavioral states, we analyzed if the time spent on "face to face meetings", "eating", "working alone", "hobbies", "resting", "traveling", "web conference", "collaborative work" and other behavioral affect the different psychological state, e.g., positive mood (morning and night), depressive mood (morning and night), and anxious mood (morning and night). In addition, "with whom the work was done" and "whether the work was standardized" were also analyzed with the different psychological states.

5 Results

We present the results from three analyses: (1) data statistics, (2) psychological index prediction performance, and (3) contributions of participants' work tasks and environment to their psychological measures: positive mood, depressive mood, and anxiety mood of the DAMS questionnaire described in Sect. 3.

5.1 *Data Statistics*

Figure 3 shows data statistics by age, gender, type of behavior, and questionnaire for the collected data. We have different work tasks (Fig. 3c), such as working alone, working via web conferencing, collaborative work, mealtime, hobbies, and so on. Working alone was the most frequent behavior label. Figure 4, represents data attributes based on work task details and work environment. Figure 4a and b are the representation of core or non-core work as well as standardized and non-standardized work. Figure 4c shows types of tasks in the office for example, office tasks, development tasks, planning tasks, manager tasks, etc. The histogram of the participants' workplaces is shown in Fig. 4d. Because these data were collected during the COVID-19 pandemic time, more data were collected at home, not in an office. Similarly, Fig. 4e depicts data counts based on the participants' roles in tasks, while Fig. 4f depicts data counts about whom the participants worked with. Our data show that the distributions of age and gender are not uniform. The participants were randomly selected, and we believe that the distributions match ones of workers who perform office work in a realistic manufacturer IT company. As seen in Fig. 4, there was imbalance in the amount of data for each task type and environment. We believe that these are also imbalances that could be expected in the real world. For example, as shown in (a), the number of core tasks was probably much higher than the number of non-core tasks, and it is easy to imagine that many office workers work alone. In addition, since the values of each data used in this study are based on the working hours worked for each variable, we believe that the difference in the amount of data between each feature is not a problem in this analysis.

5.2 *Analysis 1: Predictive Results of Psychological Indicators*

In this section, we show the results of classification prediction for each questionnaire data in binary class as shown in Sect. 4.2. For the morning questionnaire prediction, the data collected on the previous day were used for the explanatory variables, and the data collected from the night of the previous day to the morning of the previous day were used only for the sleep features.

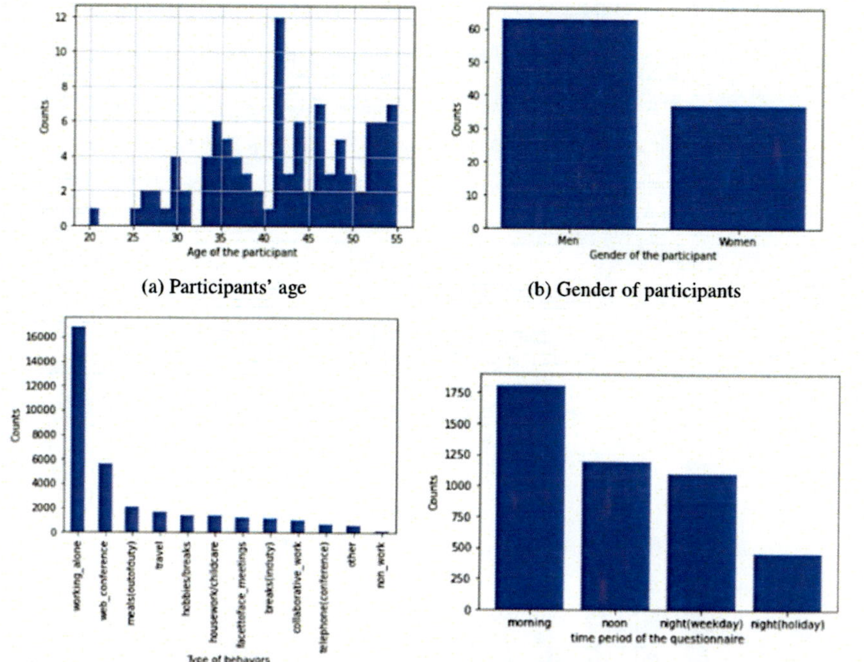

(a) Participants' age

(b) Gender of participants

(c) Behavior Labels

(d) Questionnaires filled out at different time period of the day

Fig. 3 Histograms of data collected in the experiment

The performance evaluation of the classifier was performed using Accuracy and F_1 Score. The prediction results are shown with all 75 feature values (Work task related features: 40, Participant-related features: 2, Weather: 9, Sensors: 24) as the target variables first. Then, features were selected and the result was shown with 22 target variables as we predicted 6 mental indicators on the morning questionnaire and 16 mental indicators on the evening questionnaire. The benefits of prediction with feature selection include (1) it is possible to eliminate the number of features which becomes noise and improve prediction accuracy, (2) it reduces the memory and time required for learning.

In order to see how much behavioral data, weather data, and sensor data each contribute to the prediction, we showed the prediction of positive mood index using only a single modal of data in Table 3. For example, we first used only sensor data, then work data (behavior data), and afterward we used weather data to predict positive mood. The confusion matrix is also shown in Fig. 5.

The predicted results for the morning questionnaire are shown in Table 4, and the predicted results for the evening questionnaire are shown in Table 5, where all the data collected in this study were used as input. Comparing Tables 3, 4, and 5, we can see that each type of data contributes to the prediction, and the prediction accuracy improved when multiple data were used at the same time.

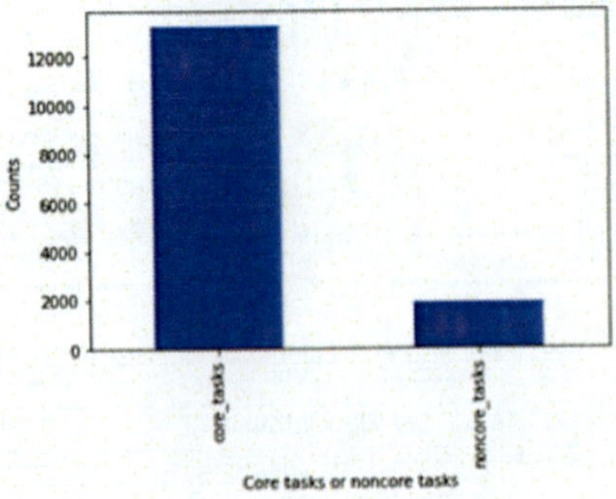

(a) Core task vs non-core tasks

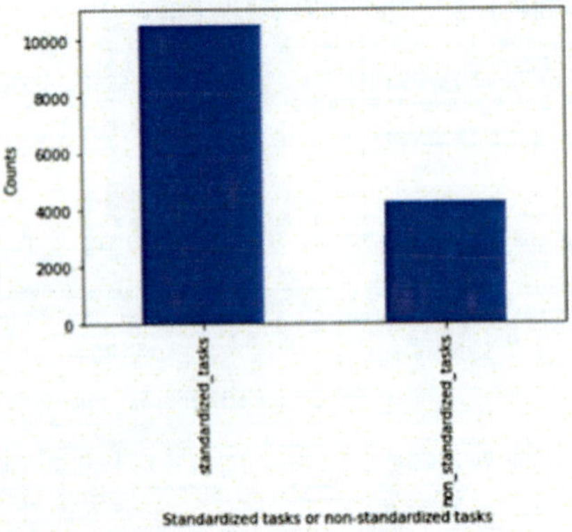

(b) Standardized vs non-standardized tasks

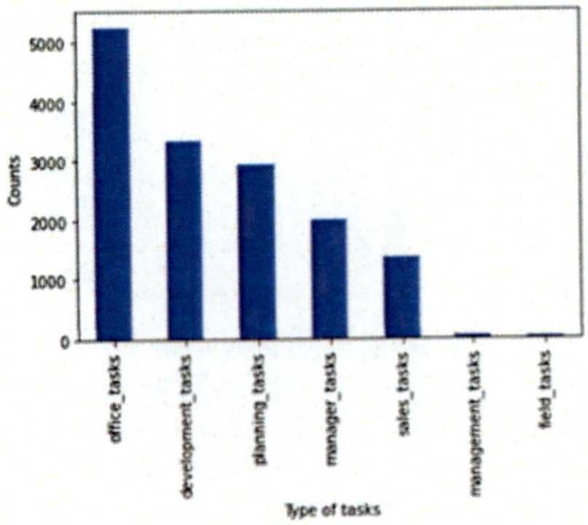

(c) Participant's task types

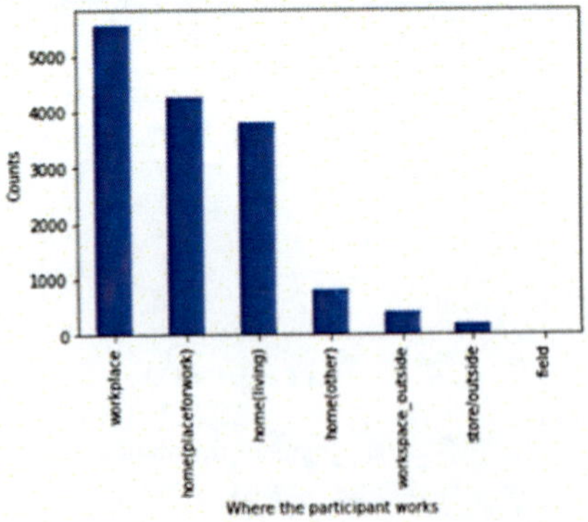

(d) Location of participants' work

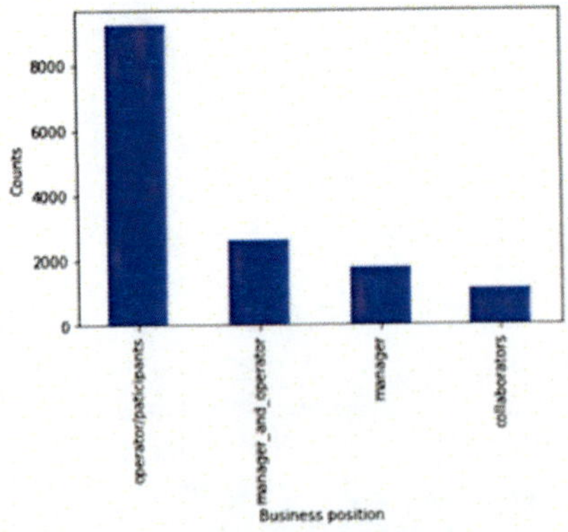

(e) Participants' business positions

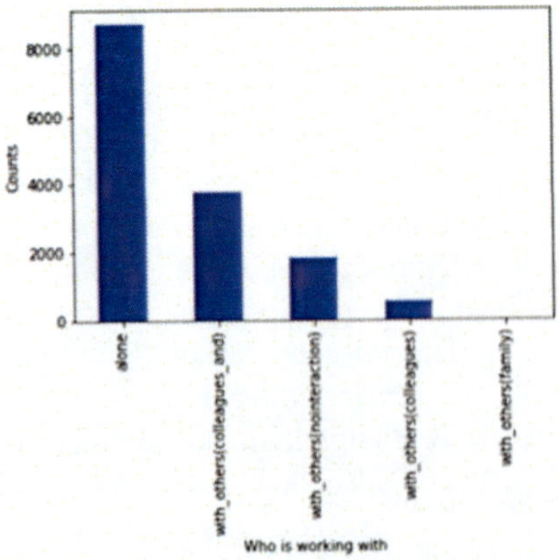

(f) Work collaborators

Fig. 4 Work details and environment

Table 3 Morning questionnaire prediction results with single modal data

Mental indicators	Objective variable	Type of data	Accuracy (%)	F_1 score (%)
DAMS	Positive mood	Behavior data	77.2	81.2
		Weather data	71.0	75.2
		Sensor data	75.2	80.0

Table 4 Morning questionnaire prediction results with all data as the target variable on the left

Mental indicators	Objective variable	Accuracy	F_1 score
DAMS	Positive mood	82.5%/83.9%	86.2%/87.2%
	Depressed mood	87.1%/88.1%	86.2%/87.2%
	Anxious mood	86.0%/89.0%	85.7%/88.7%
Subjective pain	Sleepiness	84.9%/86.3%	84.9%/86.2%
	Uncomfortable	87.1%/88.4%	86.4%/87.8%
	Sluggishness	84.6%/85.3%	82.4%/83.2%

Prediction accuracy with all data as a target variable, right side features selection. Prediction accuracy with 30 data as target variables

Table 5 Evening questionnaire prediction results with all data as a target variable

Mental indicators	Objective variable	Accuracy	F_1 score
DAMS	Positive mood	72.1%/72.1%	83.8%/83.8%
	Depressed mood	85.9%/86.8%	87.8%/88.4%
	Anxious mood	83.8%/85.0%	88.4%/89.1%
Subjective pain	Sleepiness	76.8%/77.2%	72.4%/72.1%
	Uncomfortable	83.2%/82.7%	76.1%/74.7%
	Sluggishness	81.4%/82.9%	75.6%/78.0%
Productivity	Mean score	80.3%/80.3%	79.2%/79.2%
Recovery experience	Mean score	80.4%/79.7%	80.4%/79.6%
Work engagement	Mean score	79.5%/79.4%	84.1%/84.6%
Self-evaluation of work	(1)	81.3%/81.1%	75.6%/74.5%
	(2)	82.6%/83.3%	86.2%/87.1%
	(3)	80.2%/81.5%	82.5%/83.6%
	(4)	82.3%/81.8%	85.4%/85.2%
	(5)	80.2%/81.8%	82.0%/85.2%
	(6)	80.3%/80.2%	86.3%/86.5%
	(7)	80.2%/79.7%	86.5%/81.4%

On the left side is the prediction accuracy with all data as the target variable, and on the right side is the prediction accuracy with 30 data as the target variable by feature quantity selection

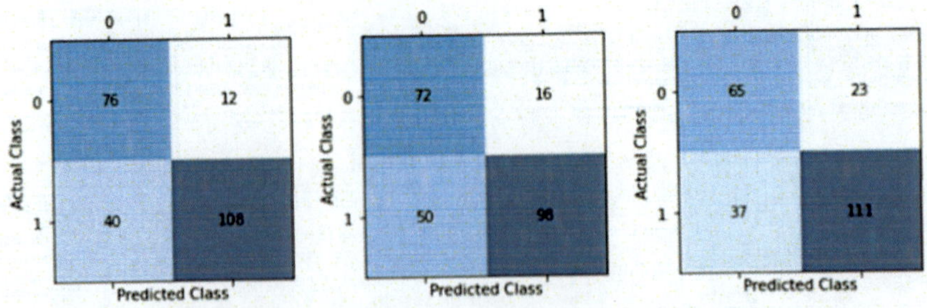

(a) Confusion matrix for predicting morning positive mood using only behavior data

(b) Confusion matrix for predicting positive morning mood using only weather data.

(c) Confusion matrix for predicting morning positive mood using only sensor data.

Fig. 5 Confusion matrix for predicting positive mood in the morning using various data

5.3 *Analysis 2: Relationship Between Psychological Indicators and Behavior*

In this study, we aim to clarify the relationship between each psychological index and the behavior of office workers. In this section, we predicted participants' mood by using behavioral data as a target variable and showed the relationship between data from the SHAP value and feature importance. The correlation between the work data and the psychological data may not have been correctly analyzed because age and gender acted as confounding factors. Therefore, only the work data and psychological data were used for Analysis 2. We built a machine learning model to predict morning and weekday night DAMS in order to calculate and analyze SHAP values. Since DAMS has three indices for "positive mood", "depressed mood", and "anxious mood", we made a total of six predictions.

In Fig. 6a and b, we showed which variables contributed to the prediction by visualizing the importance of the variables in predicting each psychological indicator. Figure 6a shows the variable importance in the prediction of the explanatory variables for the types of behaviors, where the y-axis shows the respective explanatory variables and the x-axis shows the objective variables. The variable importance was normalized for each objective variable, and the higher the value, the higher the importance and the darker the color of the heat map. Therefore, it is easy to see the importance of each explanatory variable in the prediction. Figure 6b shows results about feature importance analysis using behavioral details as explanatory variables, and shows the same heatmap of variable importance as in Fig. 6a.

Next, in order to understand the contribution and correlation of each explanatory variable to the prediction, summary plots were used to show SHAP Value as a one-axis scatter diagram for each feature quantity. Figure 7 shows a scatter chart of SHAP Value when the type of behavior of the participant was used as an explanatory variable. The features on the vertical axis were sorted by the mean absolute value of the SHAP values. Each plot shows the SHAP values, and the color indicates the

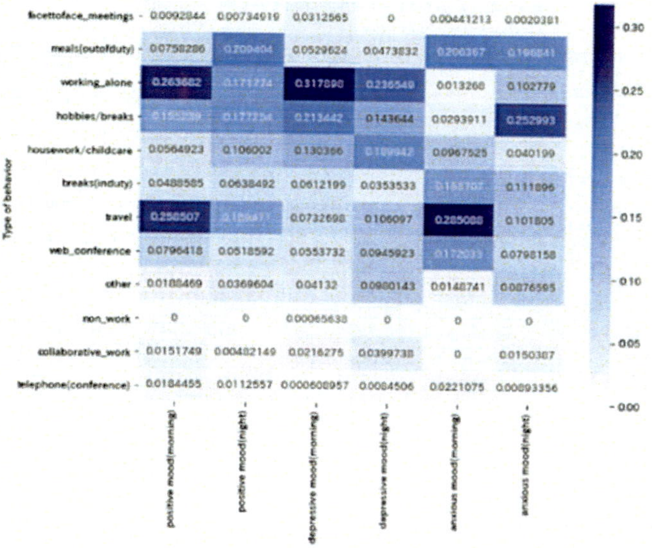

(a) Feature importance analysis for the type of behavior

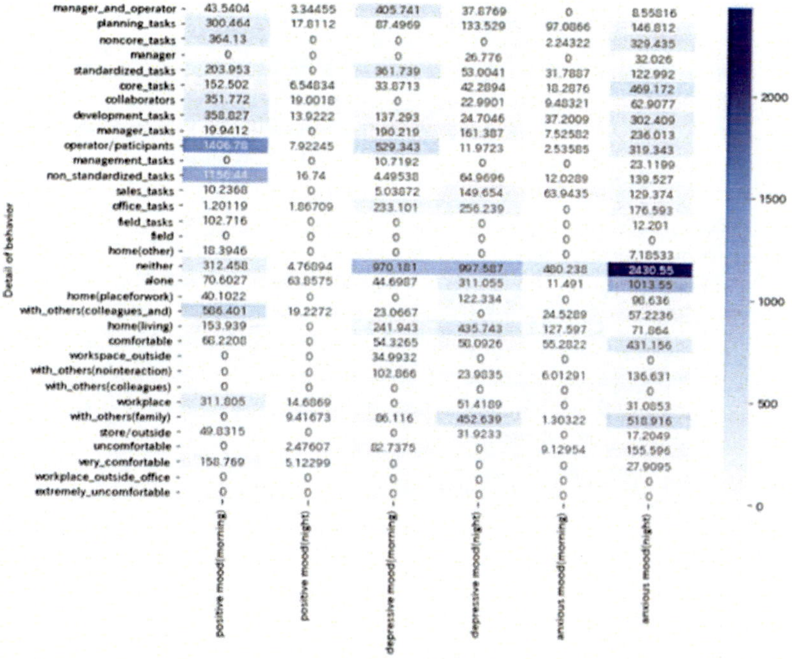

(b) Feature importance analysis with environment and details of behavior.

Fig. 6 The importance of each variable was calculated using the Gini importance. Each value was a normalized value for each classification model (Y-axis: feature used for prediction, x-axis: target variable to predict) magnitude of the feature value (blue is low, red is high). In other words, the farther the plot was from zero, the more influence it had on the inference. The features on the vertical axis were sorted by the mean absolute value of the SHAP values. By observing the color and distribution of the points, we can interpret how features affect the output. This analysis targets only continuous values of features. For example, in Fig. 7a, we observed that "participants/operator" was at the top of the list because it showed the highest average SHAP value. Also, we can see that there are many red plots in the negative direction far from 0, and many blue plots in the positive direction near 0. Therefore, the higher the value of "operator/participants", the more it influences the model in the negative direction (lower psychological score). A low SHAP value was also observed for a low "operator/participants" value that affected the model in a positive direction (higher psychological score).

6 Discussion

6.1 Discussion for Analysis 1

The prediction accuracy scores for all psychological indicators were 72–89%, which was a stable and high accuracy overall. In our findings, the prediction results for subjective pain in the night survey were lower than the prediction results for the morning survey. We believe that this may be because it takes time for a person's behavior to affect subjective pain. The pain level for the morning questionnaire was predicted based on the previous day's behavior, and the one for the night questionnaire was predicted based on the behavior of the day. Therefore, we consider that subjective pain may be more strongly influenced by the behavior of the previous day than by the behavior of the day itself. In addition, the importance of each feature amount for behavior, weather, and sensor data was found to be higher and contributing to prediction for all psychological indicators. Therefore, it is expected that better prediction accuracy can be expected if the model is made with the user's personal consideration.

Each psychological score was divided into the low and high classes using top and bottom 40% of the data, but if many of the scores distributed around the 40% boundary, the balance of the classes may be skewed: for example, the ratio of low and high score classes for morning mood was positive (57:43), depressed (51:49), and anxious (51:49). This imbalance in the data may have some effect on the accuracy, but it was not expected to be significant.

6.2 Discussion for Analysis 2

The correlation between behavior and psychological state of office workers and the factors in the workplace that affected the psychological states of office workers

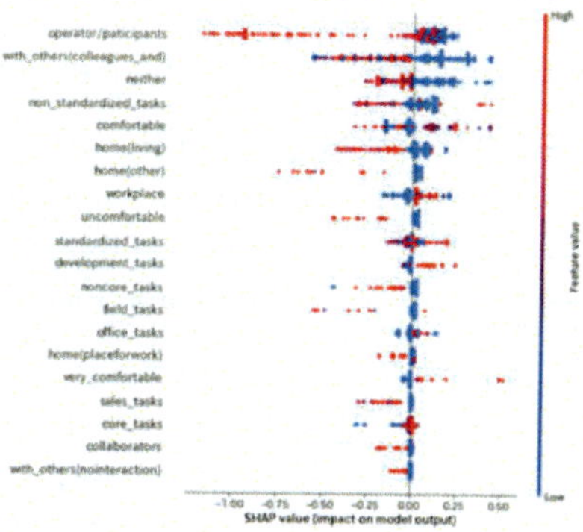

(a) positive mood prediction from the morning questionnaire

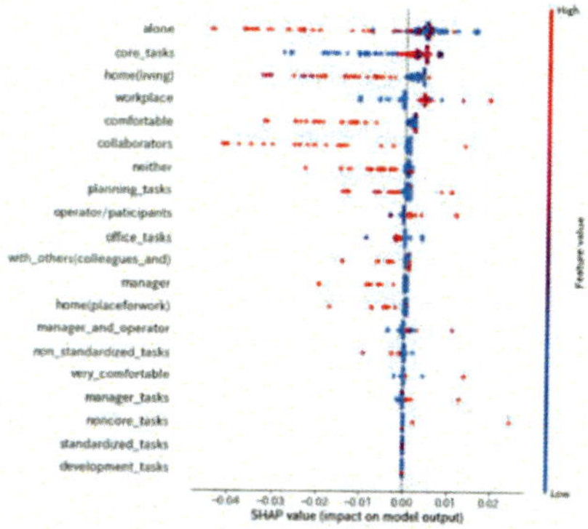

(b) positive mood prediction from the night questionnaire

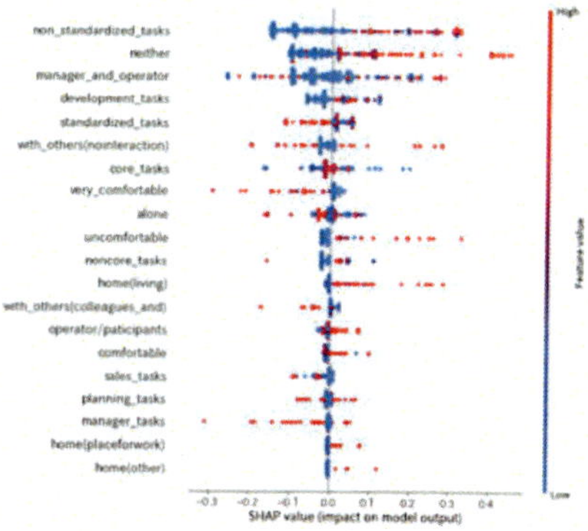

(c) depressive mood prediction from the morning questionnaire

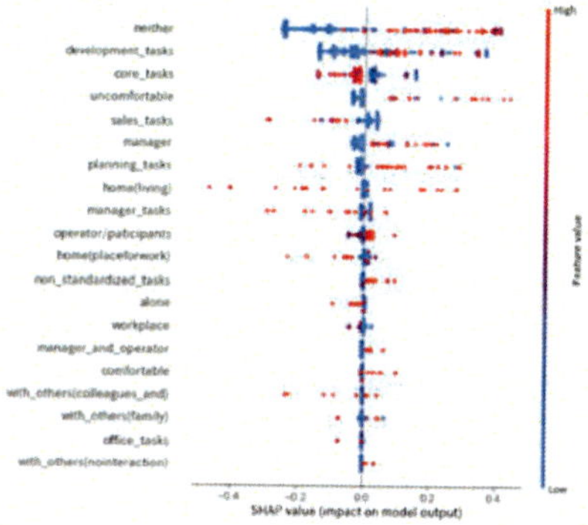

(d) depressive mood prediction from the night questionnaire

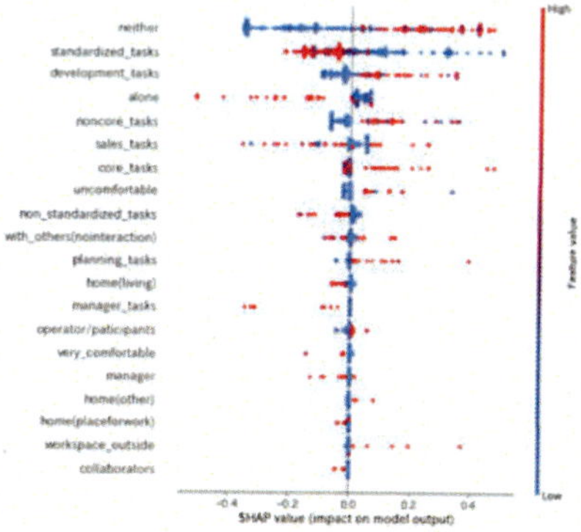

(e) anxious mood prediction from the morning questionnaire

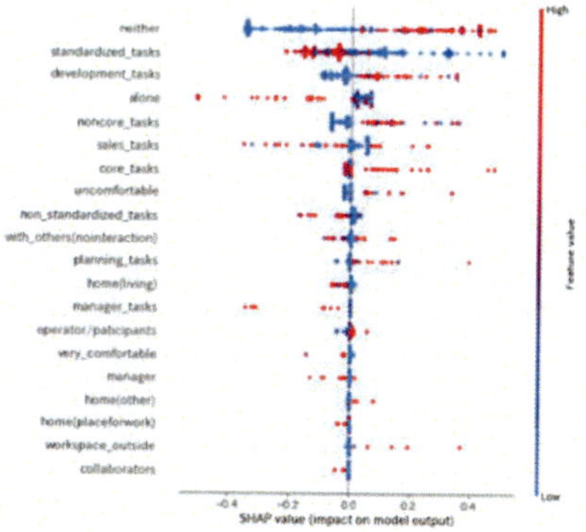

(f) anxious mood prediction from the night questionnaire

Fig. 7 Summary plots for predictive classification of positive mood, depressed mood, and anxious mood with work task details and environmental data as explanatory variables were investigated in this paper. Figure 6a, b depicted the importance of variables in predicting the DAMS score using the type of behavior and detailed data with the time of the behavior as explanatory variables. They were computed using the Gini coefficient for the classification model was trained. They were normalized for each prediction. In terms of behavioral features, the time spent on "meals", "working alone", "hobbies", "break", and "traveling" had a high effect on the psychological situation. For example, if we check working_alone behavior in Fig. 6 and its corresponding values for psychological states, then we can see that this behavior triggered depressive mood in the morning and depressive mood at night. In addition, "with whom the work was done" and "whether the work was standardized" were found to have high effects in psychological states. In addition, the relationship between each psychological index and the explanatory variable can be found in Fig. 7. In the relationship with DAMS, positive mood and depressive mood was related to features in the morning and at night. For example, positive mood was related to "independent work", "hobby/break", "movement", and depression mood was related to "independent work", "hobby/break", "housework/child-rearing". In Fig. 7c–f, the contribution of "neither" feature for the work environment comfort evaluation was high in the work content, and all of them showed positive correlation with negative mood. Participants who answered "neither" in the work environment showed a high tendency to be depressed but were accustomed to spend more time on the work. This result suggests that the amount of time spent at work may have more significant effects on the state of mood than the quality of the work environment. Negative correlations were seen with the morning depression and the morning and night anxiety. This shows that the standardized nature of work tasks has a strong influence on the anxiety and depressive psychology of employees, and the more standardized it was, the less psychological burden they had.

Regarding the work environment in telework situations, from Fig. 7a and c, there was a negative correlation between "home (living)" and positive mood at night, and there was a positive correlation with morning depression. In other words, the work environment at home also showed a strong psychological impact, and workplaces such as living tended to be prone to depression.

Using the summary plots, we also analyzed the type of work behavior and found that "web conferencing" showed a negative correlation with positive mood and a positive correlation with depressive mood. In other words, if the time of web conferencing was long, there was a high possibility that it would negatively affect the psychological state of office workers.

In the previous study [18], it was shown that subjects tended to maintain a high level of concentration when the tasks they performed were standardized..Therefore, the result that workers' psychological burden tends to be less when the tasks are standardized may be interrelated with the fact that the tasks are easy for the subjects to concentrate on. In the present analysis, days with a lot of "travel" time showed a tendency to have a lower positive mood. Previous studies have also shown that long commute times can cause stress and tension [40], which can lead to the inability to fulfill responsibilities outside of work, resulting in lower job satisfaction [41]. As far as we know, there is no past research that revealed the relationship between workers' workplace and their psychology in an environment where remote work and office work were mixed. In addition, since behaviors and work contents were collected, we were able to analyze the relationship between the work environment and situation and the psychological situation. As limitations, however, while numerous research have used sensors and behavioral data to predict psychological indicators, there have been few studies that have tested and analyzed these findings in other real-world scenario. We need to evaluate whether these findings can be generalized in other populations [42].

7 Conclusion

We conducted a 14-day experiment to collect wristband sensor data as well as behavioral and psychological questionnaire data from about 100 office workers. By designing machine learning prediction models using behavioral data, sensor data, and weather data, we were able to classify office workers' high/low six psychological indicators with 72–89% accuracy. The main findings obtained from the experiments and discussions in the paper are shown below:

- When binary classification of psychological indicators was performed using all the data collected in this experiment, the F_1 score of 17 items was 80% or more accurate in the prediction of 22 items of psychological indicators, and the accuracy was higher compared to the previous study [12, 16, 34].
- Comparing the prediction accuracy of the morning questionnaire and the evening questionnaire, the accuracy of the night subjective pain examination was significantly reduced.
- Correlations between office workers' work behavior and psychological state were also investigated to reveal the factors in the workplace that affected office workers' psychological state. As a result, we found that some factors like "web conferencing", working at "home (living room)" and "break time (work time)" had a significant impact on the psychological state. For example, "web conferencing" has a negative correlation in a positive mood and a positive correlation in a depressive mood. The correlation between "break time (work time)" and each mood was also observed.

In the future, we will understand individual differences among office workers. The information such as different personality characteristics might improve prediction accuracy. The prediction accuracy can be further improved by using a model that takes into account the time relationship of a day. Previous studies have also improved the accuracy of models that take into account the time series of sensor data and behavioral data [1, 15]. Also in this paper, we only used the duration of the behavior as features, so we will add the time-series relationship and frequency of the work behavior in the future to get more insights into the data. In the future, other machine learning models and ensemble learning approaches should be considered for prediction improvement.

Acknowledgements The experiment of this research was carried out in collaboration with companies and universities participating in the "2020 Sensing & Transformation Study Group", whose secretariat is the Applied Brain Science Consortium.

References

1. Li, B., Sano, A.: Extraction and interpretation of deep autoencoder-based temporal features from wearables for forecasting personalized mood, health, and stress. Proc. ACM Interact. Mob. Wearable Ubiquitous Technol. **4**(2) (2020)
2. Swain, V.D., Saha, K., Rajvanshy, H., Sirigiri, A., Gregg, J.M., Lin, S., Martinez, G.J., Mattingly, S.M., Mirjafari, S., Mulukutla, R., Nepal, S., Nies, K., Reddy, M.D., Robles-Granda, P., Campbell, A.T., Chawla, N.V., D'Mello, S., Dey, A.K., Jiang, K., Liu, Q., Mark, G., Moskal, E., Striegel, A., Tay, L., Abowd, G.D., De Choudhury, M.: A multisensor person-centered approach to understand the role of daily activities in job performance with organizational personas. Proc. ACM Interact. Mob. Wearable Ubiquitous Technol. **3**(4) (2019)
3. Wang, W., Mirjafari, S., Harari, G., Ben-Zeev, D., Brian, R., Choudhury, T., Hauser, M., Kane, J., Masaba, K., Nepal, S., Sano, A., Scherer, E., Tseng, V., Wang, R., Wen, H., Jialing, W., Campbell, A.: Social Sensing: Assessing Social Functioning of Patients Living with Schizophrenia Using Mobile Phone Sensing, pp. 1–15. Association for Computing Machinery, New York, NY, USA (2020)
4. Yang, F., Han, T., Deng, K., Han, Y.: The application of artificial intelligence in the mental diseases. In: Proceedings of the 2020 Conference on Artificial Intelligence and Healthcare, CAIH2020, pp. 36–40. Association for Computing Machinery, New York, NY, USA (2020)
5. Labor Ministry of Health and Welfare: Overview of the 2018 Occupational Safety and Health Survey (Fact-Finding Survey). https://www.mhlw.go.jp/toukei/list/dl/h30-46-50_gaikyo.pdf
6. Kotteeswari, M., Sharief, S.T.: Job Stress and Its Impact on Employees' Performance a Study with Reference to Employees Working in BPOS (2014)
7. Warr, P., Nielsen, K.: Wellbeing and Work Performance, 02 2018
8. Kopp, M.S., Stauder, A., Purebl, G., Janszky, I., Skrabski, A.: Work stress and mental health in a changing society. Eur. J. Public Health **18**(3), 238–244 (2007)
9. Yu, H., Itoh, A., Sakamoto, R., Shimaoka, M., Sano, A.: Forecasting Health and Wellbeing for Shift Workers Using Job-Role Based Deep Neural Network, pp. 89–103, 02 2021
10. Spathis, D., Servia-Rodriguez, S., Farrahi, K., Mascolo, C., Rentfrow, J.: Sequence multi-task learning to forecast mental wellbeing from sparse self-reported data. In: Proceedings of the 25th ACM SIGKDD International Conference on Knowledge Discovery. Data Mining, KDD'19, pp. 2886–2894. Association for Computing Machinery, New York, NY, USA (2019)
11. Sano, A., Picard, R.W.: Stress recognition using wearable sensors and mobile phones. In: Proceedings of the 2013 Humaine Association Conference on Affective Computing and Intelligent Interaction, ACII'13, pp. 671–676. IEEE Computer Society, USA (2013)
12. Koldijk, S., Neerincx, M.A., Kraaij, W.: Detecting work stress in offices by combining unobtrusive sensors. IEEE Trans. Affect. Comput. **9**(02), 227–239 (2018)
13. Alberdia, A., Aztiriaa, A., Basarabb, A., Cook, D.J.: Using Smart Offices to Predict Occupational Stress
14. Sano, A., Phillips, A., Yu, A.Z., McHill, A.W., Taylor, S., Jaques, N., Czeisler, C., Klerman, E., Picard, R.W.: Recognizing academic performance, sleep quality, stress level, and mental health using personality traits, wearable sensors and mobile phones. In: 2015 IEEE 12th International Conference on Wearable and Implantable Body Sensor Networks (BSN), pp. 1–6 (2015)
15. Robles-Granda, P., Lin, S, Wu, X., D'Mello, S., Martínez, G.J., Saha, K., Nies, K., Mark, G., Campbell, A.T., De Choudhury, M., Dey, A.D., Gregg, J.M., Grover, T., Mattingly, S.M., Mirjafari, S., Moskal, E., Striegel, A., Chawla, N.V.: Jointly predicting job performance, personality, cognitive ability, affect, and well-being. CoRR (2020). abs/2006.08364

16. Rahmani, A.M., Nejad, N.T., Perego, P.: A method for simplified HRQOL measurement by smart devices. In: Wireless Mobile Communication and Healthcare, pp. 91–98 (2017)
17. Feng, T., Booth, B., Baldwin-Rodríguez, B., Osorno, F., Narayanan, S.: A multimodal analysis of physical activity, sleep, and work shift in nurses with wearable sensor data. Sci. Rep. **11**, 04 2021
18. Lee, M.: Detecting affective flow states of knowledge workers using physiological sensors. CoRR (2020). abs/2006.10635
19. Fukuda, H., Tani, Y., Matsuda, H., Arakawa, Y., Yasumoto, K.: An analysis of the relationship between office workers' sleep status and occupational health indicators. Technical Report 22, Nara Institute of Science and Technology, Kyushu University/JST PRESTO, Nov 2019
20. Garcia-Ceja, E., Osmani, V., Mayora, O.: Automatic stress detection in working environments from smartphones' accelerometer data: a first step. IEEE J. Biomed. Health Inform. **20**(4), 1053–1060 (2016)
21. Zenonos, A., Khan, A., Kalogridis, G., Vatsikas, S., Lewis, T., Sooriyabandara, M.: HealthyOffice: Mood Recognition at Work Using Smartphones and Wearable Sensors, pp. 1–6, 03 2016
22. Mirjafari, S., Masaba, K., Grover, T., Wang, W., Audia, P., Campbell, A.T., Chawla, N.V., Das Swain, V., De Choudhury, M., Dey, A.K., D'Mello, S.K., Gao, G., Gregg, J.M., Jagannath, K., Jiang, K., Lin, S., Liu, Q., Mark, G., Martinez, G.J., Mattingly, S.M., Moskal, E., Mulukutla, R., Nepal, S., Nies, K., Reddy, M.D., Robles-Granda, P., Saha, K., Sirigiri, A., Striegel, A.: Differentiating higher and lower job performers in the workplace using mobile sensing. Proc. ACM Interact. Mob. Wearable Ubiquitous Technol. **3**(2), June 2019
23. Sano, A., Taylor, S., Mchill, A., Phillips, A., Barger, L., Klerman, E., Picard, R.: Identifying objective physiological markers and modifiable behaviors for self-reported stress and mental health status using wearable sensors and mobile phones. J. Med. Internet Res. **20**, 11 (2017)
24. Suhara, Y., Xu, Y., 'Sandy' Pentland, A.: DeepMood: forecasting depressed mood based on self-reported histories via recurrent neural networks. In: Proceedings of the 26th International Conference on World Wide Web, WWW'17, pp. 715–724. International World Wide Web Conferences Steering Committee, Republic and Canton of Geneva, CHE (2017)
25. Umematsu, T., Sano, A., Taylor, S., Tsujikawa, M., Picard, R.W.: Forecasting stress, mood, and health from daytime physiology in office workers and students. In: 2020 42nd Annual International Conference of the IEEE Engineering in Medicine Biology Society (EMBC), pp. 5953–5957 (2020)
26. Lutchyn, Y., Johns, P., Czerwinski, M., Iqbal, S., Mark, G., Sano, A.: Stress is in the eye of the beholder. In: 2015 International Conference on Affective Computing and Intelligent Interaction (ACII), pp. 119–124 (2015)
27. Shuck, B., Reio, T.: Employee engagement and well-being. J. Leadersh. Organ. Stud. **21**, 43–58 (2013)
28. Matsuda, Y., Inoue, S., Tani, Y., Fukuda, S., Arakawa, Y.: WorkerSense: mobile sensing platform for collecting physiological, mental, and environmental state of office workers. In: 2020 IEEE International Conference on Pervasive Computing and Communications Workshops (PerCom Workshops) (2020)
29. Inoue, S., Lago, P., Hossain, T., Mairittha, T., Mairittha, N.: Integrating activity recognition and nursing care records: the system, deployment, and a verification study. Proc. ACM Interact. Mob. Wearable Ubiquitous Technol. **3**(3) (2019)
30. Fukuda, I.: Attempting to develop depression and anxiety mood scale (DAMS). Action Therapy Res. **23**(2), 83–93 (1997)
31. Kubo, T., Joh, N., Takeyama, H., Makihara, T., Inoue, T., Takanishi, T., Aragomo, Y., Murazaki, M., Tetsu, I.: Examination of the Expression Pattern of Fatigue During Consecutive Night Shifts by
32. Shimazu, A., Sonnentag, S., Kubota, K., Kawakami, N.: Validation of the Japanese version of the recovery experience questionnaire. J. Occup. Health **54**, 03 (2012)
33. Barber, C., Arne, B., Berglund, P., Cleary, P.D., McKenas, D., Pronk, N., Simon, G., Stang, P., Ustun, T.B., Wang, P., Kessler, R.C.: The world health organization health and work performance questionnaire (HPQ). J. Occup. Environ. Med. **45**, 156–174 (2003)

34. Taylor, S., Jaques, N., Nosakhare, E., Sano, A., Picard, R.: Personalized multitask learning for predicting tomorrow's mood, stress, and health. IEEE Trans. Affect. Comput. **11**(2), 200–213 (2020)
35. Ke, G., Meng, Q., Finley, T., Wang, T., Chen, W., Ma, W., Ye, O., Liu, T.-Y.: LightGBM: a highly efficient gradient boosting decision tree. In: Guyon, I., Luxburg, U.V., Bengio, S., Wallach, H., Fergus, R., Vishwanathan, S., Garnett, R. (eds.) Advances in Neural Information Processing Systems, vol. 30. Curran Associates Inc. (2017)
36. Reis, J.C.S., Correia, A., Murai, F., Veloso, A., Benevenuto, F.: Explainable machine learning for fake news detection. In: Proceedings of the 10th ACM Conference on Web Science, WebSci'19, pp. 17–26. Association for Computing Machinery, New York, NY, USA (2019)
37. Bahador Parsa, A., Movahedi, A., Taghipour, H., Derrible, S., (Kouros) Mohammadian, A.: Toward safer highways, application of XGBoost and SHAP for real-time accident detection and feature analysis. Accid. Anal. Prev. **136**, 105405 (2020)
38. Lundberg, S., Lee, S.-I.: A unified approach to interpreting model predictions. CoRR (2017). abs/1705.07874
39. Lundberg, S.M., Erion, G.G., Lee, S.-I.: Consistent individualized feature attribution for tree ensembles (2019)
40. Kluger, A.N.: Commute variability and strain. J. Organ. Behav. **19**(2), 147–165 (1998)
41. Moorman, R.H.: The influence of cognitive and affective based job satisfaction measures on the relationship between satisfaction and organizational citizenship behavior. Human Relations **46**(6), 759–776 (1993)
42. Thieme, A., Belgrave, D., Doherty, G.: Machine learning in mental health: a systematic review of the HCI literature to support the development of effective and implementable ml systems. ACM Trans. Comput.-Hum. Interact. **27**(5), Aug 2020

Open-Source Data Collection for Activity Studies at Scale

Alexander Hoelzemann, Jana Sabrina Pithan, and Kristof Van Laerhoven

Abstract Activity studies range from detecting key indicators such as steps, active minutes, or sedentary bouts, to the recognition of physical activities such as specific fitness exercises. Such types of activity recognition rely on large amounts of data from multiple persons, especially with deep learning. However, current benchmark datasets rarely have more than a dozen participants. Once wearable devices are phased out, closed algorithms that operate on the sensor data are hard to reproduce and devices supply raw data. We present an open-source and cost-effective framework that is able to capture daily activities and routines and which uses publicly available algorithms, while avoiding any device-specific implementations. In a feasibility study, we were able to test our system in production mode. For this purpose, we distributed the Bangle.js smartwatch as well as our app to 12 study participants, who started the watches at a time of individual choice every day. The collected data was then transferred to the server at the end of each day.

1 Introduction

Many types of studies focus on capturing activity data from human study participants. We can distinguish these types of studies based on the measurement devices and sensors used, the carrying position of the sensors, and the domain of the data. The types of devices used go hand in hand with the sensor technology used. For example, sensors worn on the wrist offer the possibility of recording the heart rate via PPG sensors, the skin temperature with a thermometer, and the movements with

A. Hoelzemann (✉) · K. Van Laerhoven
Ubiquitous Computing, University of Siegen, Hoelderlinstr. 3, 57076 Siegen, Germany
e-mail: alexander.hoelzemann@uni-siegen.de

K. Van Laerhoven
e-mail: kvl@eti.uni-siegen.de

J. S. Pithan
Institute of Sports Science, University of Vechta, Driverstr. 22, 49377 Vechta, Germany
e-mail: jana.pithan@uni-vechta.de

M. A. R. Ahad et al. (eds.), *Sensor- and Video-Based Activity and Behavior Computing*,
Smart Innovation, Systems and Technologies 291,
https://doi.org/10.1007/978-981-19-0361-8_2

an accelerometer, gyroscope, and magnetometer. Studies in which smartphones are mainly used to record the data do not usually offer this supplementary sensor technology. Since the devices are not worn directly on the skin, the data is often limited to basic IMU sensors. In contrast, the carrying position of the sensors goes hand in hand with the specific domain of the recorded data. Sensor technology used for medical datasets is often worn on different body positions than sensor technology used for the purpose of activity recognition. As previous studies have shown, for many activities, it is often sufficient to wear the sensors only at key positions such as the wrist [24, 29]. In the medical environment, however, more complex sensors and different wearing positions are often required [1, 21] (Fig. 1).

Empirical studies for which activity plays a crucial role use indicators such as steps taken, sedentary periods, activity counts, or detected physical exercises, which often originate from closed-source algorithms. This tends to lock studies to particular devices and makes the use of other devices or comparisons difficult. In contrast, sensors such as accelerometers or inertial measurement units are already widely integrated in many wearables and tend to produce calibrated sensor data in units such as mg. Restricting studies to particular commercial wearables that also record raw inertial data have the effect that large-scale studies are only possible if the project has a high budget that allows the purchase of commercial hardware and software. In this paper, we present the ActiVatE_prevention system, which is based exclusively

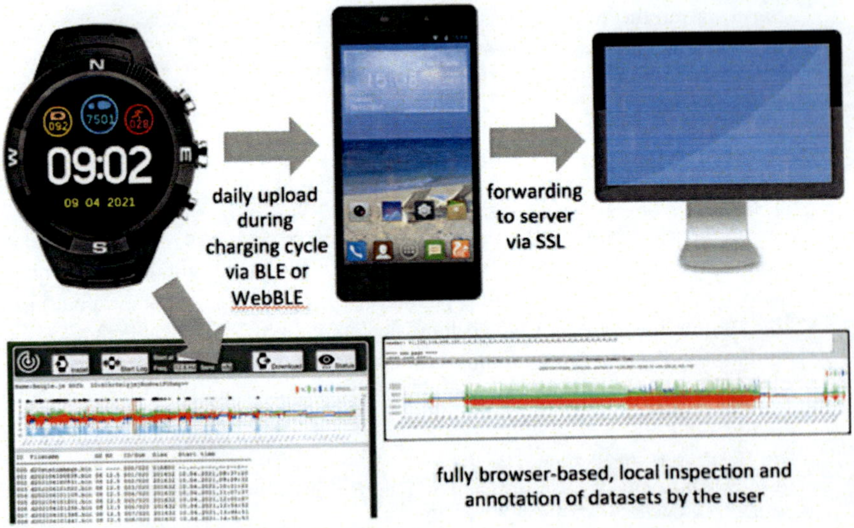

Fig. 1 Our system relies on an open-source smartwatch [37] with custom firmware, smartphone apps, and a server-side database to collect all data centrally. For participants without smartphone or in studies where users need to inspect their data or manually forward their data, a web-based suite (bottom) retrieves the data through WebBLE. The raw sensor data is frequently streamed from the smartwatch either to a nearby computer via web-based control panel or via the user's smartphone to a dedicated server

on open-source components, logs raw inertial data, and also offers subjects a similar wearing comfort as commercially manufactured products. We argue that it, therefore, lends itself well to the capturing of multiple users simultaneously for activity studies, while being an open source, replicable, and low-cost approach.

2 Related Work

Plenty of studies that log wearable inertial data to capture the activity of a user have been proposed throughout the past two decades. In human activity recognition research, for instance, recently published survey papers, such as Chen et al., Table 1, [7] or Demrozi et al., Table 6, [8], show that the same datasets, e.g., WISDM [3], OPPORTUNITY [31], PAMAP2 [30], or DSADS [2] are used for many machine learning papers published in recent years. These datasets are limited regarding their nature, in respect to scope, quality, continuity, and reliability. We extended these lists of compared datasets by adding the SHL [13] and the RealWorld (HAR) [33] datasets. Taken the numbers into account that were given by the publications, we calculate a median of about 13 activities and 12 subjects for activities of daily living. Datasets that have a significantly higher number of activities or subjects are often recorded using smartphones. However, a smartphone does not provide the same level of control to record data as our open-source operating system, since the underlying operating system is in control of when exactly an instruction is executed by the CPU. Most of the published datasets were recorded using more than one sensor attached to the body. These sensors were prototypes developed in a laboratory and, therefore, not optimized to being inconspicuous and comfortable to wear. Furthermore, study participants were always conscious of being recorded, thus (unintentionally) changing activity patterns which leads to the recorded data being biased [36].

However, in order to develop machine learning algorithms that are reliable and robust with everyday situations and data recorded in the wild, large and standardized datasets are needed. Several research projects and publications have highlighted the challenges and needs for robust and systematic collection of activity. The ActiServ project [4] presents a smartphone-based software architecture to infer activities from local sensor data and specifically designed for everyday use, enabling flexible placement of the device and requiring minimal effort from the user. The AWARE [12] framework is developed as an open-source framework which uses smartphone-integrated sensors to record human activity data. It is available for Android and iOS and comes with a server application that uses the rapid preprocessing pipeline for machine learning [35] to preprocess incoming data streams. The SPHERE sensor platform [34] is a multi-sensor fusion approach, which is deployed for health care supervision in residential housing. IMU wristbands as well as environment sensors and 3D Kinect cameras are used to supervise behaviors such as sleep, physical activity, eating, domestic chores, and social contact. The system has been deployed in about 100 households. On a smaller scale, Mairittha et al. [28] present a mobile app for crowdsourcing-labeled activity data from smartphone-integrated sensors. They recorded 1749 labeled subsets of activity data. This application is neither available on the app stores nor available on known repository platforms. E-care@home [23] is an open-source collection of software modules for data collection, labeling, and reasoning tasks, such as activity recognition or person counting in a smart home environment and is meant to be used for large-scale data acquisition in a home environment. The solution is partly open source and available to download from their GitLab repository [20]. Several sensor nodes are placed in a smart home and used to record data.

Wear OS from Google [15] was released under this name in March 2018 and also offers developers the possibility access raw sensor data. Methods for activity recognition of different sports can also be integrated via the Google FIT API [14]. For using this service, however, one is tied to Google and their contract terms.

In current publications of data collection frameworks and algorithms, the main focus has been on video and image data-based activity recognition, [6, 16, 26] or [17]. Similar open-source systems do not yet exist for IMU data, since most frameworks are either smartphone-based or the needed wearables are laboratory-made prototypes that cannot be purchased easily online.

IMUTube [25] is an algorithm that is capable of generating artificial IMU data from humans in videos. Such large and publicly available datasets do not yet exist in the area of IMU-based activity recognition.

Extensive datasets with sensor-based human activity data have been difficult to record due to the need to use specific hardware with sensors that are often difficult to start, uncomfortable to wear, or data sharing is limited for inexperienced volunteers. Therefore, researchers started to use data augmentation techniques on inertial sensor data to create synthetic data [11] or [10]. These techniques increase the size of the dataset, but they are limited if we want to increase quality and variability [18]. With the pervasiveness of inertial sensors embedded in commercial smartwatches, it has become easy to deploy applications that use inertial data locally, but longer recordings of these data in a common format (for instance, using particular sensitivities and sampling rates) remain difficult.

3 Our Proposed Approach

The design of our open-source system is shown in Figs. 2 and 3. The operating system is installed once on the Bangle.js via WebBLE, and the apps are downloadable via the Apple AppStore and the Google Play Store. The app forward the data from the smartwatch to the central server. The user interface of the app is kept simple, and the users can only select their daily activity goals and retrieve their daily activity statistics.

The sequence diagram (Fig. 3) depicts the communication in between the architecture elements. We recorded the execution time for every communication step, which is added to the diagram. On average, it takes 185 s to send one file (approx.

200 kb and 1 h of data) from the watch via BLE to the smart device. After ⌀ 45 min, the complete daily data is sent from the smartwatch to the server.
Smartwatch. To date, there are few open-source smartwatch designs that allow algorithms for detecting activities, from basic ones such as steps, sedentary bouts, and active minutes, to recognition of particular exercise repetitions, to be transparently implemented on a device with integrated inertial sensors. We used the Bangle.js [37] as an affordable (around 50 $) low-power system that is equipped with a Nordic 64 MHz nRF52832 ARM Cortex-M4 processor, inertial sensors, a PPG sensor, sufficient internal memory, and an internal BLE module. Our firmware on this open-source platform is capable of storing the sensors' raw data over a full day and integrates recognition algorithms—currently for steps, active minutes, and exercise intensities—locally on the watch. Users are expected to start the data upload process once a day, either through the web-based platform or through their smartphone or tablet app.

Since the logging of activity data requires sampling rates 10 Hz up to as high 100 Hz, depending on the activity, the recording of raw inertial data is rarely implemented in a way where local recordings are routinely synchronized and uploaded to a server. The local storage for a day's worth of inertial data and the energy footprint for sending this data tends to be substantial [5]. Instead, the early preprocessing of inertial data in the aforementioned detected features (steps, active minutes, etc.) takes place on the wearable devices, and usually, solely, these aggregated values are stored.

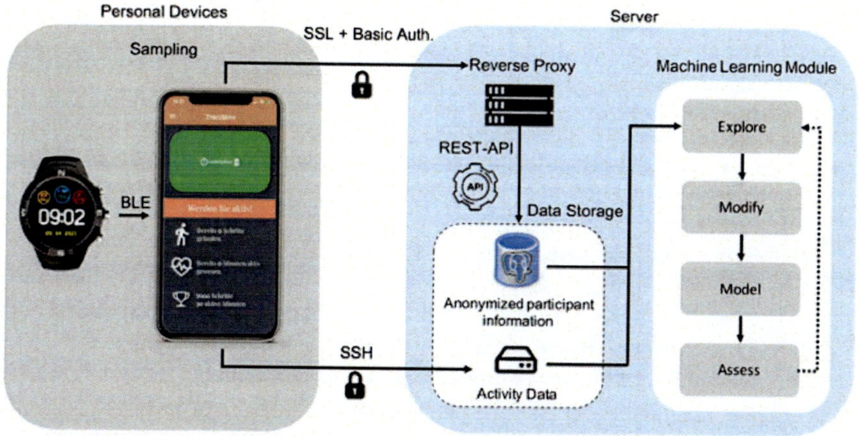

Fig. 2 Open-source client-server architecture for recording human activity data. The data is recorded by the Bangle.js smartwatch and is sent to the server daily with our app. Anonymized participant information is sent to the server via a reverse proxy that implements SSL + basic authentication. This reverse proxy communicates via a REST-API with the Postgres SQL database. The system is designed in accordance with the SEMMA data process model [32]. (1) Sampling, (2) explore, (3) modify, (4) model, and (5) asses. The model itself can be seen as a cycle

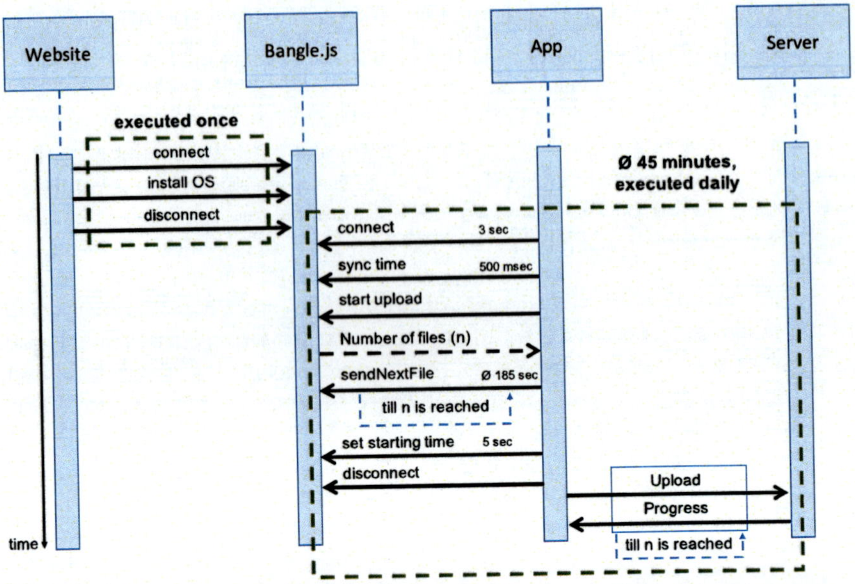

Fig. 3 Operating system is installed from our webtool via WebBLE on the Bangle.js. This needs to be executed once. The communication between Bangle.js and the app occurs on a daily basis. The procedure needs ∅ 45 min for a full day of recording (14 h of active time) and ∅ 185 s for sending one file from the watch to the smartphone. The upload to the server is executed when all files are transferred to the smartphone

Detected activity-related concepts such as active minutes [19] have been deployed locally on the Bangle.js smartwatch and are uploaded together with the raw sensor data to the server through the smartphone app (or via the browser-based tool suite) on a daily basis. We designed to fully use the watch's 4 Mb flash memory to losslessly compress 16 bit, 12.5 Hz inertial data at ±8g, along with other data such as the skin temperature and heart rate.

iOS and Android App. The activate client is implemented using Flutter. Therefore, we are able to design and implement clients for the two major operating systems, iOS and Android, at once. However, minor code changes are necessary to solve operating system specific issues, especially with regards to the BLE connection.

The interface consists of three main views and is displayed in German language. It was designed to encourage diabetes patients to perform more physical activities in their daily lives. Beyond the recording of raw inertial data, it is planned for the near future to expand this open-source app to be able to annotate and detect an arbitrary number of activities as well.

When the app starts, the participant is taken to the home screen, (1) in Fig. 4. Here, the user interface visualizes an overview of the day's accumulated number of steps taken and active minutes. When pressing the green button, the study participant saves the data on the server and sets the starting time for the following measurement

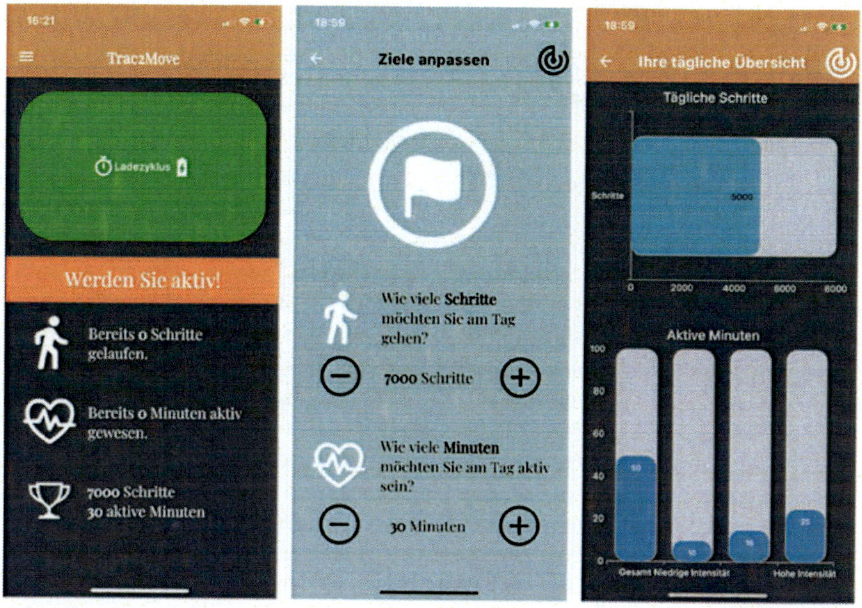

Fig. 4 Smartphone's user interface: (1) home screen, (2) setting daily activity goals, e.g., daily steps (Tägliche Schritte) and daily active minutes (Aktive Minuten), (3) graphical overview of daily activities: daily steps (Tägliche Schritte), active minutes (Aktive Minuten), devided into three intensities—low, moderate, and vigorous (niedrige, mittlere, hohe Intensität)

(typically, the next day). During the first start of the app, an anonymized user account is created and saved in a Postgres SQL database.

On the second screen in Fig. 4, the user can set their personal goals for the day within its limits. Screen (3) in Fig. 4 gives a graphical overview of the daily metrics and shows beside the total number of steps and active minutes, also the active minutes sorted by their intensities.

Server. The server communicates with the client via two channels, Fig. 2. Private information about the study participants, such as gender or age, and the confirmation of the consent form are sent via SSL and basic authentication to a reverse proxy which then sends the information to the database via local host. The information is stored in an anonymous form. The recorded activity data, as well as daily steps and active minutes, is sent via SSH to the server and stored in binary files with delta compression. The activity data can then be processed and modeled by machine learning algorithms.

Browser-based Data Analysis. The smartphone or tablet app and server software described above can be complemented with a local analysis and annotation tool that can be used by the study participants. This requires users to simply visit a Web site that can connect to the watch through WebBLE and download the watch's data locally on the computer for further inspection or manual upload to our central study server, through users' own computers without the need to install software.

4 Performance Analysis

Since our software is distributed between apps that are available as a web-based software suit or downloadable in Apple's App Store and Android's Play Store, the deployment of our system is straightforward. We gave the Bangle.js smartwatches to 12 geographically distributed study participants, recorded compliance, comfort rating, and reliability performance measures for our presented approach to illustrate the feasibility of our approach, and report our findings below.

We analyzed recordings from participants over a window of five days and decided to let them choose how many hours they recorded by letting them start and stop the smartwatch with the app at a time of their choice. This is important because of the age group and the profession of the subject, which entails certain active and inactive, as well as sleep and wake cycles [9].

During the feasibility study, we focused on detecting basic activity concepts such as steps as well as the active minutes divided into the three subclasses, low, moderate, and vigorous intensity. The participants wore the smartwatch for an average of 12 h per day. In total, we collected approx. 29 Mb (12 * 202 kb * 12 participants) of raw compressed data. Basic activity classes are already recognized on the watch without machine learning. However, since the Bangle.js has TensorFlow-Lite already implemented on the hardware, there is an opportunity to deploy a pre-trained neural network or machine learning classifier on the watch in the future. A recent article [27] demonstrates how to implement this for gesture recognition.

We can demonstrate by means of our experiment that the system we have designed can be used for data recordings in the wild without the subject being biased by the technology worn, since the smartwatch is a commercially designed product and looks and feels like a normal watch. Due to the 4 Mb memory limitation of Bangle.js, we limit the inertial measurements to a 12.5 Hz sampling rate so that a full 24-h day can still be recorded in one cycle. We consider this sampling rate acceptable, since activity detection is still possible at such a low sampling rate. Furthermore, the signal can be interpolated as part of the machine learning preprocessing, or the sampling rate can be increased at the cost of shorter recordings (100 Hz recorded dataset corresponds to about 3 h).

Occasionally, data uploads are hampered because of problems with a reliable Internet connection and the Bluetooth connection between Bangle.js and app in particular. The communication flow as depicted in Fig. 3 has, therefore, been developed for stability and has built-in recovery mechanisms that guarantee that individual files are uploaded reliably. The current version is, therefore, characterized by a high reliability and accessibility, but also relatively long upload times (around 45 min on average for a full day's dataset). However, this seems acceptable, as the download

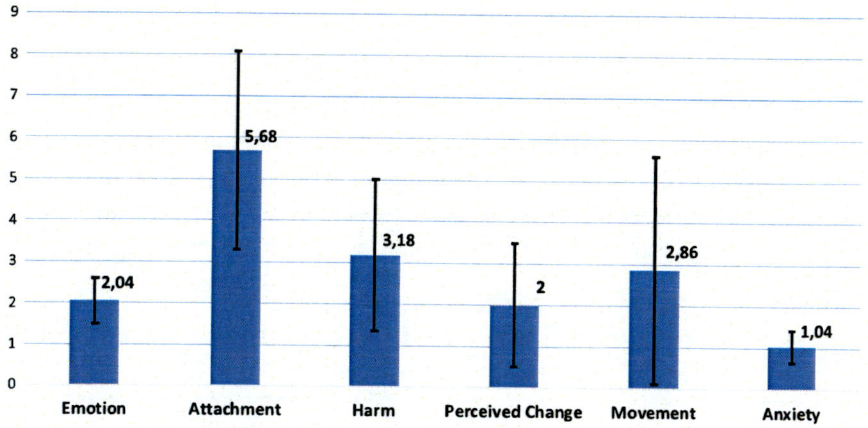

Fig. 5 CRS result means and standard deviation. Emotion: 2.04, 0.56; attachment: 5.68, 2.39; harm: 3.18, 1.84; perceived change: 2, 1.49; movement: 2.86, 2.75; anxiety: 1.04, 0.39

process has been integrated with charging the smartphone and Bangle.js smartwatch in the nightly "charging cycle".

Bangle.js Wearing Comfort. In addition to the feasibility study of our open-source architecture's ability to accommodate data over multiple users and in a distributed manner, we decided to investigate Bangle.js in terms of its comfort of use. We consider this to be important, since the success of a study is directly dependent on the acceptance of a device. We use the comfort rating scale (CRS), a questionnaire-based method proposed by Knight et al. [22], as a well-known and state-of-the-art method to evaluate the wearing comfort of wearable devices in particular.

The Bangle.js smartwatch was rated (as Fig. 5 shows) overall as comfortable to wear without restricting its users. However, users can feel the device on their wrist due to its larger size ($5 \times 5 \times 1.7$ cm case) and weight. The device is heavier and more bulky than most commercial wrist-worn products, which may lead to slightly negative wearing comfort and perhaps more difficult acceptance in larger future studies. We consider this an acceptable trade-off, as only one person in the study reported that the watch had a strong negative emotional impact on them, and that they would have liked to take it off.

5 Conclusions

The use of low-cost and open-source systems is essential for future machine learning applications. Only through the development and use of such systems, it will be possible to generate the required amount of data to train a neural network to be used in a real-world context in a generalized way. Many publications show new and exciting methods in dealing with human activity data; however, these methods are always evaluated on the same datasets mentioned before. This creates a bias in our scientific domain, which can only be eliminated by publicly available, understandable, and reusable implementations for data collection.

The already available open-source platforms and systems presented in Sect. 2 are either smartphone-based or smart home-based solutions. Smartwatch-based solutions are mostly prototypes, which are not meant to be distributed in scale and not open source. Due to its open-source architecture, the use of the Bangle.js wristwatch combines the advantages of a product while having an open architecture that is fully documented. Our custom operating system as well as the client-server architecture can serve as a starting point that can later be modified or further developed accordingly. Due to the low purchase price, the device can be used in projects with a smaller budget or in need of a larger group of users. In contrast to a self-developed prototype, where the wearing comfort is often not the main interest, the Bangle.js was confirmed to offer a high acceptance by study participants in our study using the comfort rating scale (CRS). We argue that this aspect also contributes to the long-term success of a scientific study and the scope, quality, continuity, and reliability of the produced dataset.

Commercial products tend to not open the algorithms used and do not give researchers the same insights in recorded data as a fully open-source implementation does. Therefore, we made the source code of the smartphone app as well as the smartwatch operating system available for download and inspection under the MIT license, to encourage other researchers to replicate and improve on our approach: https://github.com/ahoelzemann/activateFlutter, https://github.com/kristofvl/BangleApps/blob/master/apps/activate/app.js.

Funding

This publication is part of the project ActiVAtE_prevention which is funded by the Ministry for Science and Culture of the federal state of Lower Saxony in Germany (VW-ZN3426).

References

1. AlShorman, O., AlShorman, B., Alkhassaweneh, M., Alkahtani, F.: A review of internet of medical things (IoMT)-based remote health monitoring through wearable sensors: a case study for diabetic patients. Indonesian J. Electr. Eng. Comput. Sci. **20**(1), 414–422 (2020)
2. Altun, K., Barshan, B., Tunçel, O.: Comparative study on classifying human activities with miniature inertial and magnetic sensors. Pattern Recogn. **43**(10), 3605–3620 (2010)
3. Anguita, D., Ghio, A., Oneto, L., Parra, X., Reyes-Ortiz, J.L.: A public domain dataset for human activity recognition using smartphones. In: ESANN, vol. 3, p. 3 (2013)
4. Berchtold, M., Budde, M., Gordon, D., Schmidtke, H.R., Beigl, M.: ActiServ: activity recognition service for mobile phones. In: 2010 International Symposium on Wearable Computers

(ISWC 2010), pp. 1–8. IEEE Computer Society, Los Alamitos, CA, USA (2010). https://doi.org/10.1109/ISWC.2010.5665868
5. Berlin, E., Zittel, M., Braunlein, M., Laerhoven, K.V.: Low-power lessons from designing a wearable logger for long-term deployments. IEEE (2015). https://doi.org/10.1109/sas.2015.7133581
6. Caba Heilbron, F., Escorcia, V., Ghanem, B., Carlos Niebles, J.: ActivityNet: a large-scale video benchmark for human activity understanding. In: Proceedings of the IEEE Conference on Computer Vision and Pattern Recognition, pp. 961–970 (2015)
7. Chen, K., Zhang, D., Yao, L., Guo, B., Yu, Z., Liu, Y.: Deep learning for sensor-based human activity recognition: overview, challenges, and opportunities. ACM Comput. Surv. (CSUR) **54**(4), 1–40 (2021)
8. Demrozi, F., Pravadelli, G., Bihorac, A., Rashidi, P.: Human activity recognition using inertial, physiological and environmental sensors: a comprehensive survey. IEEE Access (2020)
9. Espiritu, J.R.D.: Aging-related sleep changes. Clin. Geriatr. Med. **24**(1), 1–14 (2008)
10. Esteban, C., Hyland, S.L., Rätsch, G.: Real-valued (medical) time series generation with recurrent conditional GANs (2017). arXiv preprint arXiv:1706.02633
11. Fawaz, H.I., Forestier, G., Weber, J., Idoumghar, L., Muller, P.-A.: Data augmentation using synthetic data for time series classification with deep residual networks (2018). arXiv preprint arXiv:1808.02455
12. Ferreira, D., Kostakos, V., Dey, A.K.: Aware: mobile context instrumentation framework. Front. ICT **2**, 6 (2015)
13. Gjoreski, H., Ciliberto, M., Wang, L., Morales, F.J.O., Mekki, S., Valentin, S., Roggen, D.: The university of Sussex-Huawei locomotion and transportation dataset for multimodal analytics with mobile devices. IEEE Access **6**, 42592–42604 (2018)
14. Google-LLC: Google Fit API
15. Google-LLC: Google Wear OS
16. Goyal, R., et al.: The "something something" video database for learning and evaluating visual common sense. In: Proceedings of the IEEE International Conference on Computer Vision, pp. 5842–5850 (2017)
17. Gtoderici: gtoderici/sports-1m-dataset
18. Hoelzemann, A., Sorathiya, N., Van Laerhoven, K.: Data augmentation strategies for human activity data using generative adversarial neural networks. In: 2021 IEEE International Conference on Pervasive Computing and Communications Workshops and Other Affiliated Events (PerCom Workshops), pp. 8–13. IEEE (2021)
19. Jetté, M., Sidney, K., Blümchen, G.: Metabolic equivalents (METS) in exercise testing, exercise prescription, and evaluation of functional capacity. Clin. Cardiol. **13**(8), 555–565 (1990). https://doi.org/10.1002/clc.4960130809
20. Kckemann, U.: Projects UWE kckemann/ecare-pub
21. Khan, Y., Ostfeld, A.E., Lochner, C.M., Pierre, A., Arias, A.C.: Monitoring of vital signs with flexible and wearable medical devices. Adv. Mater. **28**(22), 4373–4395 (2016)
22. Knight, J., Baber, C., Schwirtz, A., Bristow, H.: The comfort assessment of wearable computers. In: Sixth International Symposium on Wearable Computers (ISWC 2002). IEEE Press (2002). https://doi.org/10.1109/iswc.2002.1167220
23. Köckemann, U., Alirezaie, M., Renoux, J., Tsiftes, N., Ahmed, M.U., Morberg, D., Lindén, M., Loutfi, A.: Open-source data collection and data sets for activity recognition in smart homes. Sensors **20**(3), 879 (2020)
24. Kunze, K., Lukowicz, P.: Sensor placement variations in wearable activity recognition. IEEE Pervasive Comput. **13**(4), 32–41 (2014). https://doi.org/10.1109/mprv.2014.73
25. Kwon, H., Tong, C., Haresamudram, H., Gao, Y., Abowd, G.D., Lane, N.D., Ploetz, T.: IMU-Tube: automatic extraction of virtual on-body accelerometry from video for human activity recognition. Proc. ACM Interact. Mobile Wearable Ubiquit. Technol. **4**(3), 1–29 (2020)
26. Levine, S., Pastor, P., Krizhevsky, A., Ibarz, J., Quillen, D.: Learning hand-eye coordination for robotic grasping with deep learning and large-scale data collection. Int. J. Robot. Res. **37**(4–5), 421–436 (2018)

27. Madsen, A.: Running tensorflow lite on nodewatch/bangle.js - nearform (2020)
28. Mairittha, N., Inoue, S.: Crowdsourcing system management for activity data with mobile sensors. In: 2019 Joint 8th International Conference on Informatics, Electronics & Vision (ICIEV) and 2019 3rd International Conference on Imaging, Vision & Pattern Recognition (icIVPR), pp. 85–90. IEEE (2019)
29. Mannini, A., Intille, S.S., Rosenberger, M., Sabatini, A.M., Haskell, W.: Activity recognition using a single accelerometer placed at the wrist or ankle. Med. Sci. Sports Exerc. **45**(11), 2193 (2013)
30. Reiss, A., Stricker, D.: Introducing a new benchmarked dataset for activity monitoring. In: 2012 16th International Symposium on Wearable Computers, pp. 108–109. IEEE (2012)
31. Roggen, D., et al.: Collecting complex activity datasets in highly rich networked sensor environments. In: 2010 Seventh International Conference on Networked Sensing Systems (INSS), pp. 233–240. IEEE (2010)
32. Shafique, U., Qaiser, H.: A comparative study of data mining process models (KDD, CRISP-DM and SEMMA). Int. J. Innov. Sci. Res. **12**(1), 217–222 (2014)
33. Sztyler, T., Stuckenschmidt, H.: On-body localization of wearable devices: an investigation of position-aware activity recognition. In: 2016 IEEE International Conference on Pervasive Computing and Communications (PerCom), pp. 1–9. IEEE Computer Society (2016). https://doi.org/10.1109/PERCOM.2016.7456521, http://ieeexplore.ieee.org/xpl/articleDetails.jsp?arnumber=7456521
34. Twomey, N., et al.: The SPHERE challenge: activity recognition with multimodal sensor data (2016). arXiv preprint arXiv:1603.00797
35. Vega, J., Li, M., Aguillera, K., Goel, N., Joshi, E., Durica, K.C., Kunta, A.R., Low, C.A.: RAPIDS: reproducible analysis pipeline for data streams collected with mobile devices (Preprint) (2020). https://doi.org/10.2196/preprints.23246
36. Vickers, J., Reed, A., Decker, R., Conrad, B.P., Olegario-Nebel, M., Vincent, H.K.: Effect of investigator observation on gait parameters in individuals with and without chronic low back pain. Gait Posture **53**, 35–40 (2017)
37. Williams, G.: The world's first open source hackable smart watch, bangle.js. Hackable Smart Watch

Using LUPI to Improve Complex Activity Recognition

Kohei Adachi, Paula Lago, Yuichi Hattori, and Sozo Inoue

Abstract Sensor-based activity recognition can recognize simple activities such as walking and running with high accuracy, but it is difficult to recognize complex activities such as nursing care activities and cooking activities. One solution is to use multiple sensors, which is unrealistic in real life. Recently, learning using privileged information (LUPI) has been proposed, which enables training using additional information only in the training phase. In this paper, we used LUPI for improving the accuracy of complex activity recognition. In short, training is performed with multiple sensors during the training phase, and a single sensor is used during testing. We used four published datasets for evaluating our proposed method. As a result, our proposed method improves by up to 16% in F1-Score to 67% compared to the baseline method when we used random-split cross-validation of each subject.

1 Introduction

Human activity recognition (HAR) is a task of recognizing different types of activities from sensors or video data. This has become popular research in ubiquitous computing [1]. While simple activities such as walking, running, and sitting can be easy to recognize, complex activities such as nurse care activities and cooking activities are difficult to recognize [3, 6]. For this reason, a previous study proposed a method of HAR using multiple sensors [13]. While it is easy to collect training data

K. Adachi (✉) · Y. Hattori · S. Inoue
Kyushu Institute of Technology, Kitakyushu, Japan
e-mail: adachi@sozolab.jp

Y. Hattori
e-mail: hattori@sozolab.jp

S. Inoue
e-mail: sozo@brain.kyutech.ac.jp

P. Lago
Universidad Nacional Abierta y a Distancia, Bogota, Colombia
e-mail: paula.lago@unad.edu.co

M. A. R. Ahad et al. (eds.), *Sensor- and Video-Based Activity and Behavior Computing*,
Smart Innovation, Systems and Technologies 291,
https://doi.org/10.1007/978-981-19-0361-8_3

with multiple sensors, they are rarely used in real-life environments. In this study, we employ learning using privileged information (LUPI) [19] for HAR. LUPI is a learning paradigm based on the supposition that one may access additional information about the training samples, which is not available during testing. In classical supervised learning, the learner model is presented with the training tuple(x_i, y_i) and creates an optimization model f for predicting Y.

$$(x_i, y_i), \ldots, (x_l, x_l), x_i \in X, y_i \in \{-1, 1\}$$

On the other hand, LUPI is presented with the training tuple(x_i, x_i^*, y_i) as shown below, and X^* can be used only during training.

$$(x_i, x_i^*, y_i), \ldots, (x_l, y_l^*, x_l), x_i \in X, x_i^* \in X^*, y_i \in \{-1, 1\}$$

X^* is called privileged information(PI). In this study, we used sensors of different positions as PI. That is, we used multiple sensors during training and a single sensor during testing. The contributions of this study can be summarized as follows:

1. In sensor-based activity recognition, we show that the recognition accuracy is improved by using multiple sensors for complex activity recognition.
2. We compared the performance between LUPI and the baseline method using several situations (random-split cross-validation, leave-one-subject-out cross-validation).
3. LUPI is shown to be superior to the baseline method in a dataset containing complex activities (Fig. 1).

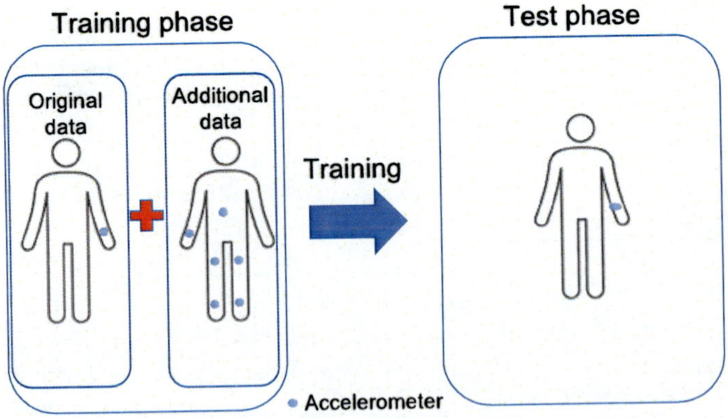

Fig. 1 Overview of our proposed method. At the time of training, training is performed with original data (single sensor) and additional data (multiple sensors), and at the time of testing, only the original data (single sensor) is used

2 Related Work

Different learning paradigms have been used in activity recognition to improve performance in real-life settings. This section describes related work about transfer learning, multi-model learning, and machine learning using LUPI.

Transfer Learning: Sensor-based activity recognition affects recognition accuracy depending on sensor orientation and subject differences in the source and target domains. To address this issue, there are proposed HAR using transfer learning [2, 15]. In this study, we handle different sets of sensors in the source domain and the target domain. Then, we aim to improve the recognition accuracy of activity recognition of complex activities that are difficult to recognize with a single sensor.

Multi-Modal Learning: In activity recognition using visual information, activity comprehension may fail due to occultation and appearance variation, but IMU sensors may be able to avoid them. For this reason, there are proposed HAR methods of combined multiple modalities such as sensor and visual information [7, 14]. Kong et al. [7] perform activity recognition using RGB Video, Keypoints, acceleration, gyroscope, orientation, Wi-Fi, and pressure signal data. They succeeded in creating a highly robust model for different subjects, viewpoints, indoor environments, and sessions in training data and test data. In this study, different position sensors worn on the body are treated as multimodal data. In our problem setting, multiple sensors are used only during training, and only a single sensor is used during the test.

Machine Learning Using LUPI: There are many studies using LUPI [5, 10, 18, 20, 21]. Gauraha et al. [5] classify MNIST and discover drugs using SVM+ with LUPI implemented, and show that it can be recognized with higher accuracy than SVM. In addition, John et al. [10] proposed a method that makes the distribution of Dropout in CNN and RNN a function of privileged information and showed that it can be recognized with higher accuracy in image recognition and machine translation than the baseline method. Michalis et al. [20, 21] use LUPI in the activity recognition of moving images and train the model by using voice, pose, and attribute data in addition to the moving image only during training. These studies use visual data instead of sensor data as this study. Lago et al. [9] use a similar problem setting for sensor-based activity recognition and improved recognition accuracy by performing feature learning using unsupervised machine learning by multiple sensors and then mapping a single sensor to the learned space. In this study, supervised learning is also used for additional information that can be used only during training.

3 Proposed Method

In this paper, we proposed a method for improved single activity recognition using LUPI. Figure 2 shows the overall proposed method. At the time of training, after feature extraction is performed from multiple sensors, the original data and additional data are trained using SVM+ [11] which is a LUPI classifier. In this study, we build

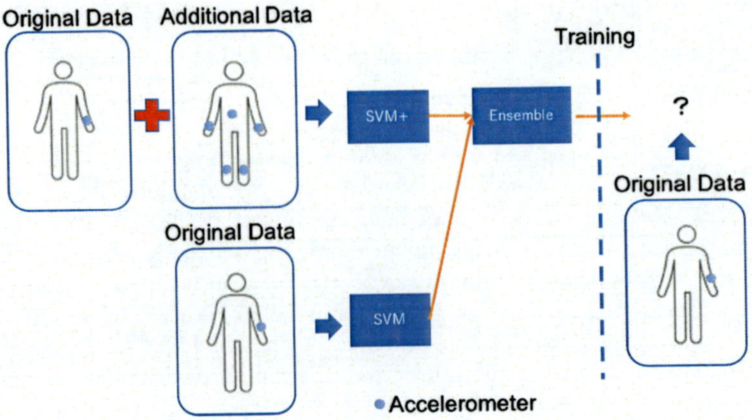

Fig. 2 Overall proposed method. We used SVM+ as a LUPI classifier. Then, we build an ensemble classifier using SVM and SVM+

the ensemble classifier that combines a LUPI classifier(SVM+) and a baseline model (SVM) trained using only a single sensor. Note that, at the time of testing, the data added during training is not used. In this section, we describe the proposed method in detail.

3.1 LUPI Classifier(SVM Plus)

We describe difference between SVM and SVM+ [11]. Both classifiers are finding some $\omega \in X$ and $b \in R$ to built according to the following rules

$$f(x) = sgn[\langle \omega, x_i \rangle + b].$$

The SVM learning method (non-separable SVM) to find ω and b to solving the following optimization problem:

$$\min \frac{1}{2}\langle \omega, \omega \rangle + C\sum_{i=1}^{m} \xi_i$$

$$s.t.\ \ y_i[\langle \omega, x_i \rangle] \geq 1 - \xi_i,\ \ i = 1, \ldots, m.$$

where C is some regularization parameter that needs to tune. And, if the slacks ξ_i are all equal to zero then we call the set of given examples separable. On other hand, SVM+ has modified the SVM formulation as follows in order to consider privileged information X^*.

$$\min \frac{1}{2}[\langle \omega, \omega \rangle + \gamma \langle \omega^*, \omega^* \rangle] + C \sum_{i=1}^{m} [\langle \omega^*, x^* \rangle + b^*]$$

$$s.t. \;\; y_i[\langle \omega, x_i \rangle + b] \geq 1 - [\langle \omega^*, x_i^* \rangle + b^*], \;\; i = 1, \ldots, m.$$

$$[\langle \omega^*, \; x_i^* \rangle + b^*] \geq 0, \;\; i = 1, \ldots, m.$$

where $\omega^* \in X^*$ and $b^* \in R$. In this problem, C and γ are hyperparameters to be tuned. The difference between SVM+ and SVM is that it uses privileged information to estimate the slack variables. Given the training tuple (x, x^*, y), SVM+ maps x to the feature space Z and x^* to a separate feature space Z^*. Then, slack variables are estimated by $\xi = \langle \omega^*, x^* \rangle + b^*$.

3.2 *Ensemble Classifier*

In this study, we combined SVM and SVM+ model to achieve better performance. We apply ensemble averaging [4] for the combination. For this, we first train the SVM using (x, y). Then we train the SVM+ using (x, x^*, y). Finally, we combined their model using ensemble averaging.

4 Experimental Evaluation

In this section, we describe datasets and evaluation method used for this experiment. The goal of the experiments is to compare the performance of the baseline method and the proposed method single sensor activity recognition in several situations.

4.1 *Dataset*

We used four datasets for evaluating our proposed method. Some important aspects of the data are summarized in Table 1. These datasets contain multiple sensor data from different placement.

4.1.1 Cooking Dataset

The Cooking Dataset [8] consists of the following main dietary activities: (i) Prepare a soup (ii) Set table. (iii) Eat meal. (iv) Clean up and put away utensils. More detailed

Table 1 Datasets used for the evaluation

Dataset (Activity type)	No. of sensors	No. of subjects	No. of classes	No. of windows
OPP HL [17] (complex activities)	5 IMUs	4	6	1745
Cooking dataset [8] (complex activities)	5 IMUs	7	16	1780
PAMAP [16] (simple activities)	3 IMUs	5	12	2569
OPP Locomotion [17] (simple activities)	5 IMUs	4	6	5461

behaviors are labeled for each dietary activity. In this study, we used the accelerometer of the IMU sensor for evaluation and we use windows of 1 s with no overlapping.

4.1.2 Opportunity Dataset

The opportunity Dataset [17] contains morning routine behaviors collected by four subjects. Activities are labeled with different types of locomotion, gestures, and high-level activities. In this study, we used high-level activities (OPP HL), which include complex activities such as relaxing, coffee (prepare and drink), sandwich (prepare and eat), early-morning (check objects in the room), and cleanup, and locomotion activities (OPP Loc) which include stand, walk, sit, and lie. As with the cooking dataset, the accelerometer of the IMU sensor was used for this dataset as well. we used a 1-second time window for simple activities and a 10-second time window for complex activities.

4.1.3 PAMAP Dataset

The Physical Activity Monitoring Dataset [16] is a benchmark dataset for monitoring physical activities. This dataset contains the activities of lie, sit, stand, walk, run, cycle, Nordic walk, iron, vacuum clean, rope jump, ascend, and descend stairs. Also, not all subjects performed all activities, so some subjects were not included in the evaluation data in this study. We also used a 5 s time window for this dataset.

4.2 *Implementation and Evaluation Metrics*

For the implementation, we used Python and Scikit-Learn. And we extracted max, min, average, and standard deviation of each segment for each axis. For evaluation protocol, we used a random-split cross-validation(each subject and entire data) and leave-one-subject-out cross-validation (user-independent models). As evaluation metrics, we used F1-score to compare the performance between our proposed method and the baseline method.

4.3 *Result*

We present the results of the evaluation. We first show the results of comparing activity recognition performance between a single sensor and multiple sensors (Sect. 4.3.1). Then, we show results of our proposed method using three cross-validations, namely random-split cross-validation using each subject (Sect. 4.3.2), random-split cross-validation using entire dataset (Sect. 4.3.3), and leave-one-subject-out cross-validation (Sect. 4.3.4).

4.3.1 Measuring the Gap Between Single-sensor and Multi-sensor Activity Recognition Performance

Figures 3 and 4 show the results of comparing the recognition accuracy of activity recognition using a single sensor and the accuracy using multiple sensors for the four datasets. We used SVM after the feature extraction, use leave-one-subject-out cross-validation for evaluation. As we can see, recognition accuracy is higher when multiple sensors are used in most cases. Especially in the case of complex activities of the cooking dataset and opportunity dataset (Fig. 4a, b), it can be seen that the recognition accuracy is relatively high when using multiple sensors. This experiment validates the hypothesis that using multiple sensors improves the accuracy of activity recognition. Therefore, multiple sensors can be used as additional information during training.

4.3.2 Validation Results Using Additional Information During Training (Random-Split Cross-Validation of Each Subject)

Figure 5 shows the results showing the average value of F1-score using random-split cross-validation of each subject. Since the number of labels for one subject was small and it was impossible to properly divide it into training data and test data, the cooking dataset was excluded from this validation.

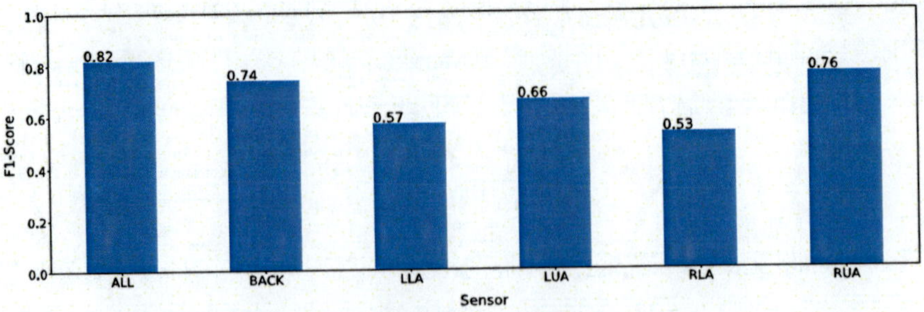

(a) Opportunity dataset

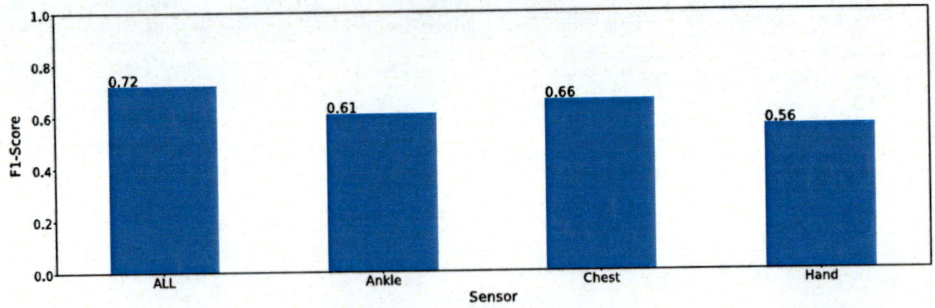

(b) PAMAP dataset

Fig. 3 Comparison of recognition accuracy of activity recognition with a single sensor and multiple sensors (simple activity). "ALL" used multiple sensors, others used a single sensor

Figure 5a shows the results using the PAMAP dataset. This dataset can use 5 subjects and 3 IMU sensors. Therefore, we validated 15 cases combinations of subjects and sensors in total. From the figure, it can be seen that the average value of F1-Score is improved compared to the baseline method in all cases.

Figure 5b shows the validation results using simple activities dataset in the opportunity dataset. This dataset can use 4 subjects and 5 IMU sensors. Therefore, we validated 20 cases combinations of subjects and sensors in total. From the figure, it can be seen that the average value of F1-Score is improved in 2 out of 5 cases compared to the baseline method.

Figure 5c shows the validation results when using the complex activities dataset of the opportunity dataset. This dataset can use 4 subjects and 5 IMU sensors. Therefore, we validated 20 cases combinations of subjects and sensors in total. From this figure, it can be seen that the average value of the F1-score is improved compared to the baseline method in each case.

Table 2 shows the number of improvements and the number of deteriorations between SVM (baseline) and ensemble for each dataset in this validation. From the table, it can be seen that the number of improvements is greater than the number of deteriorations in all datasets. In addition, it can be seen that the F1-score of the complex activity type dataset is improved compared to the simple activity type dataset.

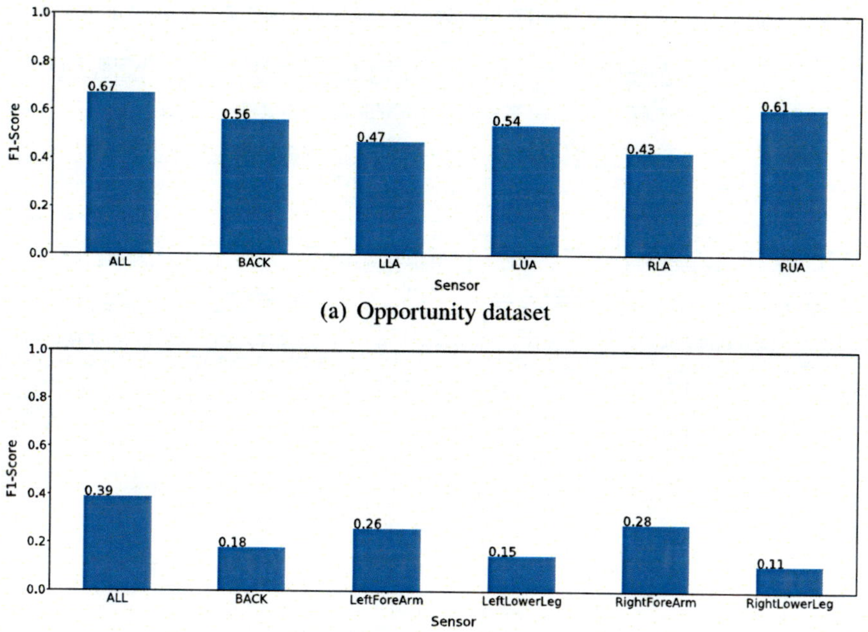

(a) Opportunity dataset

(b) Cooking dataset

Fig. 4 Comparison of recognition accuracy of activity recognition with a single sensor and multiple sensors (complex activity) “ALL” used multiple sensors, others used a single sensor

4.3.3 Validation Results Using Additional Information During Training (Random-Split Cross-Validation of the Entire Data)

Figures 6 and 7 show that the results of validation by randomly setting 80% of the training data and 20% of the test data for each dataset.

Figure 6a shows that results of using a simple activities dataset in the opportunity dataset are shown. This dataset contains 5 sensors, we validated 5 cases in total. The figure shows that the F1-score was improved compared to the baseline method in 3 out of 5 cases.

Figure 6b shows the results of validation using the PAMAP dataset. This dataset contains 3 sensors, we validated 3 cases in total. From the figure, the F1-score was improved compared to the baseline method (SVM) when hand and ankle are used for X.

Figure 7a shows the results when using a dataset of complex activities in the opportunity dataset. This dataset contains 5 sensors, we validated 5 cases in total. From the figure, it can be seen that the F1-score was improved compared to the baseline method in 4 out of 5 cases.

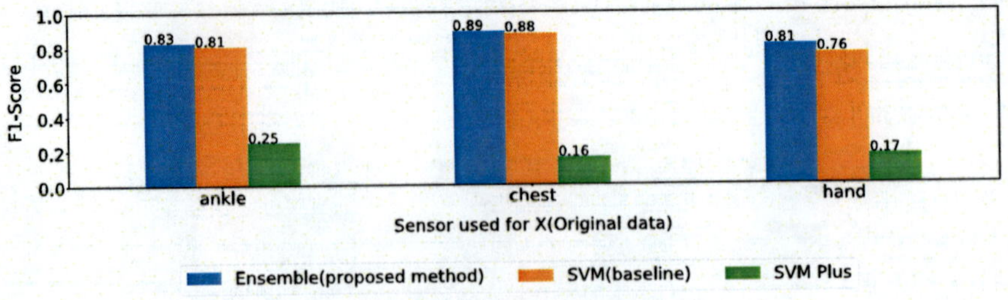

(a) PAMAP Dataset

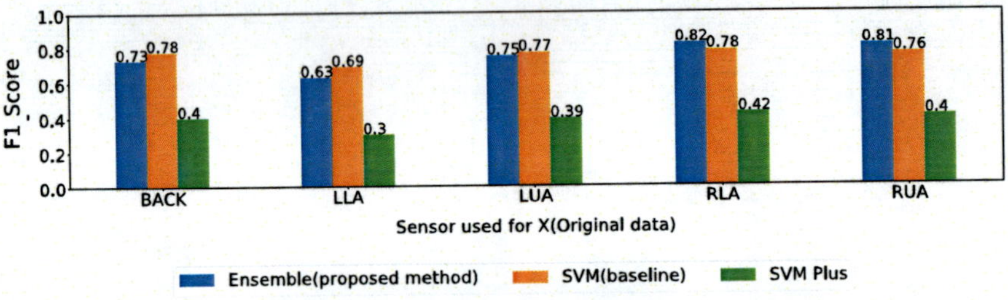

(b) Opportunity Dataset(simple activate)

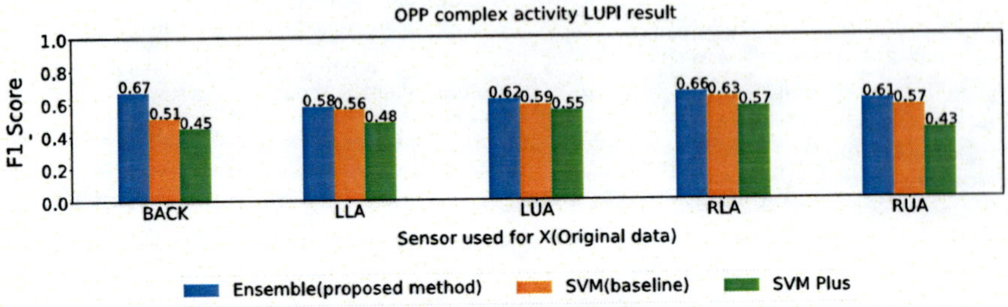

(c) Opportunity Dataset(complex activities)

Fig. 5 Validation result of the each subject using random-split cross-validation (train:80% test:20%)

Table 2 Total number of improvements and degradations between SVM (baseline) and ensemble was validated using random-split cross-validation of each subject using three datasets

	Total number of cases	Number of improvements	Number of deteriorations
PAMAP	15	14	1
OPP HL	20	18	2
OPP Locomotion	20	11	9

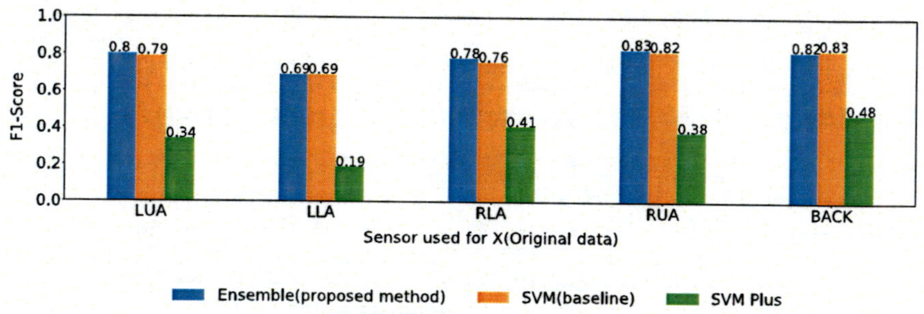

(a) Opportunity Dataset

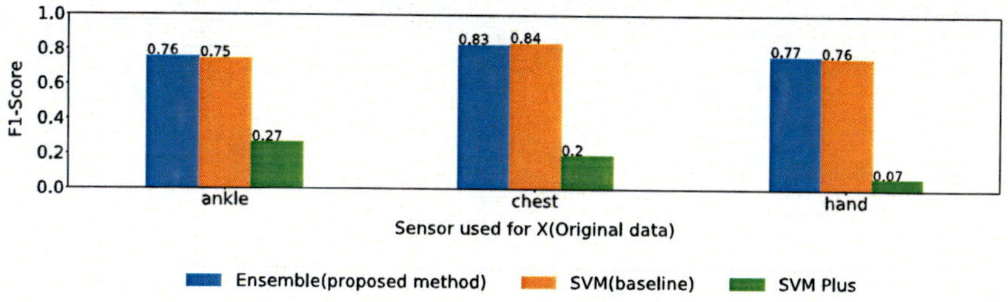

(b) PAMAP Dataset

Fig. 6 Validation result of the entire dataset (simple activities) using random cross-validation (train:80% test:20%)

Figure 7b shows the validation results using the cooking dataset. From this figure, it can be seen that the F1-score was improved compared to the baseline method (SVM) in all cases.

Table 3 shows the number of improvements and the number of deteriorations between SVM (baseline) and ensemble for each dataset in this validation. From the table, the number of improvements is greater than the number of deteriorations in all datasets

4.3.4 Validation Results Using Additional Information During Training (Leave-One-Subject-Out Cross-Validation)

Figures 8 and 9 show the results of leave-one-subject-out cross-validation. These figures show the average value of the F1-score when cross-validation was performed.

Figure 8a shows the results when a simple activities dataset in the opportunity dataset is used. This dataset can use 4 subjects and 5 IMU sensors. Therefore, we validated 20 cases combinations of subjects and sensors in total (4 cross-validation patterns $\times$ 5 combination patterns of X and X^*). The figure shows that the average value of F1-Score is improved in 2 out of 5 cases compared to the baseline method.

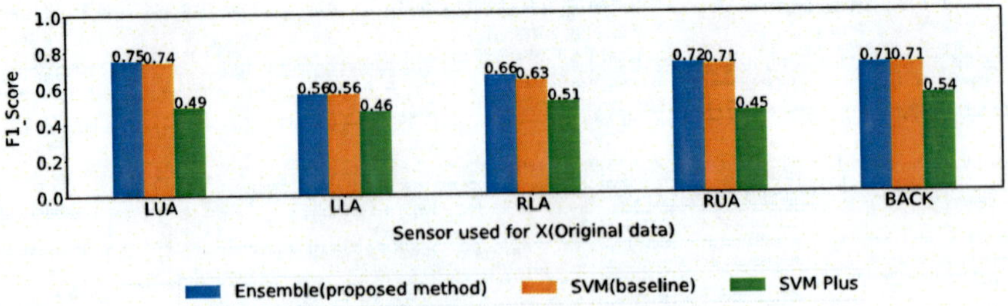

(a) Opportunity dataset

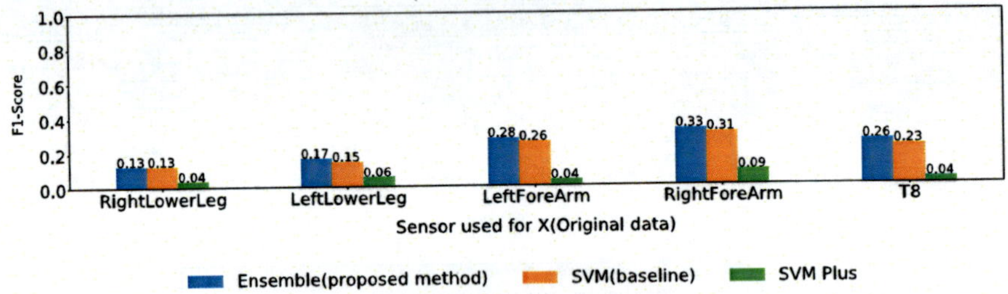

(b) Cooking dataset

Fig. 7 Validation result of the entire dataset (complex activities) using random cross-validation (train:80% test:20%)

Table 3 Total number of improvements and degradations between SVM (baseline) and ensemble was validated using random cross-validation using four datasets

	Total number of cases	Number of improvements	Number of deteriorations
Cooking	5	5	0
PAMAP	3	2	1
OPP HL	5	4	1
OPP Locomotion	5	3	2

Figure 8b shows the results of validation using the PAMAP dataset. This dataset can use 5 subjects and 3 IMU sensors. Therefore, we validated 15 cases combinations of subjects and sensors in total (5 cross-validation patterns × 3 combination patterns of X and X^*). The figure shows that the average value of F1-Score is improved in 2 out of 3 cases compared to the baseline method.

Figure 9a shows the results of using the complex activities dataset in the opportunity dataset. This dataset can use 4 subjects and 5 IMU sensors. Therefore, we validated 20 cases combinations of subjects and sensors in total (5 cross-validation patterns × 3 combination patterns of X and X^*). The figure shows that the average value of F1-score is improved in 2 out of 5 cases compared to the baseline method.

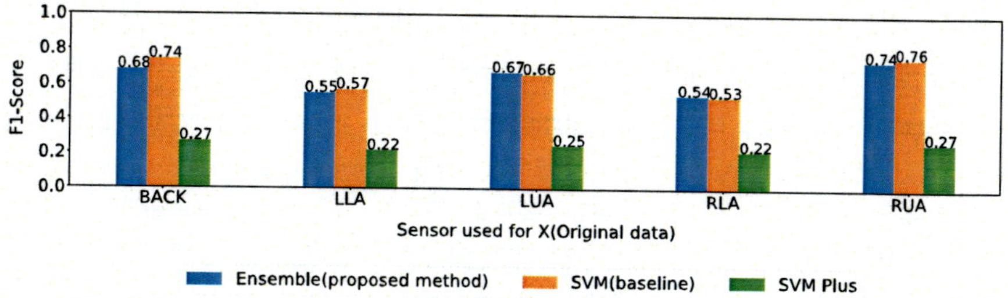

(a) Opportunity dataset

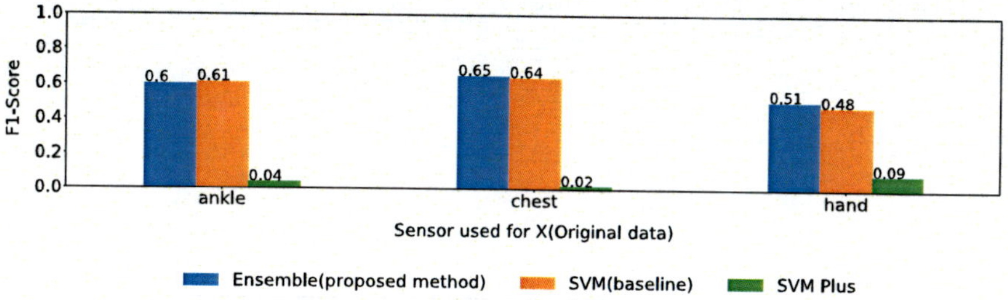

(b) PAMAP dataset

Fig. 8 Validation result using leave-subject-out cross-validation(simple activities)

Figure 9b shows the results of validation using the Cooking dataset. This dataset can use 7 subjects and 5 IMU sensors. Therefore, we validated 35 cases combinations of subjects and sensors in total (7 cross-validation patterns × 5 combination patterns of X and X^*). From the figure, it can be seen that the average value of F1-Score is improved in recognition accuracy in 1 case out of 5 cases compared to the baseline method.

Table 4 shows the number of improvements and the number of deteriorations between SVM(baseline) and ensemble for each dataset in this validation. From the table, it can be seen that the number of deteriorations is higher than the number of improvements, except for the datasets of complex activities types of PAMAP and opportunity dataset.

5 Discussion

In this section, we consider the following based on the results of the previous section.

- Improvement of recognition accuracy by using additional training information
- Deterioration of recognition accuracy due to the use of additional training information

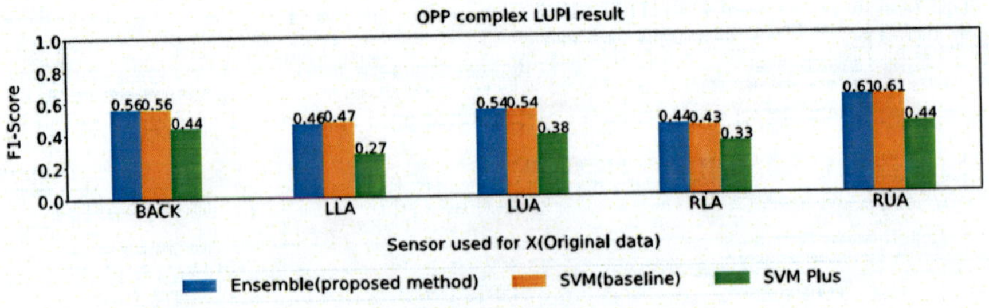

(a) Opportunity dataset

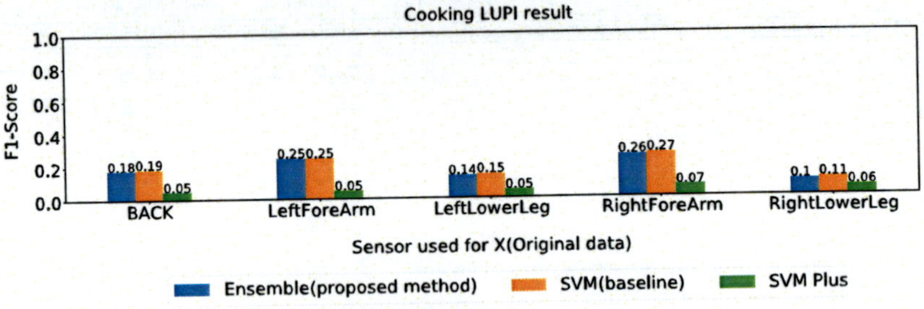

(b) Cooking dataset

Fig. 9 Validation result using leave-subject-out cross-validation (complex activities)

Table 4 Total number of improvements and degradations between SVM (baseline) and ensemble was validated using leave-one-subject-out cross-validation using four datasets

	Total number of cases	Number of improvements	Number of deteriorations
Cooking	35	15	20
PAMAP	15	8	7
OPP HL	20	9	11
OPP Locomotion	20	13	7

5.1 Improvement of Recognition Accuracy by Using Additional Learning Information

From the results of Table 3, it can be said that the recognition accuracy can be improved when training with additional information that can be used only during training. In particular, as we can see, it is effective for the datasets containing complex activities such as the opportunity dataset (Fig. 7a) and the cooking dataset (Fig. 7b).

5.2 *Deterioration of Recognition Accuracy Due to the Use of Additional Training Information*

From Table 4, it was found that when the subjects are different between the training data and the test data, there are more cases of deterioration than improvement. Therefore, in order to apply this method to such cases, it is necessary to consider the difference in the features of each subject. In addition, it can be said that the recognition accuracy of SVM+ is lower than that of the baseline method as a whole, which is the cause of the low recognition accuracy even when combined as an ensemble. As a feature of SVM+, additional information is assumed trained as accurate information, so even if it is not accurate information, it is treated as correct information, which is thought to have led to a decrease in recognition accuracy. Furthermore, the previous research [12] studies sensor-based activity recognition using SVM+. But, the same IMU sensor information has been used. In short, the accelerometer sensor is used as original data, the gyroscope sensor is used as additional data.

6 Conclusion

In this paper, in order to improve the accuracy of complex activity recognition, we employ ensemble learning which combined baseline (SVM) and LUPI (SVM+) classifier. We used four published datasets for evaluating our proposed method using random-split cross-validation and leave-one-subject-out cross-validation. As a result, the proposed method improved by up to 16% in F1-score to 67% compared to baseline method when we used random-split cross-validation of each subject. However, when we used leave-one-subject-out cross-validation, the recognition accuracy is worse than the baseline method. In addition, it is different features between sensor positions and affects recognition accuracy. Another major reason is that SVM + has lower accuracy than SVM. Unfortunately, our work does not show a benefit of LUPI, with the performance of SMV+ significantly lower than the baseline SVM. The performance of the ensemble is slightly higher than SVM. While this might indicate that a combination of classical SVM and SVM with LUPI could lead to better ensembles, it does not rule out that the improvement observed comes from using an ensemble at all. In order to elucidate this question, other ensembles should be assessed (e.g., SVM and KNN). Based on the above, As future work, we would like to study the following:

- Examining methods for extracting common features from different sensors.
- Examining feature extraction methods that do not depend on the subject.
- Comparing ensemble learning with other classifiers to use in combination with SVM+.

References

1. Bulling, A., Blanke, U., Schiele, B.: A tutorial on human activity recognition using body-worn inertial sensors. ACM Comput. Surv. **46**(3) (2014). https://doi.org/10.1145/2499621
2. Chang, Y., Mathur, A., Isopoussu, A., Song, J., Kawsar, F.: A systematic study of unsupervised domain adaptation for robust human-activity recognition. Proc. ACM Interact. Mob. Wearable Ubiquitous Technol. **4**(1) (2020). https://doi.org/10.1145/3380985
3. Dernbach, S., Das, B., Krishnan, N.C., Thomas, B.L., Cook, D.J.: Simple and complex activity recognition through smart phones. In: 2012 Eighth International Conference on Intelligent Environments, pp. 214–221 (2012). https://doi.org/10.1109/IE.2012.39
4. Dietterich, T.G.: Ensemble methods in machine learning. In: Multiple Classifier Systems, pp. 1–15. Springer, Heidelberg (2000)
5. Gauraha, N., Carlsson, L., Spjuth, O.: Conformal prediction in learning under privileged information paradigm with applications in drug discovery. In: Gammerman, A., Vovk, V., Luo, Z., Smirnov, E., Peeters, R. (eds.) Proceedings of the Seventh Workshop on Conformal and Probabilistic Prediction and Applications, *Proceedings of Machine Learning Research*, vol. 91, pp. 147–156. PMLR (2018). http://proceedings.mlr.press/v91/gauraha18a.html
6. Inoue, S., Ueda, N., Nohara, Y., Nakashima, N.: Mobile activity recognition for a whole day: Recognizing real nursing activities with big dataset. In: Proceedings of the 2015 ACM International Joint Conference on Pervasive and Ubiquitous Computing, UbiComp '15, pp. 1269–1280. Association for Computing Machinery, New York, NY, USA (2015). https://doi.org/10.1145/2750858.2807533
7. Kong, Q., Wu, Z., Deng, Z., Klinkigt, M., Tong, B., Murakami, T.: Mmact: A large-scale dataset for cross modal human action understanding. In: 2019 IEEE/CVF International Conference on Computer Vision (ICCV), pp. 8657–8666 (2019). https://doi.org/10.1109/ICCV.2019.00875
8. Krüger, F., Nyolt, M., Yordanova, K., Hein, A., Kirste, T.: Computational state space models for activity and intention recognition. a feasibility study. PLOS ONE **9**(11), 1–24 (2014). https://doi.org/10.1371/journal.pone.0109381
9. Lago, P.A., Matsuki, M., Inoue, S.: Achieving single-sensor complex activity recognition from multi-sensor training data. ArXiv abs/2002.11284 (2020)
10. Lambert, J., Sener, O., Savarese, S.: Deep learning under privileged information using heteroscedastic dropout. In: The IEEE Conference on Computer Vision and Pattern Recognition (CVPR) (2018)
11. Lapin, M., Hein, M., Schiele, B.: Learning using privileged information: Svm+ and weighted svm. Neural Netw. **53**, 95–108 (2014). https://doi.org/10.1016/j.neunet.2014.02.002. https://www.sciencedirect.com/science/article/pii/S0893608014000306
12. Li, X., Du, B., Xu, C., Zhang, Y., Zhang, L., Tao, D.: Robust learning with imperfect privileged information. Artificial Intelligence **282**, 103246 (2020). https://doi.org/10.1016/j.artint.2020.103246. https://www.sciencedirect.com/science/article/pii/S0004370220300114
13. Liu, L., Peng, Y., Wang, S., Liu, M., Huang, Z.: Complex activity recognition using time series pattern dictionary learned from ubiquitous sensors. Information Sci. **340–341**, 41–57 (2016). https://doi.org/10.1016/j.ins.2016.01.020. https://www.sciencedirect.com/science/article/pii/S0020025516000311
14. Mao, D., Lin, X., Liu, Y., Xu, M., Wang, G., Chen, J., Zhang, W.: Activity Recognition from Skeleton and Acceleration Data Using CNN and GCN, pp. 15–25. Springer, Singapore (2021). https://doi.org/10.1007/978-981-15-8269-1_2
15. Morales, F.J.O.N., Roggen, D.: Deep convolutional feature transfer across mobile activity recognition domains, sensor modalities and locations. In: Proceedings of the 2016 ACM International Symposium on Wearable Computers, ISWC '16, pp. 92–99. Association for Computing Machinery, New York, NY, USA (2016). https://doi.org/10.1145/2971763.2971764
16. Reiss, A., Stricker, D.: Introducing a new benchmarked dataset for activity monitoring. In: 2012 16th International Symposium on Wearable Computers, pp. 108–109 (2012). https://doi.org/10.1109/ISWC.2012.13

17. Roggen, D., Calatroni, A., Rossi, M., Holleczek, T., Förster, K., Tröster, G., Lukowicz, P., Bannach, D., Pirkl, G., Ferscha, A., Doppler, J., Holzmann, C., Kurz, M., Holl, G., Chavarriaga, R., Sagha, H., Bayati, H., Creatura, M., Millán, J.d.R.: Collecting complex activity datasets in highly rich networked sensor environments. In: 2010 Seventh International Conference on Networked Sensing Systems (INSS), pp. 233–240 (2010). https://doi.org/10.1109/INSS.2010.5573462
18. Tang, F., Xiao, C., Wang, F., Zhou, J., Lehman, L.w.H.: Retaining privileged information for multi-task learning. In: Proceedings of the 25th ACM SIGKDD International Conference on Knowledge Discovery & ; Data Mining, KDD '19, pp. 1369–1377. Association for Computing Machinery, New York, NY, USA (2019). https://doi.org/10.1145/3292500.3330907
19. Vapnik, V., Izmailov, R.: Learning using privileged information: similarity control and knowledge transfer. J. Mach. Learn. Res. **16**(61), 2023–2049 (2015). http://jmlr.org/papers/v16/vapnik15b.html
20. Vrigkas, M., Kazakos, E., Nikou, C., Kakadiaris, I.: Human activity recognition using robust adaptive privileged probabilistic learning. In: Pattern Analysis and Applications (2021). https://doi.org/10.1007/s10044-020-00953-x
21. Vrigkas, M., Kazakos, E., Nikou, C., Kakadiaris, I.A.: Inferring human activities using robust privileged probabilistic learning. In: 2017 IEEE International Conference on Computer Vision Workshops (ICCVW), pp. 2658–2665 (2017). https://doi.org/10.1109/ICCVW.2017.307

Attempts Toward Behavior Recognition of the Asian Black Bears Using an Accelerometer

Kaori Fujinami, Tomoko Naganuma, Yushin Shinoda, Koji Yamazaki, and Shinsuke Koike

Abstract The miniaturizations of sensing units, the increase in storage capacity, and the longevity of batteries, as well as the advancement of big-data processing technologies, are making it possible to recognize animal behaviors. This allows researchers to understand animal space use patterns, social interactions, habitats, etc. In this study, we focused on the behavior recognition of Asian black bears (*Ursus thibetanus*) using a three-axis accelerometer embedded in collars attached to their necks, where approximately 1% of data obtained from four bears over an average of 42 d were used. A machine learning was used to recognize seven bear behaviors, where oversampling and extension of labels to the period adjacent to the labeled period were applied to overcome data imbalance across classes and insufficient data in some classes. Experimental results showed the effectiveness of oversampling and a large difference in individual bears. Effective feature sets vary by experimental conditions. However, a tendency of features calculated from the magnitude of the three axes contributing to classification performance was confirmed.

1 Introduction

Noninvasive monitoring of human activities using mobile and wearable devices has been gaining considerable attention in various application domains such as fitness and sports [1], health care [2], and work performance management [3] due to the improvement of the computational and processing capabilities of these devices. Meanwhile, the use of sensors on animals has been employed for ecological research of various animals such as birds, fish, and mammals using electronic tags [4, 5].

K. Fujinami (✉) · T. Naganuma · Y. Shinoda · S. Koike
Tokyo University of Agriculture and Technology, Tokyo, Japan
e-mail: fujinami@cc.tuat.ac.jp

S. Koike
e-mail: koikes@cc.tuat.ac.jp

K. Yamazaki
Tokyo University of Agriculture, Tokyo, Japan
e-mail: yamako@j.email.ne.jp

M. A. R. Ahad et al. (eds.), *Sensor- and Video-Based Activity and Behavior Computing*, Smart Innovation, Systems and Technologies 291,
https://doi.org/10.1007/978-981-19-0361-8_4

In recent years, the miniaturization of measurement units, the increase in storage capacity, and the longevity of batteries have made it possible to mount various sensors, such as inertial sensors, proximity sensors, magnetic sensors, temperature sensors, and cameras, on animals and to record a large amount of data for a long period. Such sensor data analysis has also been improved by the advancement of data processing technologies such as machine learning (ML), which enables automated analysis, resulting in human-independent large-scale analysis in the research community. This has allowed researchers to study and better understand animal movements, space use patterns, physiology, social interactions, and habitats [6, 7]. Knowledge obtained from this analysis is intended to be used in the conservation and management of wild animals [8, 9], welfare and production management of livestock [10, 11], and health care and communication with humans and pets [12, 13].

In this study, we focus on behavior recognition of Asian black bears (*Ursus thibetanus*) (hereinafter simply called "bears") using a collar-mounted accelerometer. Since the beginning of the 2000s, the range of bears has expanded, and their habitat has been confirmed in the vicinity of villages, making it easier for bears and humans to encounter each other. This has increased the number of conflicts between humans and bears, causing human casualties and damage to agriculture and forestry [14, 15]. Attempts have been made to understand seasonal movements and inhabiting patterns through the GPS [16, 17]. In addition, an "activity sensor" based on an accelerometer is combined with GPS to distinguish between active and inactive states, which is difficult to achieve with only GPS [14]. This suggests that deeper understanding of the ecology of bears is possible by combining movement information from GPS with behavioral information from an accelerometer.

Cattle [18, 19], other livestock such as sheep [10, 20] and chickens [21], and pets such as dogs [13, 22] are popular in behavior recognition research because of the ease of data collection and the size of the market, where a variety of behaviors are targets for recognition: foraging, ruminating, resting, traveling, and other behaviors for cattle [19]; barking, chewing, digging, drinking, and other 12 behaviors for dogs [22]; and pecking, preening, and dust bathing for chickens [11]. However, to the best of our knowledge regarding bears, there are no other studies that deal with more complex behavior recognition than discriminating between active and inactive states, except for the work by Pagano et al.[23]. In their work, ten behaviors of wild polar bears, i.e., resting, walking, swimming, eating, running, pouncing, grooming, digging, head shaking, and rolling, were recognized by a random forest classifier with data obtained from a three-axis accelerometer and conductivity sensor. In this study, seven classes are subject to classification, including resting, feeding, sniffing, foraging, traveling, socializing, and others, with some overlaps, excesses, and deficiencies between the work of Pagano et al. and ours. Our work is considered the first attempt to recognize the behaviors of bears using a three-axis accelerometer. The contributions of our work are summarized as follows:

- A classification method for recognizing seven behaviors is presented, where variation classifier models and classification features are evaluated.

- Oversampling and a technique that assigns the same label to the period adjacent to the labeled period are used to overcome the impact of imbalanced and small amounts of data.

The remainder of this paper is organized as follows. Section 2 describes the dataset. The behavior recognition method is presented in Sect. 3, followed by experiments to understand the suitable classifier model and feature set, as well as training data configuration and generalizability. Section 5 concludes the study.

2 Dataset

In this section, the information regarding the dataset used in this study is presented.

2.1 Basic Information

The data were originally collected for a study to better understand the mating system of wild bears in 2018 [24], where four adult bears (two males and two females) were captured and attached GPS collars equipped with cameras (VERTEX Plus Iridium camera [25], 1.2 kg) from May to July 2018 in Okutama, Tokyo. The duration of data collection varied for each bear and was 42 d on average (41, 45, 36, and 45 d) each.

A GPS receiver, a video recorder, and a three-axis accelerometer were integrated into the collar. In this study, signals from the three-axis accelerometer sampled 8 Hz were used to model bears behavior based on the force and gravity given to the sensor. Pagano et al. [23] showed that there is no difference between the predictability at 8 and 16 Hz even though the predictability 4 Hz was lower than that 8 Hz. Thus, we believe that 8 Hz is reasonable for our case. The orientation of the axes of the accelerometer is shown in Fig. 1a, where the x-, y-, and z-axes denote surge, sway, and heave, respectively. However, because the collar can rotate around the neck, the orientation of the y- and z-axes might be interchangeable.

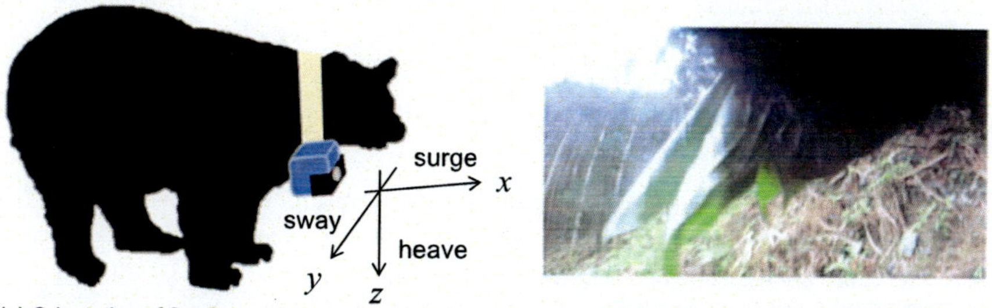

(a) Orientation of 3-axis accelerometer and camera (b) Snapshot of video data (feeding)

Fig. 1 Sensor placement and axis orientation. Note that the collar can rotate around the neck

Table 1 Behavior classes distinguished on collar-mounted videos

Behavior	Description
Resting	No movement, e.g., sleeping, grooming, scratching, staying, and lying down
Feeding	Eating something, e.g., chewing and licking
Sniffing	Sniffing something, excluding food items, e.g., air, ground, shrub, tree, decayed tree, under-forestry herb, and artificial objects
Foraging	Searching for food items, e.g., digging the ground, breaking decayed trees, sniffing or touching food items, and moving or breaking branches on the tree with food items
Traveling	Movement on land such as running or walking
Socializing	Interacting with other individuals, e.g., social engagement, mating
Others	Other behaviors (approx. 3.1% of all data), e.g., bedding, drinking, moving on trees rubbing on trees, swimming, shaking head, and unknown due to unclear image

Video data were recorded for 10 s every 15 min from 5:00 to 18:00, which was leveraged for labeling even though it was originally the main study material in [24]. A snapshot of a captured video is also shown in Fig. 1b. Note that the recording period (10 s), interval (15 min), and duty cycle (13 h on and 11 h off) were determined by the limitations of the battery and storage capacity of the device, as well as the requirement of the original study to record daytime behaviors. For more details regarding data collection, please refer to [24].

2.2 *Data Labeling*

By referring to the work on behavior classification of polar bears [23] and taking into account the ecology of bears, we classified their behaviors into seven classes (Table 1), where each class contained concrete behaviors. For example, "resting" may indicate that a bear is sleeping, grooming, scratching, or having a break. Acceleration signals were labeled with one of the seven classes by watching video clips (e.g., Fig. 1b). Note that labeling was performed by a person familiar with bear behaviors. Major waveforms in each behavior class are shown in Fig. 2.

3 Behavior Recognition Method

Figure 3 shows the pipeline of behavior recognition, where a supervised ML model is used, with the procedure of the training phase presented. The basic components consist of windowing, feature calculations, training, and classification, and label extension, oversampling, and scaling which are options, depending on experimental conditions. In the following subsections, each component is described.

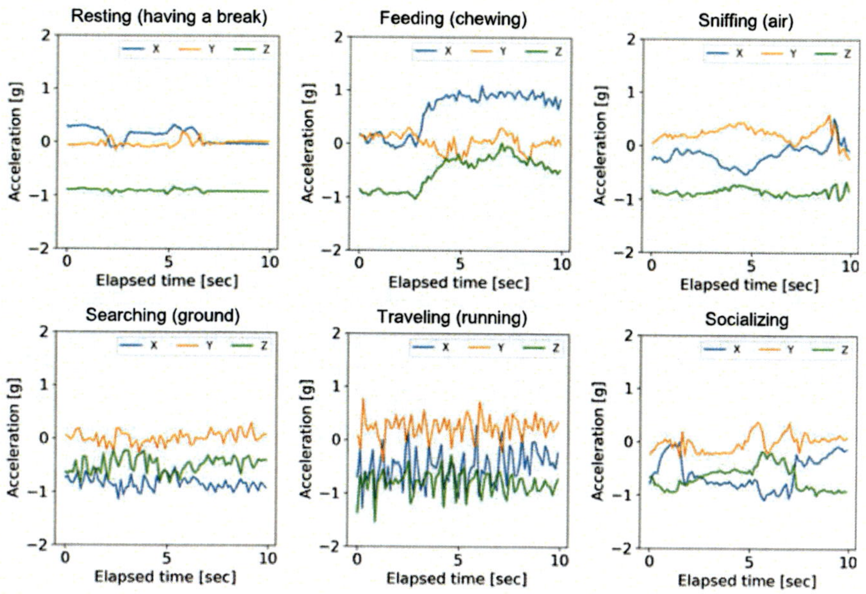

Fig. 2 Waveforms of major instances from each behavior class except for class "Others"

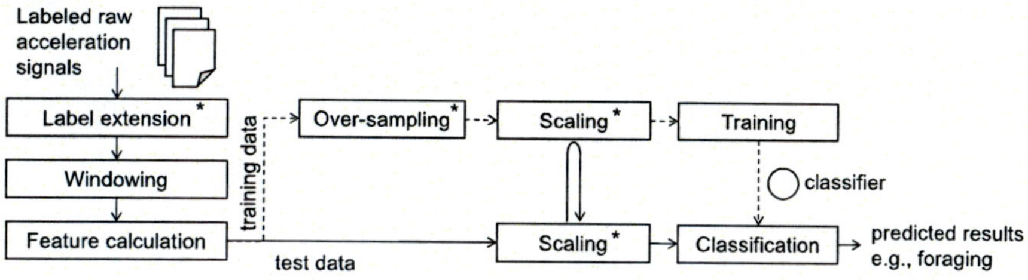

Fig. 3 Processing pipeline. The asterisks indicate options in particular experimental conditions

3.1 Windowing

In windowing, windows of 64 (=8 s) samples are generated from a labeled period. A large window contains much behavioral information. However, because fast Fourier transform (FFT) requires the number of samples to be a power of two for feature calculations, 64 samples are the upper limit in the labeled period of 80 samples. A sliding width of 16 samples (=2 s, 3/4 overlapped) was used. A small sliding width is undesirable in terms of bias of training data because it generates training data that reflect characteristics of samples near the center of the labeled period of 80 samples. Meanwhile, if the window is 64 samples, only 16 samples will remain. Thus, we set the sliding width to 16 samples. If the time difference between two consecutive samples is more than 250 ms due to data loss, the window is discarded.

3.2 Classification Features

Classification features play a critical role in determining the performance of a recognition system. In this section, we describe the definition of features. In addition to the three axes, i.e., x, y, and z, we introduce the magnitude of the acceleration signal (m) as the fourth dimension (Eq. (1)), where $i \in \{1, \ldots, N\}$ and N indicates the number of samples in a calculation window.

$$m_i = \sqrt{x_i^2 + y_i^2 + z_i^2} \tag{1}$$

Here, 74 features are specified from four types of information conveyed by features, as summarized in Table 2. The BASIC features are basic statistics calculated for each axis. The DOMI features represent the acceleration dominance of a particular axis against the magnitude of acceleration (m), consisting of the level of the acceleration dominance of the three axes and the name of the dominant axis. The DOMI features are considered to represent the axis of the sensor to which the most force (including gravity) is applied. Pearson's correlation coefficient (CORR) represents the relationship between two axes and is considered especially useful for differentiating among activities with transition in simply one or multiple axes [26]. The BASIC, DOMI, and CORR features are calculated from the time-domain signal. By contrast, the FREQ features are obtained from the frequency-domain via FFT with which 20 features are specified. Except for DOMI features, the other features are popularly used in animal behavior recognition [10, 20, 23] and for humans [26, 27]. The effectiveness of the feature types and individual features is evaluated in Sect. 4.4. Because the scales of the features are different among various features, scaling should be performed before training a classifier and using (testing) the trained one, except for a decision tree-based classification model.

3.3 Classification

A supervised ML technique is applied, where an ML classifier is trained using feature vectors with labels, and unlabeled new feature vectors are given to the classifier to identify (predict) the labels. For evaluation, we use parts of labeled data as unlabeled data. We will compare the effectiveness of various classification models in predictability in Sect. 4.2.

3.4 Label Extension and Oversampling

As described in Sect. 2.2, raw data were labeled by watching a video clip recorded for 10 s every 15 min, which indicates that the data for the remaining 14 min and 50 s

Table 2 Classification features, where $a \in \{x, y, z, m\}$ and $b \in \{x, y, z\}$

Name	Type	Number	Description or Formula
$mean_a$	BASIC	4	Average of time-series data
$stdev_a$	BASIC	4	Standard deviation of time-series data
$skew_a$	BASIC	4	Skewness of time-series data, i.e., $\frac{1}{N}\sum_{i=1}^{N}(a_i - mean_a)^3/stdev_a^3$
$kurto_a$	BASIC	4	Kurtosis of time-series data, i.e., $\frac{1}{N}\sum_{i=1}^{N}(a_i - mean_a)^4/stdev_a^4$
min_a	BASIC	4	Minimum value of time-series data
$1^{st}Q_a$	BASIC	4	1st quartile (1/4 smallest value) of time-series data
$median_a$	BASIC	4	Median value of time-series data
$3^{rd}Q_a$	BASIC	4	3rd quartile (3/4 smallest value) of time-series data
max_a	BASIC	4	Maximum value of time-series data
IQR_a	BASIC	4	Interquartile range of time-series data, i.e., $3^{rd}Q_a - 1^{st}Q_a$
$meanCrs_a$	BASIC	4	The number of crossing the mean value ($mean_a$)
$domi_b$	DOMI	3	Level of acceleration dominance, i.e., $\frac{1}{N}\sum_{i=1}^{N} b_i/m_i$
$dAxis$	DOMI	1	The axis with the largest $domi_b$
$corr_{st}$	CORR	6	Pearson's correlation coefficient of signals from two axes (s and t) in time-series data, where $s, t \in \{x, y, z, m\}, s \neq t$
$energy_a$	FREQ	4	Sum of energy spectrum, i.e., $\sum_{i=2}^{N/2} {f_{a,i}}^2$
$entropy_a$	FREQ	4	Frequency entropy, i.e., $-\sum_{i=2}^{N/2} p_{a,i} \times log_2 p_{a,i}$, where $p_{a,i} = {f_{a,i}}^2/\sum_{i=2}^{N/2} {f_{a,i}}^2$
$maxAmp_a$	FREQ	4	Maximum amplitude in the frequency spectrum
$maxF_a$	FREQ	4	Frequency that gives $maxAmp_a$
$meanF_a$	FREQ	4	Mean frequency, i.e., $\frac{\Delta f}{N/2}\sum_{i=2}^{N/2}(f_{a,i} \times i)$, where Δf is the sampling interval

Note In the calculation of frequency-domain features, the direct current component is eliminated by starting with $i = 2$.

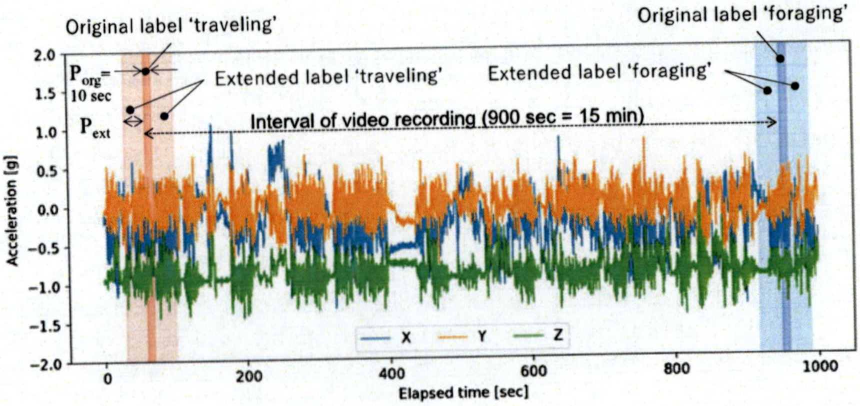

Fig. 4 Notion of label extension, where the P_{ext}-second periods on either side of the originally labeled period are labeled with the same label as the adjacent one

cannot be used in model training because of the lack of ground truth information, but it is natural to assume that samples temporally adjacent to the labeled interval have the same behavior. Thus, periods of P_{ext} sec adjacent to the originally labeled period are automatically labeled with the same label, which we call *label extension*. Figure 4 illustrates the notion of label extension with two 10-s periods of original labels, i.e., "traveling" and "foraging" drawn in red and blue, respectively, and corresponding extended periods in light colors. Note that data with extended labels are used only as training data.

The number of feature vectors n (hereinafter, simply called "data") in P-second period is represented by Eq. (2), where P, w, and s are the period with a label, regardless of whether it is original or extended, the window size, and sliding width in seconds, respectively. The symbols $\lfloor \cdot \rfloor$ indicate the floor function.

$$n = \left\lfloor \frac{P - w}{s} + 1 \right\rfloor \tag{2}$$

As described in Sect. 3.1, the originally labeled period, the window size, and the sliding width are 80 samples ($P_{org} = 10$), 64 samples ($w = 8$), and 16 samples ($s = 2$), respectively. Thus, the number of data points (n_{org}) obtained from the originally labeled period is two. The larger size of extension P_{ext} increases the number of training data points, but the actual label may be different from the extended one if s is too large. In this paper, we set P_{ext} to 32 s because we considered it reasonable to expect 74 s for a behavior although there is a little possibility to include different behavior in the extended period, which implies that the number of windows with extended labels on one side (n_{ext}) is 13. Thus, the number theoretically increases 13 times ($= 2 \times n_{ext}/n_{org}$) from the original on both sides.

Class imbalance is not addressed even though label extension increases the number of data points, i.e., feature vectors. To balance the number of data points, we apply the synthetic minority oversampling technique (SMOTE) [28] that generates data of minority classes by interpolating the nearest samples as one of the most popular oversampling methods. Similar to data extension, oversampled data are used only as training data. In the experiment, we evaluate the effect of data extension and oversampling by switching on and off these functionalities.

4 Experiment

In this section, we present experiments from the following aspects: (1) classification models, (2) individual differences in bears, (3) amount of data and data imbalance, and (4) classification features.

4.1 Common Settings

4.1.1 Implementation of the Experimental System

The experimental system was implemented using scikit-learn 0.24.2, a Python-based ML library, on Python 3.7.10. Furthermore, imbalanced-learn 0.8.0 was used to balance the number of classes by SMOTE. Feature scaling was realized by `RobustScaler` in scikit-learn.

4.1.2 Evaluation Methods

Tenfold cross-validation (CV) (10fold-CV) was adopted to understand basic predictability, which used 9/10 of the entire data for training a classifier and 1/10 for testing the classifier and was iterated 10 times by changing the training and test data. Generally, 10fold-CV tends to result in high predictability because the training data contains 1/4 of data from each of the four bears in theory, and hence, the classifier "knows" about the providers of the test data in advance. Note that the folds were made by preserving the percentage of samples for each class by applying `StratifiedKFold` class in scikit-learn.

By contrast, leave-one-bear-out CV (LOBO-CV)[1] was used to assess generalizability, which was performed by testing a dataset from a particular bear using a classifier trained without a dataset from the bear. LOBO-CV is regarded as a fair and practical test method because the classifier does not know the provider of the test data if the number of bears in the training dataset is sufficiently large and heterogeneous to represent the population. In this study, the number of bears was four, and thus, it is

[1] In human behavior recognition, it is called leave-one-subject-out CV or leave-one-person-out CV.

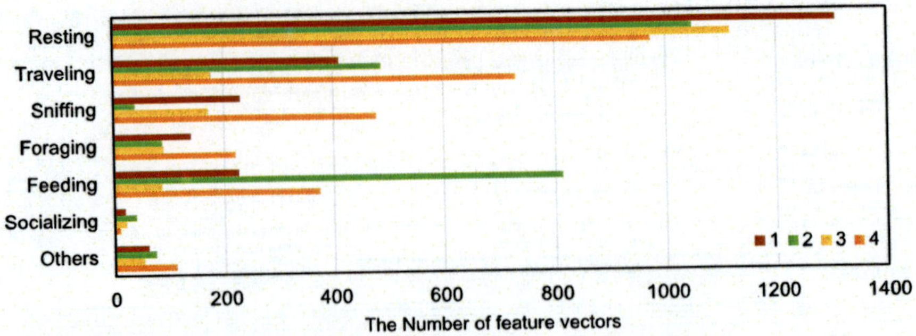

Fig. 5 Distribution of the number of feature vectors per class and individual bear with IDs 1 to 4

too small to represent the population. However, we consider that the obtained result would help in understanding individual differences.

As shown in Fig. 5, there is a large difference in the number of data per class. To cope with class imbalance [29], we calculated the *macro average* of predictability metrics. Macro-average is the arithmetic average of the metric of each class. We used F1-score as a predictability metric. The F1-score of $class_i \in$ {"resting," ..., "others"} is represented by Eq. (3), which is a harmonic mean between recall and precision defined by Eqs. (4) and (5), respectively. Here, $N_{correct_i}$, N_{tested_i}, and N_{judged_i} represent the number of data points correctly classified into $class_i$, the number of test data points in $class_i$, and the number of data points classified into $class_i$, respectively.

$$F1 - score_i = \frac{2}{1/recall_i + 1/precision_i} \quad (3)$$

$$recall_i = \frac{N_{correct_i}}{N_{tested_i}} \quad (4)$$

$$precision_i = \frac{N_{correct_i}}{N_{judged_i}} \quad (5)$$

4.1.3 Distribution of Data per Class in Different Experimental Conditions

The distribution of the number of data points per class and bear is shown in Fig. 5, where the number of data points per class largely varies among classes, e.g., "socializing" has only 89 instances and is approximately 1/50 of "resting." In addition, another imbalance can be seen among individual bears; e.g., the number of data points of bear 4 in "sniffing" is approximately 12 times larger than that of bear 1.

To increase the amount of training data and handle data imbalance in training data, the original data are extended and oversampled, as described in Sect. 3.4. Tables 3 and

Table 3 Average number of data points in training and test data per class in 10fold-CV

Evaluation	Condition	Resting	Feeding	Sniffing	Foraging	Traveling	Socializing	Other
Training	ORG_IMB	4001.4	1350.9	959.4	486.9	1627.2	80.1	285.3
	ORG_OVER	4001.4	4001.4	4001.4	4001.4	4001.4	4001.4	4001.4
	ORG_OVER+	78597.0	78597.0	78597.0	78597.0	78597.0	78597.0	78597.0
	EXT_IMB	78597.0	25112.7	26118.9	10233.9	36073.8	1629.0	6321.6
	EXT_OVER	78597.0	78597.0	78597.0	78597.0	78597.0	78597.0	78597.0
Test	ORG	444.6	150.1	106.6	54.1	180.8	8.9	31.7
	EXT	439.0	149.0	104.8	53.5	178.3	8.8	31.5

Table 4 Average number of data points in training and test data per class in LOBO-CV

Evaluation	Condition	Resting	Feeding	Sniffing	Foraging	Traveling	Socializing	Other
Training	ORG_IMB	3334.5	1125.8	799.5	405.8	1356.0	66.8	237.8
	ORG_OVER	3334.5	3334.5	3334.5	3334.5	3334.5	3334.5	3334.5
	ORG_OVER+	67857.0	67857.0	67857.0	67857.0	67857.0	67857.0	67857.0
	EXT_IMB	65497.5	20927.3	21765.8	8528.3	30061.5	1357.5	5268.0
	EXT_OVER	65497.5	65497.5	65497.5	65497.5	65497.5	65497.5	65497.5
Test	all	1111.5	375.3	229.8	135.3	452.0	22.3	75.3

4 show the average number of data points in training and test data per class in 10fold-CV and LOBO-CV, respectively. In the tables, the column "Condition" indicates the condition of the experiment in the processing of the training data. ORG, EXT, IMB, and OVER denote the original (=nonextended), extended, imbalanced, and over-sampled (=balanced) data, respectively. Thus, for example, ORG_IMB represents the original data without any data processing. By contrast, the original training data are extended and oversampled to be equal to the maximum number in the classes in EXT_OVER. In the data, "Resting" is the largest majority. Thus, in any case of OVER in the training data, the number of data points in the other classes is matched to that of "Resting." Additionally, OVER+ represents a condition in which the original data are oversampled to the same number of extended ones. In LOBO-CV, the number of data points in ORG_OVER+ (67857.0) is matched to the largest number in the classes of four bears. OVER+ is intended to evaluate the effectiveness of data extension by comparing it with EXT.

Although the training data are extended and/or oversampled, these processing techniques are not applied to the test data. Because the random seed in making folds in 10fold-CV is fixed, the test data are identical in various conditions so that predictability could be compared against the same test data. Note that the slight differences in the number of data points in the ORG (444.6) and EXT (439.0) conditions in Table 3 came from the difference in our implementation of data sampling. Therefore, the test data of ORG and EXT are not identical. Regarding LOBO-CV, the test data are obtained from a particular bear. Thus, the numbers in Table 4 are averages of four bears. Furthermore, the ratio of the extension defined by dividing the number of data points of OVER by that of IMB is larger than that estimated (13.0) in Sect. 3.4, where it is 19.6 in the case of "Resting" of EXT_IMB and ORG_IMB. We consider that the major reason for this is that the originally labeled period was less than 80 s in some cases, which made the number of data points with the original label be 0 or 1, thereby increasing the ratio.

4.2 *Experiment: Difference in Classifier*

The difference in classifiers was examined.

4.2.1 Method

The following five classifier models were evaluated: (1) k-nearest neighbor (kNN) as an instance-based method, (2) naïve Bayes (NB) as a probabilistic method, (3) a support vector machine (SVM) classifier as a kernel-based method, (4) multilayer perceptron (MLP) as an artificial neural network-based method, and (5) random forest (RF) as an ensemble learning method. Each classifier has inherent parameters that should be optimized to achieve the best performance; however, we used the

Table 5 Classifiers and their main parameter values in scikit-learn

Classifier	Abbreviation	Major parameters in scikit-learn
k-Nearest Neighbor	kNN	`n_neighbors=5`, i.e., 5NN
Näive Bayes	NB	–
Support Vector Machines	SVM	`C=1.0, kernel='rbf', gamma='scale'`
Multilayer Perceptron	MLP	`hidden_layer_sizes=100`, i.e., one hidden-layer with 100 neurons
RandomForest	RF	`n_estimator=100`

Table 6 Abbreviations of feature sets and the number of features in a set. The concrete features in BASIC (B), DOMI (D), CORR (C), FREQ (F), and ALL are shown in Table 2

Abbreviation	B	BD	BC	BDC	F	ALL
Feature set	{B}	{B, D}	{B, C}	{B, D, C}	{F}	{B, D, C, F}
Number	44	48	50	54	20	74

default parameters specified in scikit-learn ver. 0.24.2. The main parameter values are summarized in Table 5.

In this experiment, data extension was not performed, and the original imbalanced data (ORG_IMB) and balanced data by oversampling (ORG_OVER) were used. 10fold-CV was applied to evaluate basic performance. Regarding classification features, six combinations (sets) of 74 features were used, as shown in Table 6. For each classification method, the average of the performance metrics of six sets was calculated as a summary of the predictability of classifiers.

4.2.2 Result

Figure 6 summarizes F1-scores obtained by the classifier models, where RF showed the highest values in both imbalanced and balanced data conditions. Although there is a possibility of reversing the ranking by other classifiers based on hyperparameter tuning, RF was chosen as a classifier in further experiments because of the simplicity of tuning.

4.3 *Experiment: Individual Dependency and Training Data Type*

Differences in the training data conditions were examined. In addition, the dependency of data on an individual bear was evaluated.

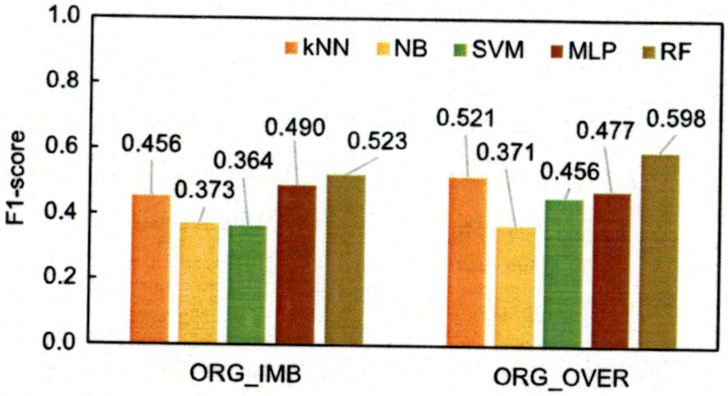

Fig. 6 Average F1-scores of various classifiers trained with imbalanced and balanced (oversampled) data in 10fold-CV

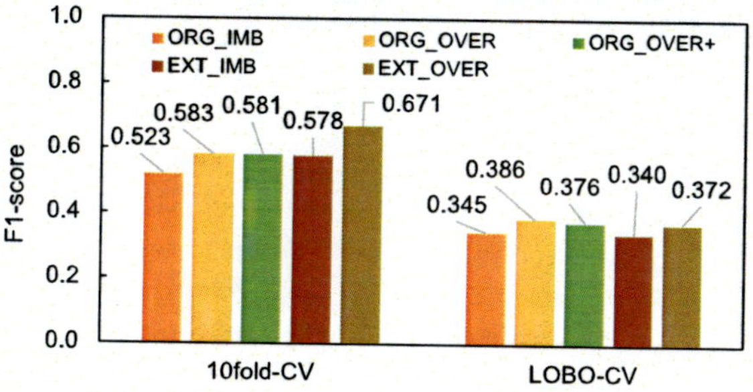

Fig. 7 F1-scores averaged over various feature sets under different training data conditions

4.3.1 Method

The original data with and without oversampling, i.e., ORG_OVER and ORG_IMB, respectively, were used to train the classifiers. Six classifiers were trained with six sets of features (see Table 6). In addition to 10fold-CV, LOBO-CV was adopted to understand the individual dependency of data.

4.3.2 Result

Figure 7 shows the F1-scores averaged over six sets of features per training data condition in two experimental methods. In the figure, we can confirm differences in F1-scores in 10fold-CV and LOBO-CV and in training data conditions, which are analyzed in Sects. 4.3.3 and 4.3.4, respectively.

4.3.3 Analysis: Individual Dependency of Classification

In the training data of 10fold-CV, one-fourth of each bear's data were included, whereas no particular bears data were tested in LOBO-CV. Individual dependency is small if the difference in predictability between 10fold-CV and LOBO-CV is close to zero because predictability is constant, regardless of the presence of particular individual's data. By comparing the values corresponding to each data condition

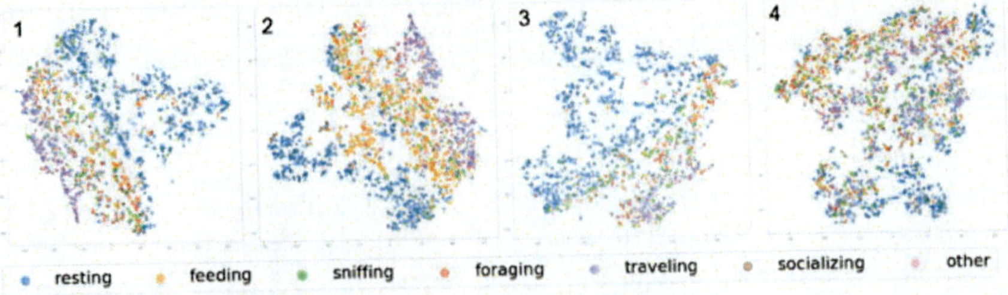

Fig. 8 t-SNE visualization of the distribution of classes by individual bear in ORG_IMB condition

between 10fold-CV and LOBO-CV in Fig. 7, large individual dependencies were confirmed.

Figure 8 shows two-dimensional (2D) mappings of 74 features using t-distributed stochastic neighbor embedding (t-SNE) [30]. t-SNE is a nonlinear dimensionality reduction method that preserves the local structure of high-dimensional data very well and captures global structures as much as possible. If 2D visualizations of individual bears look similar, the distributions in the actual feature space are also similar, indicating that the individual difference is small. In Fig. 8, the distributions of plots for the four bears appear different, especially those of bears 2 and 4 look different. Thus, from the viewpoint of the feature, a large decrease in F1-score is considered reasonable.

4.3.4 Analysis: Differences in Training Data Conditions

In Fig. 7, F1-scores vary in the training data conditions, ranging from 0.523 (ORG_IMB) to 0.671 (EXT_OVER) in 10fold-CV and 0.340 (EXT_IMB) to 0.386 (ORG_OVER) in LOBO-CV. By comparing the values of IMB and OVER in ORG, EXT, 10fold-CV, and LOBO-CV, the values of OVER were larger than those of IMB in either case. For example, the simplest case of balancing the number of data points by oversampling without label expansion (ORG_OVER) in 10fold-CV increased F1-score from 0.523 to 0.583. Such an increase in F1-score indicates that balancing data with oversampling was effective in improving predictability.

The effect of balancing can also be found by breaking down the classification results. Figure 9 shows the confusion matrices of (a) imbalanced (ORG_IMB) and (b) balanced (ORG_OVER) conditions in LOBO-CV, where the feature set "B" was used and showed the highest F1-scores (0.390) in ORG_OVER (Sect. 4.4). Note that the values in each row were normalized by the sum of the number of classified samples in the row. The element $[i, j]$ indicates the ratio of $class_i$ classified into $class_j$. Thus, the diagonal element $[i, i]$ represents the ratio of samples correctly classified as $class_i$ and $recall_i$ in Eq. (4), whereas the nondiagonal element indicates the missclassification of $class_i$ into $class_{j(\neq i)}$. Comparing (b) with (a) of

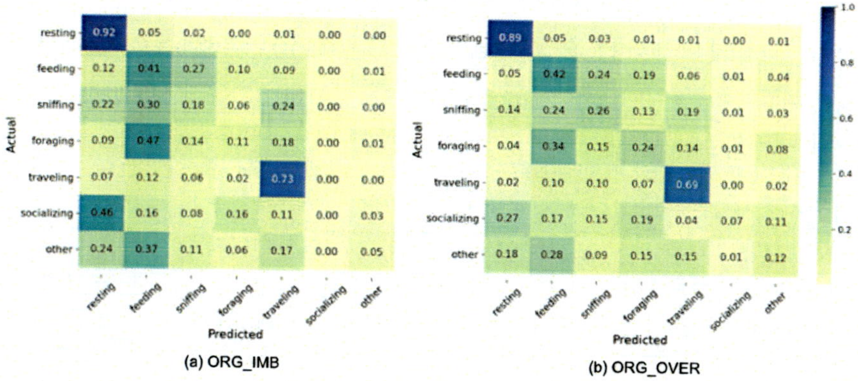

Fig. 9 Normalized confusion matrices of classification results trained with **a** imbalanced (ORG_IMB) and **b** balanced (ORG_OVER) data in LOBO-CV. Feature set B was used

Fig. 9, the missclassification of the minority classes such as "socializing," "others," and "foraging" into the majority class such as "resting," "traveling," and "feeding" decreased even though the correct classification of "resting" and "traveling" also decreased. Balancing with oversampling was considered to improve the recall of the minority classes.

Regarding label extension, the improvement was limited to the case with 10fold-CV, where increases in IMB and OVER were 0.055 and 0.088, respectively. Comparing the results for each feature set, the highest value (0.726) was obtained when the feature set BC was used in EXT_OVER. As shown in Table 3, the average ratio of an increase in labels in EXT_IMB to that of ORG_IMB is 21.6. In addition, the ratio in the case of ORG_OVER to EXT_OVER is 19.6. Thus, the heterogeneity of the training data was thought to be sufficiently increased to enable the classifier to learn decision boundaries more robustly. However, we consider that the label extension caused overfitting in LOBO-CV. That is, there was a decrease in F1-score from ORG_IMB to EXT_IMB and from ORG_OVER to EXT_OVER. As discussed in Sect. 4.3.3, individual dependency was found. Because the training data for a particular classifier were obtained from different individual bears than the one from which the test data were obtained, regardless of the extent to which heterogeneity was increased by label extension, it did not decrease individual differences but rather increased it.

The condition OVER+ was introduced to validate the effectiveness of label extension by comparing it with EXT_OVER. EXT_OVER was generated by extending the label, followed by oversampling to the largest number of data points in the seven classes. Thus, the number of data points in both conditions was almost the same, as shown in Tables 3 and 4, which indicates that the comparison allows highlighting the effectiveness of label extension under balanced data conditions. In 10fold-CV shown in Fig. 7, the value of ORG_OVER+ was smaller than that of EXT_OVER by 0.090, indicating the superiority of label extension. However, in LOBO-CV, ORG_OVER+

was larger, and the difference of 0.004 was almost negligible. Meanwhile, the comparison between ORG_OVER and ORG_OVER+ shows the reduction of ORG_OVER+ by 0.010 even though ORG_OVER+ has 19.6 times more data than ORG_OVER. We consider that excessive oversampling increased the discrepancy between the training and test data.

4.4 Experiment: Effectiveness of Features

4.4.1 Method

The RF classifier was trained using balanced and imbalanced original data consisting of various feature sets. Two evaluation methods, i.e., 10fold-CV and LOBO-CV, were used. Data extension was not applied.

4.4.2 Result and Analysis

Table 7 summarizes the results. In the columns of 10fold-CV, the feature set BC had the highest F1-scores in all training data conditions, i.e., ORG_IMB and ORG_OVER, with the highest average F1-score of 0.597. The fact that BDC also showed remarkably higher F1-scores than ALL in the two conditions suggests that F did not perform properly. In LOBO-CV, the differences between data conditions were not sufficiently large as in 10fold-CV, i.e., 0.023 in ORG_IMG and 0.010 in ORG_OVER, even though ALL showed the highest average F1-score of 0.370.

Table 8 shows the breakdown of the classification results per class and feature set in ORG_OVER of LOBO-CV. The highest values in each class differ by feature set. For example, F had the highest value in "Traveling" even though it had the lowest in "Socializing." Thus, it is difficult to discuss the effectiveness of feature sets in general. In ORG_IMB of LOBO-CV, we confirm a similar tendency. However, in the two conditions of 10fold-CV, effective feature sets were almost constant; i.e., six of seven classes in ORG_IMB and five of seven classes in ORG_OVER had the highest BC values. We consider that the reason for the large variation in LOBO-CV is caused by individual differences in the way of performing each behavior.

To understand the effectiveness of individual features, the Gini importance or mean decrease in impurity (MDI) was evaluated, which is calculated as the total reduction of impurity caused by a particular feature [31]. In scikit-learn, MDI is obtained by the `feature_importances_` attribute of `RandomForestClassifier` class in a normalized form. Note that the values of importance are computed from the training dataset and thus do not necessarily represent importance because of classifying the training dataset. Figure 10 shows the importance of all features in different experimental conditions. Because EXT extends the data of ORG, we only visualize the values of ORG. In the figure, the importance in different experimental conditions seems to be highly correlated.

Table 7 F1-scores by the RF classifier trained with balanced and imbalanced data consisting of various feature sets

	10fold-CV			LOBO-CV		
	ORG_IMB	ORG_OVER	average	ORG_IMB	ORG_OVER	average
ALL	0.400	0.605	0.503	**0.353**	0.387	**0.370**
B	0.548	0.628	0.588	0.344	**0.390**	0.367
BD	0.550	0.550	0.550	0.346	0.388	0.367
BC	**0.562**	**0.632**	**0.597**	0.348	0.380	0.364
BDC	0.561	0.630	0.595	0.352	0.386	0.369
F	0.516	0.452	0.484	0.330	0.387	0.358
average	0.523	0.583	0.553	0.345	0.386	0.366

Bold type indicates the maximum value in each column

Table 8 F1-scores per class and feature sets in ORG_OVER of LOBO-CV

	Resting	Traveling	Sniffing	Foraging	Feeding	Socializing	Other	average
ALL	0.898	0.725	**0.277**	0.207	0.399	0.070	0.131	0.387
B	0.898	0.725	0.269	0.198	**0.417**	**0.084**	0.136	**0.390**
BD	0.898	0.728	0.268	0.198	0.397	0.078	0.146	0.388
BC	**0.899**	0.724	0.269	0.193	0.399	0.054	0.126	0.380
BDC	**0.899**	0.733	0.269	0.203	0.401	0.049	**0.148**	0.386
F	**0.899**	**0.736**	0.270	**0.209**	0.416	0.033	0.146	0.387
average	0.898	0.728	0.270	0.201	0.405	0.061	0.139	0.386

Bold type indicates the maximum value in each column

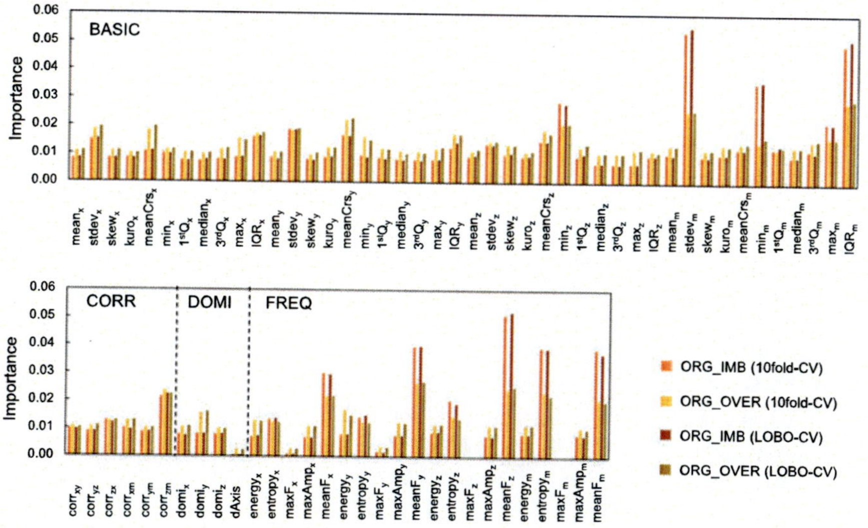

Fig. 10 Feature importance measures of various training data conditions

Table 9 Average importance aggregated by axes

Axis	10fold-CV ORG_IMB	ORG_OVER	LOBO-CV ORG_IMB	ORG_OVER
x	0.0100	0.0121	0.0100	0.0122
y	0.0107	0.0130	0.0107	0.0129
z	0.0126	0.0127	0.0127	0.0127
m	**0.0173**	**0.0144**	**0.0173**	**0.0143**

Bold type indicates the maximum value in each column

The top 10 most important features are almost fixed in the four conditions: min_z, IQR_m, $stdev_m$, $meanF_x$, $meanF_y$, $meanF_z$, $meanF_m$, $entropy_m$ (four times all), $corr_{zm}$ (three times), $meanCrs_y$, min_m (twice), and max_m (once). Note that features in the FREQ group (F) are included in the top 10 groups even though we previously discussed that F is ineffective in the experiment by 10fold-CV. By contrast, features with the five least important features are common in the four conditions: four from FREQ ($maxF_x$, $maxF_y$, $maxF_z$, and $maxF_m$) and one from DOMI ($dAxis$). This implies that these features degraded the effectiveness of other frequency-domain features and decreased the effectiveness of F overall.

To further understand the effective axis of an accelerometer, importance was aggregated for each axis in different experimental conditions. As shown in Table 2, features are calculated not only by a single axis such as $mean_x$ and $engergy_x$ but also by more than two axes such as $corr_{xy}$ and $domi_x$. In the case of such multiaxis features, all related axes are used for calculating aggregated values. Note that the magnitude m is also calculated from three axes. However, we regarded m as a single independent axis rather than depending on x-, y-, and z-axes. Table 9 shows the result, where the magnitude m showed the highest values in the four axes for each experimental condition. The magnitude m does not have an orientation, unlike other axes. Instead, it presents the amount of force applied to the sensor, including gravity. Thus, we consider that this characteristic may work effectively in a case in which the sensor-embedded collar can rotate around the body's axis and axes y and z are interchangeable.

We initially considered that the x axis (surge) is more effective than y (sway) and z (heave), but the result contradicted the expectation. One possible reason for this is that behaviors with one common behavior label may be performed in a way that the x-axis has a different orientation. For example, a bear looks upward when sniffing the air but downward when sniffing the ground. In such a case, rather than initially labeling on the basis of the commonality of intentions of behaviors, e.g., sniffing, predictability might be improved by first labeling and classifying in detail based on the posture and way of performing the behavior, e.g., sniffing the air and sniffing the ground, and then merging by the commonality.

5 Conclusion

We presented a method for recognizing seven classes of behaviors of wild bears using data obtained from a three-axis accelerometer embedded in collars. Approximately 1% of the data obtained from the four bears over an average of 42 d were labeled by watching 10-s video clips, and various experiments were conducted. The findings are summarized below:

- In the classifiers kNN, NB, SVM, RF, and MLP, RF had the highest predictability (F1-score) of behaviors in both imbalanced and balanced training data conditions of 10fold-CV, where the highest value was 0.726 (EXT_OVER, using the feature set BC). In LOBO-CV, it was 0.390 (ORG_OVER, using the feature set B).
- Balancing the training data by oversampling (SMOTE) to the majority class improved predictability, where the classification of the minority class was particularly improved.
- Label extension was ineffective in LOBO-CV because it seems to enhance the individual difference. By contrast, predictability was improved in 10fold-CV.
- A large difference in predictability was found between the evaluation methods, i.e., 10fold-CV and LOBO-CV, implying a large dependency of trained classifiers on an individual bear.
- The effective feature sets varied in the evaluation methods and balanced and imbalanced training data conditions, as well as in the behavior classes. In general, the features calculated from the magnitude of the three axes contributed to classification performance, and the frequency-domain features were ineffective in classification performance improvement in 10fold-CV evaluation, as in LOBO-CV.

Unlike in livestock, very few efforts have been made to recognize the behaviors of wild animals, especially bears. Several ecological differences exist in the genus of bears such as food sources and consequently foraging behaviors. This makes the recognition target different, and suitable recognition methods can vary. Thus, this work is the first step toward understanding the ecology of bears and the coexistence of bears and humans. As next steps, we will attempt to improve predictability by hierarchical classification and "detail classification first and merge by behavioral intentions" approach. Furthermore, deep learning-based classification will be investigated, which eliminates the need to design classification features. Data augmentation will also be applied to increase training data with heterogeneity sufficient for unknown individuals.

Acknowledgements This work was supported fully by TAMAGO program of Tokyo University of Agriculture and Technology and partly by JSPS KAKENHI Grant (Number 17H05971).

References

1. Jones, M., Walker, C., Anderson, Z., Thatcher, L.: Automatic setection of Alpine Ski turns in sensor data. In: Proceedings of the 2016 ACM International Joint Conference on Pervasive and Ubiquitous Computing and Proceedings of the 2017 ACM International Symposium on Wearable Computers: Adjunct, pp. 856–860 (2016)
2. Gjoreski, M., Gjoreski, H., Lutrek, M., Gams, M.: How accurately can your wrist device recognize daily activities and detect falls? Sensors **16**(6) (2016)
3. Inoue, S., Ueda, N., Nohara, Y., Nakashima, N.: Mobile activity recognition for a whole day: recognizing real nursing activities with big dataset. In: Proceedings of the 2015 ACM International Joint Conference on Pervasive and Ubiquitous Computing, UbiComp '15, pp. 1269–1280 (2015)
4. Hussey, N.E., Kessel, S.T., Aarestrup, K., Cooke, S.J., Cowley, P.D., Fisk, A.T., Harcourt, R.G., Holland, K.N., Iverson, S.J., Kocik, J.F., Mills Flemming, J.E., Whoriskey, F.G.: Aquatic animal telemetry: a panoramic window into the underwater world. Science **348**(6240) (2015)
5. Kays, R., Crofoot, M.C., Jetz, W., Wikelski, M.: Terrestrial animal tracking as an eye on life and planet. Science **348**(6240) (2015)
6. Brown, D.D., Kays, R., Wikelski, M., Wilson, R., Klimley, A.P.: Observing the unwatchable through acceleration logging of animal behavior. Animal Biotelemetry **1**(20), 1–16 (2013)
7. Neethirajan, S.: Recent advances in wearable sensors for animal health management. Sensing Bio-Sensing Res. **12**, 15–29 (2017)
8. Brown, D.D., LaPoint, S., Kays, R., Heidrich, W., Kümmeth, F., Wikelski, M.: Accelerometer-informed GPS telemetry: reducing the trade-off between resolution and longevity. Wildlife Soc. Bull. **36**(1), 139–146 (2012)
9. Graf, P.M., Wilson, R.P., Qasem, L., Hackländer, K., Rosell, F.: The use of acceleration to code for animal behaviours; A case study in free-ranging Eurasian beavers. Castor fiber. PLOS ONE **10**(8), 1–17 (2015)
10. Mansbridge, N., Mitsch, J., Bollard, N., Ellis, K., Miguel-Pacheco, G.G., Dottorini, T., Kaler, J.: Feature selection and comparison of machine learning algorithms in classification of grazing and rumination behaviour in sheep. Sensors **18**(10) (2018)
11. Abdoli, A., Alaee, S., Imani, S., Murillo, A., Gerry, A., Hickle, L., Keogh, E.: Fitbit for chickens? Time series data mining can increase the productivity of poultry farms. In: Proceedings of the 26th ACM SIGKDD International Conference on Knowledge Discovery and Data Mining, KDD'20, pp. 3328–3336 (2020)
12. Ladha, C., Hoffman, C.L.: A combined approach to predicting rest in dogs using accelerometers. Sensors **18**(8) (2018)
13. Kumpulainen, P., Valldeoriola, A., Somppi, S., Törnqvist, H., Väätäjä, H., Majaranta, P., Surakka, V., Vainio, O., Kujala, M.V., Gizatdinova, Y., Vehkaoja, A.: Dog activity classification with movement sensor placed on the collar. In: Proceedings of the Fifth International Conference on Animal-Computer Interaction, ACI '18 (2018)
14. Furusaka, S., Tochigi, K., Yamazaki, K., Naganuma, T., Inagaki, A., Koike, S.: Estimating the seasonal energy balance in Asian black bears and associated factors. Ecosphere **10**(10), e02891 (2019)
15. Oi, T., Yamazaki, K. (eds.).: The status of Asiatic black bears in Japan. In: Understanding Asian Bears to Secure Their Future, Chapter 16.2, pp. 122–133. Japan Bear Network (2006)
16. Kozakai, C., Yamazaki, K., Nemoto, Y., Nakajima, A., Koike, S., Abe, S., Masaki, T., Kaji, K.: Effect of Mast production on home range use of Japanese black bears. J. Wildlife Manage. **75**(4), 867–875 (2011)
17. Takahata, C., Takii, A., Izumiyama, S.: Seasonspecific habitat restriction in Asiatic black bears, Japan. J. Wildlife Manage. **81**, 1254–1265 (2017)
18. Dutta, R., Smith, D., Rawnsley, R., Bishop-Hurley, G., Hills, J., Timms, G., Henry, D.: Dynamic cattle behavioural classification using supervised ensemble classifiers. Comput. Electronics Agric. **111**, 18–28 (2015)

19. González, L.A., Bishop-Hurley, G.J., Handcock, R.N., Crossman, C.: Behavioral classification of data from collars containing motion sensors in grazing cattle. Comput. Electronics Agric. **110**, 91–102 (2015)
20. Kamminga, J.W., Bisby, H.C., Le, D.V., Meratnia, N., Havinga, P.J.M.: Generic online animal activity recognition on collar tags. In: Proceedings of the 2017 ACM International Joint Conference on Pervasive and Ubiquitous Computing and Proceedings of the 2017 ACM International Symposium on Wearable Computers: Adjunct, pp. 597–606 (2017)
21. Abdoli, A., Murillo, A.C., Yeh, C.-C.M., Gerry, A.C., Keogh, E.J.: Time series classification to improve poultry welfare. In: Proceedings of the 2018 17th IEEE International Conference on Machine Learning and Applications (ICMLA), pp. 635–642 (2018)
22. Ladha, C., Hammerla, N., Hughes, E., Olivier, P., Ploetz, T.: Dog's life: wearable activity recognition for dogs. In: Proceedings of the 2013 ACM International Joint Conference on Pervasive and Ubiquitous Computing, pp. 415–418 (2013)
23. Pagano, A.M., Rode, K.D., Cutting, A., Owen, M.A., Jensen, S., Ware, J.V., Robbins, C.T., Durner, G.M., Atwood, T.C., Obbard, M.E., et al.: Using tri-axial accelerometers to identify wild polar bear behaviors. Endangered Species Res. **32**, 19–33 (2017)
24. Naganuma, T., Tanaka, M., Tezuka, S., Steyaert, S.M.J.G., Tochigi, K., Inagaki, A., Myojo, H., Yamazaki, K., Koike, S.: Animal-borne video systems provide insight into the reproductive behavior of the Asian black bear. Ecol. Evol. **11**(14), 9182–9190 (2021)
25. Vectronic Aerospace GmbH.: VERTEX PLUS collars. https://www.vectronic-aerospace.com/vertex-plus-collar/. Accessed 13 August 2021
26. Reiss, A., Stricker, D.: Creating and benchmarking a new dataset for physical activity monitoring. In: Proceedings of the 5th International Conference on PErvasive Technologies Related to Assistive Environments, PETRA '12, Article 40 (2012)
27. Pirttikangas, S., Fujinami, K., Nakajima, T.: Feature selection and activity recognition from wearable sensors. In: Proceedings of the 2006 International Symposium on Ubiquitous Computing Systems, UCS'06, pp. 516–527 (2006)
28. Chawla, N.V., Bowyer, K.W., Hall, L.O., Kegelmeyer, W.P.: SMOTE: synthetic minority oversampling technique. J. Artif. Intelligence Res. **16**, 321–357 (2002)
29. He, H., Ma, Y.: Imbalanced Learning: Foundations, Algorithms, and Applications. John Wiley and Sons (2013)
30. van der Maaten, L., Hinton, G.: Visualizing Data using t-SNE. J. Mach. Learn. Res. **9**(86), 2579–2605 (2008)
31. Louppe, G.: Understanding Random Forests: From Theory to Practice. *arXiv preprint* arXiv:1407.7502 (2014)

Using Human Body Capacitance Sensing to Monitor Leg Motion Dominated Activities with a Wrist Worn Device

Sizhen Bian, Siyu Yuan, Vitor Fortes Rey, and Paul Lukowicz

Abstract Inertial measurement unit (IMU) is currently the dominant sensing modality in sensor-based wearable human activity recognition. In this work, we explored an alternative wearable motion-sensing approach: inferring motion information of various body parts from the human body capacitance (HBC). While being less robust in tracking the body motions, HBC has a property that makes it complementary to IMU: It does not require the sensor to be placed directly on the moving part of the body of which the motion needs to be tracked. To demonstrate the value of HBC, we performed exercise recognition and counting of seven machine-free leg-alone exercises. The HBC sensing shows significant advantages over the IMU signals in both classification(0.89 vs 0.78 in F-score) and counting.

1 Introduction

Inertial measurement unit (IMU) is currently playing the key(even unique) role in wearable sensor-based motion monitoring. This is on one hand due to the fact that the motion of body parts is a defining characteristic of many human activities. On the other hand, there is broad availability in unobtrusive form factor including all sorts of consumer electronic "gadgets." An obvious yet little considered weakness of IMU is the fact that in most scenarios to get acceptable signal quality, the sensor needs to be directly attached to the body part that it should monitor. This restricts the scope

S. Bian (✉) · V. F. Rey · P. Lukowicz
DFKI, Kaiserslautern, Germany
e-mail: sizhen.bian@dfki.de

V. F. Rey
e-mail: vitor.fortes_rey@dfki.de

P. Lukowicz
e-mail: paul.lukowicz@dfki.de

S. Yuan
TU Kaiserslautern, Kaiserslautern, Germany
e-mail: yuan@eit.uni-kl.de

M. A. R. Ahad et al. (eds.), *Sensor- and Video-Based Activity and Behavior Computing*, Smart Innovation, Systems and Technologies 291,
https://doi.org/10.1007/978-981-19-0361-8_5

of applications for which sensors are integrated into devices in popular unobtrusive locations such as the wrist (smartwatch, fitness tracker) or on the hip (phone in the pocket). Thus, for example, physical exercises defined by certain specific leg motions are difficult to recognize using a wrist-worn fitness tracker (which is what most people use). Leg motions, in particular more forceful ones do propagate through the entire body, but in passing through several joints until reaching the wrist a lot of information is lost.

In this paper, we investigate how human body capacitance(HBC) sensing could contribute to the solution of this problem: both as an alternative and as addition to IMU. We exploit the fact that the human body can be seen as a conductive plate of a capacitor isolated from the ground (which is the "other" plate) by air, shoes, clothing, etc., Fig. 1, [1]. What makes HBC an attractive alternative/complement to IMU motion sensing is:

1. The capacitance value of a capacitor depends on the size and shape of the electrodes and on the extend and material in the "gap" that isolates the plates from each other. This means that any changes in body shape (in particular distance between bid parts to each other and to objects connected to ground) and especially lifting and putting feet on the ground results in measurable changes in the capacitance. In other words, changes in body capacitance are an indication of body motion and posture change.
2. All that is needed to measure the capacitance value is electrical contact *anywhere* on the plate. This means that no matter where on the body we place a sensor, it will be able to measure the capacitance change, no matter which part of the body caused that change. In other words, we can sense motion of different body parts without having to place a sensor on the specific body part [2].

1.1 Related Work

HBC describes the body's ability to store electrons. Studies [3–5] show that the value of body capacitance ranges in 100−400pF. Since the surrounding varies in practical scenarios, the HBC is not a constant value. Body postures [6], garment

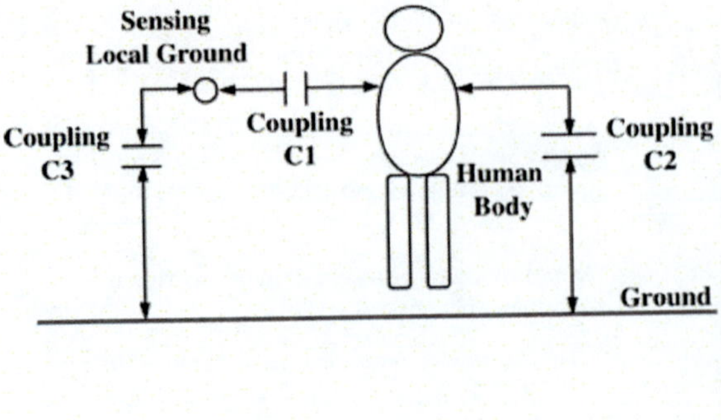

Fig. 1 Capacitive coupling among ground, human body, and sensing hardware's local ground

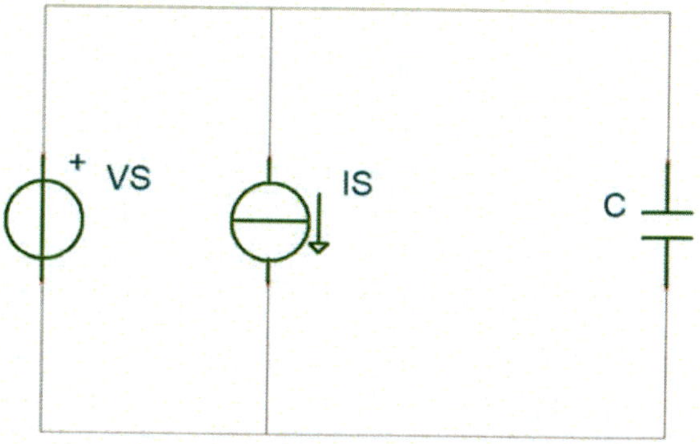

Fig. 2 Basic structure of the body capacitance sensing method

[7], skin state(moisture, etc.) [8, 9], etc., are all potential influence factors to the HBC. Wearable capacitive sensing goes back to early work on capacitive intra-body personal area networks [10]. Based on HBC or related, works also include proximity sensing [11], communication[12], cooperation detection [2]. Although most of those works utilized the conductivity feature of human body, the body–environment interaction features were not widely and deeply explored. A previous work [13] has demonstrated the overall feasibility of HBC for human activity recognition, where the authors had looked at recognition and counting of gym exercises performed on fitness equipment such as adductor machine. In this paper, we take the idea further looking at free fitness exercises and focusing on types of exercises that are difficult to recognize using an arm-based IMU and investigating in detail how HBC sensing can complement IMU. Available HBC-related motion-sensing works were either based on capacitance variation of local body part (like neck [14] and wrist [15]) or full-body capacitance for proximity or motion sensing. For example, Arshad et al. [16] designed a floor sensing system leveraging active capacitance variation caused by body intrusiveness to monitor the motion of elderly patients. Marco et al. [14] presented a textile capacitive neckband for head gesture recognition. Cohn et al. [12] showed a prototype to detect the arm movement by supplying a conductive ground plane near the wrist. However, the benefits of HBC for body activity recognition are still less explored compared with the widely used IMU. This work aims to present the advantages of HBC for human activity recognition over IMU with leg-alone exercises, where the IMU was traditionally deployed for such fitness monitoring [17, 18].

2 Physical Background and Sensing Prototype

Assuming that the charge on a human body is Q_B and the direct capacitance between body and ground is C_B, the potential of the body U_B can be expressed as $U_B = Q_B/C_B$. Where C_B is depicted as $C2$ in Fig. 1, describing the capacitance between body and surroundings. $C1$ and $C3$ describe the coupling between the human body and wearable devices' local ground and the coupling between ground and devices' local ground. $C2$ dominates the motion signal since $C1$ is a constant value when the devices are worn on wrist and $C3$ is insignificant because of the large distance to "real ground." Since the actual capacitance is difficult to measure directly, we continuously measure the electrical potential of the body. Variation in C_B in the interface between the body and ground (e.g., lifting a foot) and in body shape (pose change) leads to potential variations. Figure 2 shows the basic principle of our sensing design. C is basically the sum of $C1$, $C2$, $C3$ from Fig. 1. The voltage source maintains the potential level of the body at the measurement position; the current source supplies electrons to C. When C changes, a potential variation will occur immediately. After a while the potential level returns to the level of VS with the complement of the electrons from IS. In essence, we are looking at a series of charging and discharging processes. Figure 3 shows our prototype for body motion tracking. The prototype consists of a battery charging module, an ESP32 processing unit with integrated WIFI and BLE units, a 24 bits high-resolution ADC, an IMU, and a HBC sensing part composed of several discrete components. The discrete components include two nF-level capacitors and four up to Mohm-level resistors, which makes the sensing unit low-cost, compact, and power-efficient. We used the standard 43mm ECG electrode as the connection medium between our prototype and the human body.

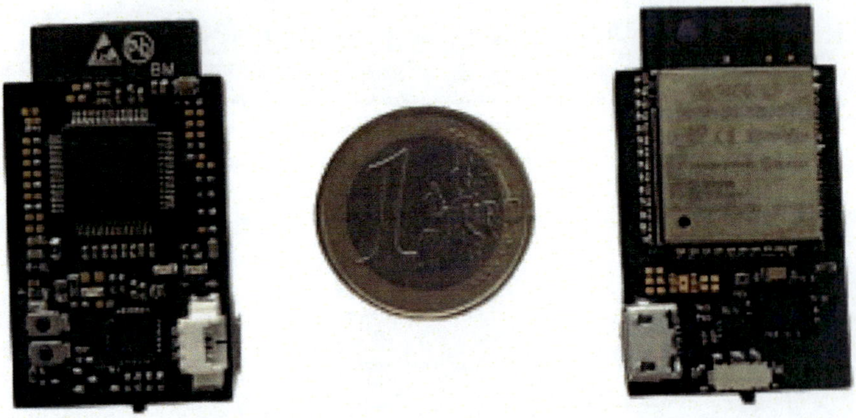

Fig. 3 A prototype for body motion sensing with IMU and HBC sensing integrated

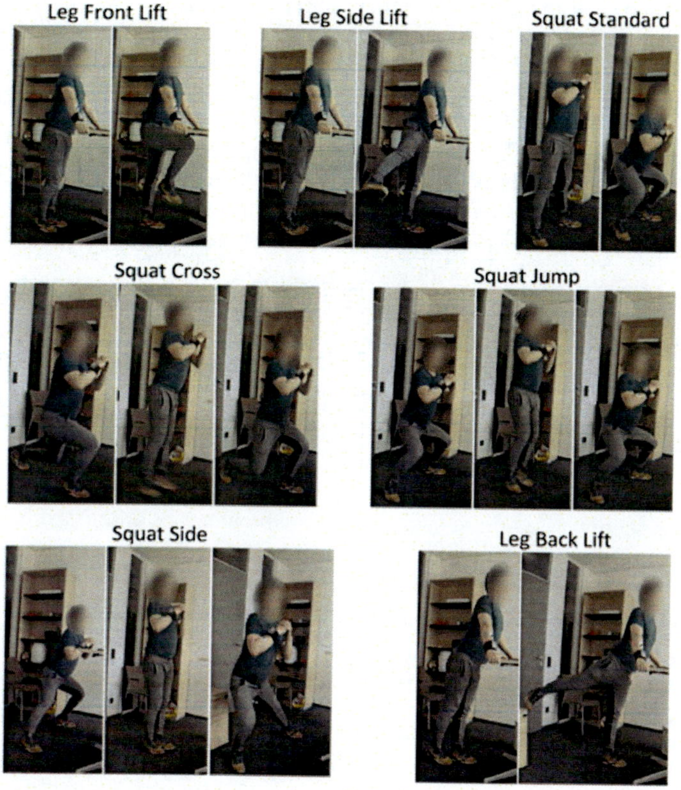

Fig. 4 Seven leg exercises where leg front/side/back lift with hands grasping the table for balance and squat standard/cross/jump/side with crossed hands in front of chest. The developed prototype worn on wrist collects both HBC and IMU signals

3 Activity Recognition Exploration

3.1 Experiment Setup

To demonstrate the potential of HBC-based motion sensing and show how it complements traditional IMU-based method, we performed an experiment where five volunteers performed seven machine-free leg exercises in our laboratory: leg-front-lift, leg-side-lift, leg-back-lift, standard-squat, cross-squat, jump-squat, and side-squat. As Fig. 4 depicts, while doing the first three lift-related leg exercises, the volunteers held the desk for balance(with the wrist in a relatively static state but still vibrated slightly while the leg actions occur). The lifted foot fully touched the ground at the end of each repetition in the exercise of leg-front-lift. For leg-side-lift, the lifted foot was always in the air during the repetitions. For leg-back-lift, the lifted foot touched the ground with tiptoes. For the rest four squat-related activities, the volunteer's hands were crossed in front of the chest, and the feet were all fully touching the ground in each foot-ground contact. The prototype was worn on the wrist, forwarding both HBC and IMU data from the local hardware to the computer through Bluetooth. Since the selected exercises were physically strenuous, especially the cross- and jump-squat, all five volunteers were fitness enthusiasts aged 25 to 32 (by chance all recruits were male, given COVID circumstances we did manage not to recruit more subjects). They performed the exercises with their preferred speed and sequence and worn their daily sports clothes in the experiment.

Figure 5 shows one session of the experiment with both HBC signal (interpreted by the sensed potential variation in the unit of uV after detrending) and IMU signals(three-axis accelerometer and three-axis gyroscope). The exercise types are labeled with arrows in the subplot. It can be seen that HBC gives a more recognizable motion signal for all the seven exercises than the IMUs. However, since HBC has a high cross-sensitivity, factors like the soles could impact the signal so that, for example, different sessions could have different amplitudes of the HBC signals. In this section, we ignore such variation which can be addressed by normalization or using appropriately broad training data sets for the later recognition stage. A close look of each exercise is depicted in Fig. 6. The sensed capacitance signal could obviously capture the leg's repetitions, especially for the three leg-lift exercises where it is hard to get a sufficient signal from the IMU(which gives mostly an irregular vibration signal). The variation pattern of the capacitance signals also shows its potential ability for exercise recognition. Overall we collected ten sessions data, including

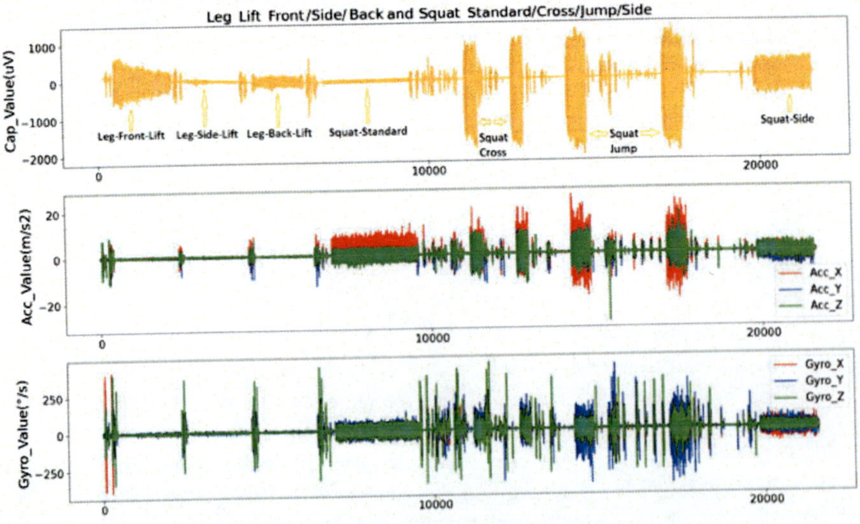

Fig. 5 A Full session of HBC and IMU signals while doing the seven leg exercises, a much more recognizable motion signal was captured by the HBC sensing module than the IMU while doing the leg-lift exercises with hands in the relatively static state

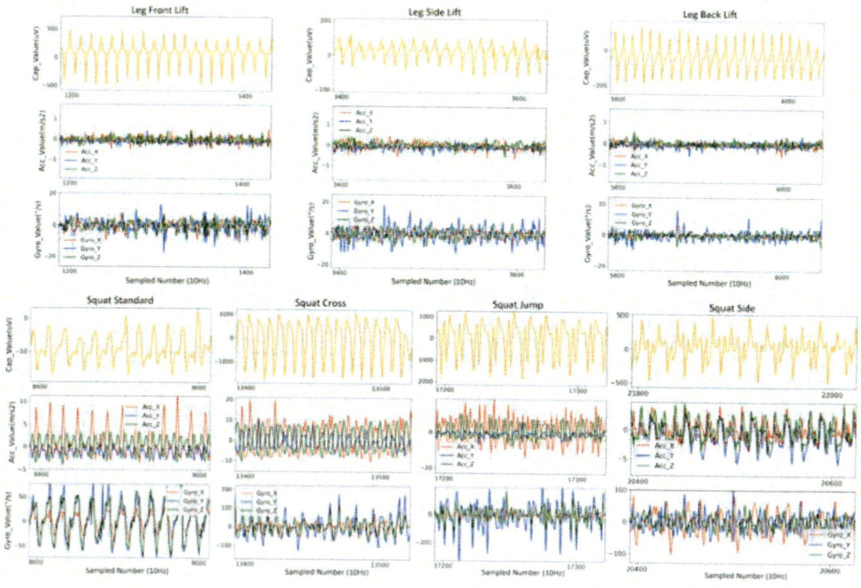

Fig. 6 A close look of HBC and IMU signals for the seven leg exercises, respectively, in one session. (To have a better view of the raw signals, scale of the y-axis was not uniformed.)

1500 leg-front-lift, 1500 leg-side-lift, 1500 leg-back-lift, 1500 standard-squat, 1000 cross-squat, 1000 jump-squat, and 1000 side-squat.

3.2 Exercise Classification with RF and DNN

Classical approaches to classify sequences of sensor data involve two steps. Firstly, handcraft the features from the time series data with sliding/event windows. Secondly, feed the models with the features and train the models. Our work evaluated a diverse set of machine learning models, including k-nearest neighbors, support vector machine, gradient boosting machine, random forest, adaptive boosting, etc. The random forest provided the best performance. As a classifier for human activity recognition, the random forest model outperforms in plenty of related work from the literature [19–22]. In this leg-exercise classification task, we firstly split each session data with four seconds sliding window (two seconds overlap), then abstract the features from each instance, and finally, feed the feature instances into the random forest model with grid-searched hyper-parameters (tree numbers with 20 and tree depth with 15). The features we used are:

- mean, standard deviation, max, min, difference between max and min
- mad: Median absolute deviation

- energy: Sum of the squares divided by the number of values.
- IQR: Interquartile range
- Minimum distance of neighbor Peaks

We deduced altogether 14 variations from the original seven signals:

- Cap, Acc/Gyro_XYZ
- Cap_Jerk, Acc/Gyro_Jerk_XYZ

In total, we utilized 18 features per window for HBC-based exercises classification, and 108 features per window for the IMU-based. The minimum distance of neighbor peaks was calculated by firstly detecting the peaks in each window by a peak detection [23] approach, then picking out the minimum distance of the neighbor peaks, which was proved to be helpful for the distinction of exercises when multiple peaks are generated in each repetition, like the exercise of the squat-jump. The selected hyper-parameters for the peak detection were prominence, distance, and width (3, None, 1 for the HBC signal, 3, 5, 1 for the accelerometer signal, and 20, 5, 2 for the gyroscope signal, respectively). Since we had unbalanced data for each exercise, we balanced the training data before feeding it into the model with the method of SMOTE [24].

To examine the robustness of the HBC signal against user specific variations, influence of clothing, etc., we performed five-folds leave-one-user-out and ten-folds leave-one-session-out cross-validation. This also helps prevent over-fitting. Before the cross-validation, we normalized the HBC signal of each session so that the leg-front-lift has the same minimal and maximal signal(-500 uV and 500 uV). The classification results are depicted in Fig. 7(leave one user out) and Fig. 8(leave-one-session-out). Obviously, HBC gives better recognition results for almost every class than IMU, especially for the three leg-lift exercises, demonstrating the ability of HBC for full-body motion sensing. For squat-cross and squat-jump, HBC also shows a much better recognition rate in between, benefiting from its high sensitivity in distinct leg-ground actions. Only the recognition of Squat-Cross in the leave-one-user-out situation, the IMU gives a better result. Combining both signal sources does not supply a better classification than the HBC alone. Overall, we could conclude that the HBC outperforms in the machine-free leg exercise classification(0.89 vs. 0.78 in F-score).

Note that the above result is due to the fact that we were using wrist-worn devices (simulating, e.g., a smartwatch) to recognize exercises that are defined mainly by leg motions. In the IMU signals, what we registered are vibrations propagated through several joints, which means that they have little information and much noise. By contrast, the HBC signal comes from the change in distance between legs and the ground/body, which is the main source of the capacitive signal.

Besides the classical models, plenty of deep models have been investigated to recognize activities from sensor data and achieved impressive result, as summarized by Chen et al. [25]. An example is the Sussex-Huawei Transportation-Locomotion (SHL) recognition challenge [26–28], which intends to recognize eight locomotion and transportation activities from the inertial sensor data of a smartphone. Forty-eight

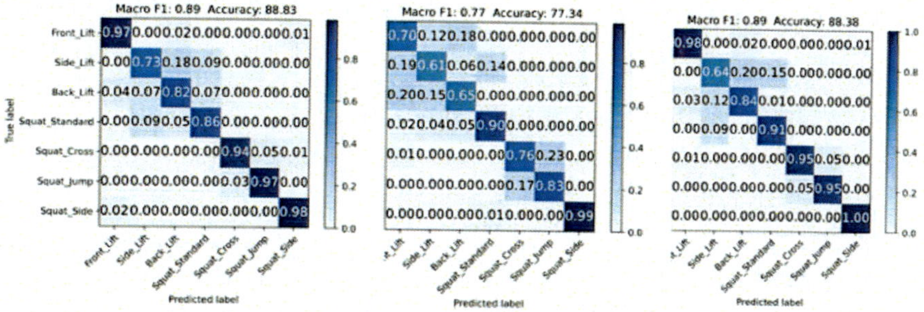

Fig. 7 Classification result with five-folds cross-validation with features from HBC, IMU, and both(from left to right), respectively. (Leave one person out)

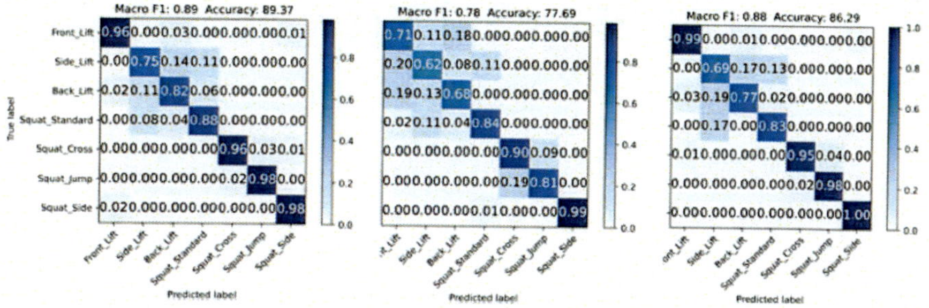

Fig. 8 Classification result with ten-folds cross-validation with features from HBC, IMU, and both(from left to right), respectively. (Leave-one-session-out)

teams submitted their exploration in the last three years with classical machine learning models like the random forest, XGBoost, and SVM, and deep neural network-based models like CNN, RNN, and CNN+LSTM. The data volume increased each year, and the best result was achieved by different models on the three years' data sets (winner of 2018: an ensemble way; winner of 2019: random forest; winner of 2020: CNN), which indicates that the HAR result is mostly data-dependent and the best way to get the outperformed classification is to try different models. Thus, we also tried two popular deep models that gave the state-of-the-art recognition result in other data set.

The first model is named with "DeepConvLSTM" by Francisco et al. [29]. The model is composed of four CNN and two LSTM layers and outperforms in two public data set (OPPORTUNITY [30] and Skoda [31]). The convolutional layers act as feature extractors and provide abstract representations of the input sensor data in feature maps. The recurrent layers model the temporal dynamics of the feature maps. Thus, this hybrid framework exploits both spatial and temporal information from the raw sensor data. The hyper-parameters used in the model are described in the paper, and we trained our data with the lasagna-backend code published by the authors [32]. The second model is a deep residual network inspired by the work from Qin et al. [33], where the authors firstly encode the time series of sensor data as images, then

Table 1 Classification result with ResNet model: F-score/accuracy

Deep model	Test approach	HBC	IMU	$HBC+IMU$
DeepConvLSTM	Leave one user out	0.76/0.73	0.75/0.73	0.77/0.73
	Leave one session out	0.74/0.70	0.76/0.73	0.75/0.72
Resnet 21	Leave one user out	0.75/0.75	0.65/0.65	0.71/0.74
	Leave one session out	0.76/0.77	0.60/0.61	0.69/0.72

leverage these transformed images to retain the necessary features for human activity recognition. In our residual networks, instead of feeding the model with the serial data transformed two-dimensional images, we used the 1D convolutional neural networks supplied by Keras [34] directly to extract features from data sequences and map the internal features of the sequence, which has been proved effective in related works [35, 36]. One-dimensional CNN is proved to be an effective way for deriving features from a fixed-length segment of the overall data set, where the location of the feature in the segment is not so important [37, 38].

The classification results of both deep models are listed in Table 1 with an F-score around 0.75 and accuracy around 0.72 from the signal source of HBC, IMU, and the combination. Compared to the previously presented random forest performance, the deep neural network results are less competitive. Sensor-based human activity recognition is a task that is highly user- and sensor-dependent. Variables, including the dynamic activity complexity, sensor orientation and position, data quality, etc., will cause an unsatisfactory performance of proved models, especially the neural network-based ones, where the models struggle more for generalization with an end-to-end structure for instances with large data volume.

3.3 Exercise Counting

Besides the significant contribution of HBC for leg-exercise recognition, HBC also contributes significantly to the exercise counting. Since the signals show clear waves while doing the leg movement repetition with the prototype worn on the wrist, we used the peak detection [23] approach to count the exercise. The classification shows great recognition between the three leg-lift exercises and the four squat-related exercises, thus we use different parameters(prominence and distance) for the two groups. Peaks were counted from the raw data of HBC signal, noise-filtered Z-axis of accelerometer, and noise-filtered Y-axis of the gyroscope (both axes provide the best result compared to the other two).

Figure 9 uses Boxplot to show the counting accuracy of each exercise with different signal sources. For the leg-lift exercises, the wrist-worn IMU couldn't deliver helpful repetition information at all, but irregular micro-vibrations. In contrast, the HBC could produce a reliable count number with over 95% accuracy. HBC signal also outperforms in counting the four squat-related exercises since the foot-to-ground, and leg-to-leg distance variations result in significant variation of the HBC signal. For IMU, on one side, it is so motion-sensitive that the signal contains many noises. On the other side, it has to be worn on the moving body part to get a piece of clear moving information. Table 2 lists the averaged counting accuracy with the source of HBC and IMU. With an averaged counting accuracy of 98.2%, HBC shows an impressive contribution in leg-exercise counting.

4 Limitation and Future Work

We have demonstrated that certain physical activities determined predominately by leg motions can be recognized and analyzed (repetition counting) reliably from the

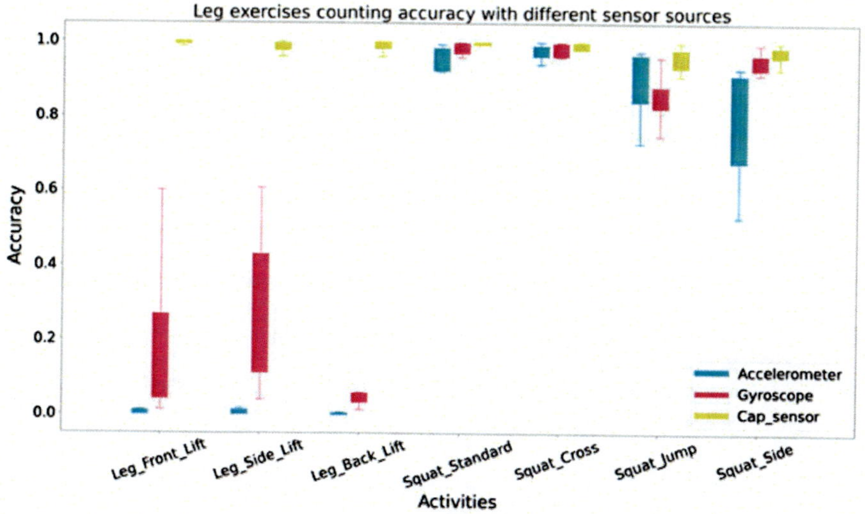

Fig. 9 Counting accuracy of the seven leg exercises with signal source of HBC and IMU, where HBC signal outperforms in all performed exercises with significant advantage

Table 2 Counting accuracy with signal of HBC(all seven exercises) and IMU(only four squat-related exercises)

Signal source	Acc	Gyro	HBC
Mean Accuracy(std)	0.891 ± 0.119	0.938 ± 0.066	**0.982** ± 0.022

wrist using HBC. By contrast, as expected, wrist-worn IMUs perform poorly for such exercises. The relevance of this result stems from the popularity of wrist-worn fitness trackers and smartwatches. Integrating HBC in such devices could significantly enlarge the class of activities monitored by them.

However, there are a few limitations on HBC-based motion sensing. Firstly, since HBC is describing the capacitance between the body and surroundings, which means that environmental changes will also cause the signal variation, like the intruder of another body(within a range of around 1.5 m), which means that during the exercises, a stable environment is needed to keep a noiseless signal. To address this limitation, a shielding layer at the hardware side needs to considered. Secondly, although the classification result is attractive, the HBC value in real-life scenarios is subtle and could be affected by clothing(like shoes), skin conditions(like moisture), action speed and scale, which means there is always a different bias in the signal. As we stated above, HBC is not fully explored to bring it into real life with reliability. Thus, a rich amount of future work needs to be performed to get a better understanding of it.

An interesting question that we will investigate in the future is if HBC can be used to recognize activities performed by the user's dominant hand from a smartwatch worn on the non-dominant wrist. The fact that watches are mostly worn on the non-dominant hand is a well-known problem of smartwatch-based activity recognition. We will also examine in more detail activities that involve a mix of leg and other motions with respect to the fusion of information from IMUs and HBC.

References

1. Presta, E., Wang, J., Harrison, G.G., Björntorp, P., Harker, W.H., Van Itallie, T.B.: Measurement of total body electrical conductivity: a new method for estimation of body composition. Am. J. Clin. Nutrition **37**(5), 735–739 (1983)
2. Bian, S., Rey, V.F., Younas, J., Lukowicz, P.: Wrist-worn capacitive sensor for activity and physical collaboration recognition. In: 2019 IEEE International Conference on Pervasive Computing and Communications Workshops (PerCom Workshops), pp. 261–266. IEEE (2019)
3. Bonet, C.A., Areny, R.P.: A fast method to estimate body capacitance to ground. In: Proceedings of XX IMEKO World Congress 2012, September 9-14, Busan South Korea, pp. 1–4 (2012)
4. Greason, W.D.: Quasi-static analysis of electrostatic discharge (esd) and the human body using a capacitance model. J. Electrostatics **35**(4), 349–371 (1995)
5. Bian, S., Lukowicz, P.: A systematic study of the influence of various user specific and environmental factors on wearable human body capacitance sensing. In: EAI International Conference on Body Area Networks. Springer, Berlin (2021)
6. Osamu Fujiwara and Takanori Ikawa. Numerical calculation of human-body capacitance by surface charge method. *Electronics and Communications in Japan (Part I: Communications)*, 85(12):38–44, 2002
7. Jonassen, N.: Human body capacitance: static or dynamic concept?[esd]. In: Electrical Overstress/Electrostatic Discharge Symposium Proceedings. 1998 (Cat. No. 98TH8347), pp. 111–117. IEEE (1998)
8. Goad, N., Gawkrodger, D.J.: Ambient humidity and the skin: The impact of air humidity in healthy and diseased states. Journal of the European Academy of Dermatology and Venereology 30(8), 1285–1294 (2016)

9. Egawa, Mariko, Oguri, Motoki, Kuwahara, Tomohiro, Takahashi, Motoji: Effect of exposure of human skin to a dry environment. Skin Research and Technology 8(4), 212–218 (2002)
10. Zimmerman, T.G.: Personal area networks: near-field intrabody communication. IBM Syst. J. **35**(3.4), 609–617 (1996)
11. Zimmerman, T.G., Smith, J.R., Paradiso, J.A., Allport, D., Gershenfeld, N.: Applying electric field sensing to human-computer interfaces. In: CHI, vol. 95, pp. 280–287. Citeseer (1995)
12. Cohn, G., Morris, D., Patel, S., Tan, D.: Humantenna: using the body as an antenna for real-time whole-body interaction. In: Proceedings of the SIGCHI Conference on Human Factors in Computing Systems, pp. 1901–1910. ACM (2012)
13. Bian, S., Rey, V.F., Hevesi, P., Lukowicz, P.: Passive capacitive based approach for full body gym workout recognition and counting. In: 2019 IEEE International Conference on Pervasive Computing and Communications (PerCom), pp. 1–10. IEEE (2019)
14. Hirsch, M., Cheng, J., Reiss, A., Sundholm, M., Lukowicz, P., Amft, O.: Hands-free gesture control with a capacitive textile neckband. In: Proceedings of the 2014 ACM International Symposium on Wearable Computers, pp. 55–58 (2014)
15. Sizhen, B., Lukowicz, P.: Capacitive sensing based on-board hand gesture recognition with tinyml. In: Adjunct Proceedings of the 2021 ACM International Joint Conference on Pervasive and Ubiquitous Computing and Proceedings of the 2021 ACM International Symposium on Wearable Computers (2021)
16. Arshad, A., Khan, S., Zahirul Alam, A.H.M., Abdul Kadir, K., Tasnim, R., Ismail, A.F.: A capacitive proximity sensing scheme for human motion detection. In: 2017 IEEE International Instrumentation and Measurement Technology Conference (I2MTC), pp. 1–5. IEEE (2017)
17. Wahjudi, F., Lin, F.J.: Imu-based walking workouts recognition. In: 2019 IEEE 5th World Forum on Internet of Things (WF-IoT), pp. 251–256. IEEE (2019)
18. Chang, K.-H., Chen, M.Y., Canny, J.: Tracking free-weight exercises. In: International Conference on Ubiquitous Computing, pp. 19–37. Springer, Berlin (2007)
19. Casale, P., Pujol, O., Radeva, P.: Human activity recognition from accelerometer data using a wearable device. In: Iberian Conference on Pattern Recognition and Image Analysis, pp. 289–296. Springer, Berlin (2011)
20. Feng, Z., Mo, L., Li, M.: A random forest-based ensemble method for activity recognition. In: 2015 37th Annual International Conference of the IEEE Engineering in Medicine and Biology Society (EMBC), pp. 5074–5077. IEEE (2015)
21. Bayat, A., Pomplun, M., Tran, D.A.: A study on human activity recognition using accelerometer data from smartphones. Proc. Comput. Sci. **34**, 450–457 (2014)
22. Nurwulan, N.R., Selamaj, G.: Random forest for human daily activity recognition. J. Phys.: Conf. Ser. **1655**, 012087 (IOP Publishing, 2020)
23. SciPy.org. Find peaks inside a signal based on peak properties
24. Chawla, N.V., Bowyer, K.W., Hall, L.O., Kegelmeyer, W.P.: Smote. synthetic minority over-sampling technique. J. Artif. Intelligence Res. **16**, 321–357 (2002)
25. Chen, K., Zhang, D., Yao, L., Guo, B., Yu, Z., Liu, Y.: Deep learning for sensor-based human activity recognition: overview, challenges and opportunities. arXiv preprint arXiv:2001.07416 (2020)
26. Wang, L., Gjoreskia, H., Murao, K., Okita, T., Roggen, D.: Summary of the sussex-huawei locomotion-transportation recognition challenge. In: Proceedings of the 2018 ACM international joint conference and 2018 international symposium on pervasive and ubiquitous computing and wearable computers, pp. 1521–1530 (2018)
27. Wang, L., Gjoreskia, H., Mathias, C., Paula, L., Kazuya, M., Tsuyoshi, O., Roggen, D.: Summary of the sussex-huawei locomotion-transportation recognition challenge 2019. In: Adjunct Proceedings of the 2019 ACM International Joint Conference on Pervasive and Ubiquitous Computing and Proceedings of the 2019 ACM International Symposium on Wearable Computers, pp. 849–856 (2019)
28. Wang, L., Gjoreski, H., Ciliberto, M., Lago, P., Murao, K., Okita, T., Roggen, D.: Summary of the sussex-huawei locomotion-transportation recognition challenge 2020. In: Adjunct Proceedings of the 2020 ACM International Joint Conference on Pervasive and Ubiquitous Computing

and Proceedings of the 2020 ACM International Symposium on Wearable Computers, pp. 351–358 (2020)
29. Ordóñez, F., Roggen, D.: Deep convolutional and lstm recurrent neural networks for multimodal wearable activity recognition. Sensors **16**(1), 115 (2016)
30. Roggen, D., Calatroni, A., Rossi, M., Holleczek, T., Förster, K., Tröster, G., Lukowicz, P., Bannach, D., Pirkl, G., Ferscha, A., et al.: Collecting complex activity datasets in highly rich networked sensor environments. In: 2010 Seventh International Conference on Networked Sensing Systems (INSS), pp. 233–240. IEEE (2010)
31. Zappi, P., Lombriser, C., Stiefmeier, T., Farella, E., Roggen, D., Benini, L., Tröster, G.: Activity recognition from on-body sensors: accuracy-power trade-off by dynamic sensor selection. In: European Conference on Wireless Sensor Networks, pp. 17–33. Springer, Berlin (2008)
32. STRCWearlab. Deepconvlstm
33. Qin, Z., Zhang, Y., Meng, S., Qin, z., Choo, K.-K.R.: Imaging and fusing time series for wearable sensor-based human activity recognition. Information Fusion **53**, 80–87 (2020)
34. Chollet, F., et al.: Keras. https://keras.io (2015)
35. Cho, H., Yoon, S.: Divide and conquer-based 1d cnn human activity recognition using test data sharpening. Sensors **18**(4), 1055 (2018)
36. Cruciani, F., Vafeiadis, A., Nugent, C., Cleland, I., McCullagh, P., Votis, K., Giakoumis, D., Tzovaras, D., Chen, L., Hamzaoui, R.: Feature learning for human activity recognition using convolutional neural networks. CCF Trans. Pervasive Comput. Interaction **2**(1), 18–32 (2020)
37. TensorFlow Teams. https://tf.keras.layers.conv1d
38. Missinglink.ai. Keras conv1d: Working with 1d convolutional neural networks in keras

BoxerSense: Punch Detection and Classification Using IMUs

Yoshinori Hanada, Tahera Hossain, Anna Yokokubo, and Guillaume Lopez

Abstract Physical exercise is essential for living a healthy life since it has substantial physical and mental health benefits. For this purpose, wearable equipment and sensing devices have exploded in popularity in recent years for monitoring physical activity, whether for well-being, sports monitoring, or medical rehabilitation. In this regard, this paper focuses on introducing sensor-based punch detection and classification methods toward boxing supporting system which is popular not only as a competitive sport but also as a fitness standard for people who wish to keep fit and healthy. The proposed method is evaluated on 10 participants where we achieved 98.8% detection accuracy, 98.9% classification accuracy with SVM in-person-dependent (PD) cases, and 91.1% classification accuracy with SVM in person-independent (PI) cases. In addition, we conducted a preliminary experiment for classifying six different types of punches performed from both hands for two different sensor positions (right wrist and upper back). The result suggested that using an IMU on the upper back is more suited for classifying both hand punches than an IMU on the right wrist. To provide feedback in real time, we estimated the real-time performance of each classification method and found out all our methods could classify a single punch in less than 0.1 s. The paper also discussed some points of improvement toward a practical boxing supporting system.

Y. Hanada (✉) · T. Hossain · A. Yokokubo · G. Lopez
Aoyama Gakuin University, Kanagawa, Japan
e-mail: yhanada@wil-aoyama.jp

T. Hossain
e-mail: tahera@wil-aoyama.jp

A. Yokokubo
e-mail: yokokubo@it.aoyama.ac.jp

G. Lopez
e-mail: guillaume@it.aoyama.ac.jp

M. A. R. Ahad et al. (eds.), *Sensor- and Video-Based Activity and Behavior Computing*, Smart Innovation, Systems and Technologies 291,
https://doi.org/10.1007/978-981-19-0361-8_6

1 Introduction

Encouraging people to perform physical exercise regularly plays a key role in maintaining health and quality of life. Hammer et al. [1] found out that frequent physical exercise in a week reduces the risk of psychological distress. However, in practice, maintaining regular physical exercise as a lifelong habit is challenging [2, 3]. As a result, many people failed to maintain the recommended levels of exercise [4]. Some hindrances include location and time constraints, a lack of knowledge on appropriate exercise intensity, and poor performance and motivation due to monotony and fatigue. Wearable technology can assist in resolving these difficulties.

In recent years, the number of low-cost wearable devices has increased. This promoted the development of applications for tracking exercise to support people's health. Aside from that, the rapid progress in smart wearable and portable electronics, as well as the high-quality embedded sensors within smartphones, is acting as a further boost in monitoring people's daily activity efficiently [5, 6]. The inertial sensor data based on accelerometer and gyroscope signals which can be collected from an inertial measurement unit (IMU) are the most important source for state-of-the-art motion analysis for sports science [7]. As an example, a physical exercise tracking application on the smartphone, 'Adidas Running' is one of the successful apps to track running [8]. It uses an embedded pedometer and global positioning system (GPS) in smartphones to track walking and running and, it allows the users to keep track of their exercise plan and share their activity results on social network system (SNS).

The smartwatch is also a wearable computing device that runs various applications to tracking exercise. In recent years, due to the growth in technologies such as the long-lasting rechargeable battery, high-performance central unit (CPU), and graphic processing unit (GPU), it has become possible to embed high-performance computers in watches making the demand for smartwatches increased. The smartwatch is embedded with sensors that provide fitness or healthcare-related functionality, e.g., exercise tracking such as swimming, running, and cycling. As an example of exercise tracking application of smartwatch, Kim et al. [9] introduced 'StretchArm' which is a system to promote stretching exercise. The system regularly notifies the user to stretch, guides the stretching motion, evaluates how correctly the stretching motion is made, and provides feedback for the user with gamification elements.

Although the state-of-the-art exercise tracking applications in smartwatches and smartphones and other wearable technologies can track exercise intensity from the pedometer and heart-rate monitor, however, there are still a limited number of applications for boxing, which is popular not only as a competitive sport but also as a fitness standard for people who wish to keep fit and healthy [10]. In this paper, we focused on boxing for punch detection. We propose a method for detecting and classifying shadow-boxing punches using IMUs toward boxing supporting system to provide useful feedback in real time and non-real time for the user to improve boxing skills and increase the motivation for boxing.

To validate the proposed method, we hired ten participants and detect and classify three different basic punches of boxing (straights, hooks, and uppercuts) using several algorithms. As a result, we achieved 98.8% detection accuracy, 98.9% classification accuracy with SVM in-person-dependent (PD) cases, and 91.1% classification accuracy with SVM in person-independent (PI) cases. In addition, we conducted a preliminary experiment with 1 participant to see the difference in classification accuracy between an IMU worn on the right wrist and upper part of the back for classifying six different types of punches performed from both hands. The result suggested that using an IMU on the upper part of the back is more suited for classifying both hand punches than an IMU on the right wrist.

2 Related Work

In this chapter, we introduce related works including physical exercise recognition and existing boxing supporting system.

2.1 *Vision-Based Exercise Recognition*

Vision-based exercise and sensor-based exercise recognition are the two types of research studies used to evaluate exercise quality quantitatively. For a long time, vision-based technology of three-dimensional (3D) image analysis has been taken the principal role of exercise recognition due to its high accuracy to recognize dynamic joint motions of body movement. As an example of three-dimensional (3 D) image analysis, Antón et al. introduced vision-based tel-rehabilitation [11]. They proposed a very accurate Kinect-based algorithm to monitor physical rehabilitation exercise in real time. Their algorithm is consist of posture classification method and the exercise recognition method. They first tested their algorithm with real movement performed by volunteers. As a result, they achieved 91.9% accuracy in posture classification and 93.75% accuracy in exercise recognition. They also tested whether the algorithm can process the data in real time and found out that the algorithm could process more than 20000 postures per second and required exercise data series in real time. Finally, they carried out two clinical trials with patients who suffered shoulder disorders and achieve monitoring accuracy of 95.16%, which was considered adequate by the physiotherapists that supervised the clinical trials.

2.2 *Sensor-Based Exercise Recognition*

Although vision-based approaches are generally more accurate exercise recognition results than sensor-based exercise recognition, the use of exercise recognition system is limited to dedicated location and not suited to process large number of subjects which makes image analysis too complicated. Sensor-based approach can cover these disadvantages with its ability to process large numbers of data regardless of location by attaching tiny inertial sensor to the users body or gear. As a matter of fact, Tubez et al. [12] showed the great prospect offered by inertial measurement units for tennis serve evaluation.

As an example of sensor-based exercise recognition, Ishii et al. [13, 14] introduce a real-time segmentation and classification algorithm that recognize five different indoor and outdoor exercise (push-ups, running, walking, jumping, and sit-ups). They used correlation-based method instead of commonly used machine learning methods to reduce the needs of collecting large numbers of sample data required in machine learning to only one sample of motion data of each target exercises. As a result, they achieved 95% classification accuracy, including segmentation error outperforming previous works.

2.3 *Recognition of Movement Repetition Based Exercises*

Since boxing includes repetitive shadow-boxing punches, it can be categorized as a repetition exercise. One of the previous related works for repetition exercise recognition is that of Dan et al. [15] who introduced RecoFit, a system for automatically tracking repetitive exercises such as weight training and calisthenics using an arm-worn inertial sensor. Their goal is to provide real-time and post-workout feedback, with no user-specific training and no intervention during workouts. They addressed three challenges to achieve the goal: (1) segmenting exercise from intermittent non-exercise periods, (2) recognizing which exercise is being performed, and (3) counting repetitions. They achieved precision and recall greater than 95% in identifying exercise periods, recognition of 99%, 98%, and 96% on circuits of 4, 7, and 13 exercises, respectively, and counting that is accurate to ± 1 repetition 93% of the time.

Although these results suggested that their approach enables a new category of fitness tracking devices, their method is only optimized for exercises that are performed at regular intervals. Since shadow-boxing punches do not repeat with the same interval, which implies demands for other methods specifically for punches.

2.4 *Recognition of Fast Movement*

Unlike exercises such as push-up and sit-up which are recognized in research of Ishii et al.[13], boxing involves relatively fast movement of hand speed. Therefore, we assumed that a specific algorithm for fast speed is needed. One of the relevant previous works which recognize fast exercise movement is that of Blank et al. who introduced a sensor-based table tennis stroke detection and classification system [16]. They attached inertial sensors to table tennis rackets and collected eight different basic stroke types. As a result, they achieved 95.7% stroke detection accuracy and 96.7% classification accuracy. Therefore, they proved the validity of their method and show that the system has the potential to be implemented as an embedded real-time application, to analyze training exercise and present match statistics to support the athletes' training. Although table tennis involves similar speed with punching motion in boxing, punching motion involves different dynamic movement of fists and body. Thus, algorithm that is specific to detect and recognize punch motion is needed.

One of the relevant previous works for punch recognition is that of Ovalle et al. [17], who classified four different taekwondo punches from IMU sensors attached to a right-hand wrist and a microphone. In this research, they investigate if it is possible to recognize punches with bare hands and increase the recognition rate by adding audio input that is produced by hitting the mitt. They achieve 94.4% accuracy when using only the IMU sensor. However, the audio signal did not improve its performance. Even though they achieved high accuracy, they only had three participants and did not investigate person-dependent case. Therefore, their research lacks credibility in punch recognition accuracy. They also used wired communication to transfer the data, which makes the system difficult to apply to real-world applications. In addition, they did not proposed algorithm to detect the punch automatically.

Another previous work for punch recognition is that of Tobias et al. [18], who introduced a system consisting of smartwatch as a measuring device and server sided machine learning classification models to classify four different classes of punch motion: frontal punch, hook, uppercut, and no-action. They conducted experiment with 7600 punches performed by eight different athletes to evaluate their classification models. As a result, they achieved accuracy of 98.68% for the punch type classification. However, they achieved high accuracy, their research lacks credibility in evaluation of the models because they did not test the result in person-independent case and include other important indices to evaluate the model such as recall, precision, and F1-score. In addition, they did not proposed method to automatically detect a single punch and estimate real-time performance of classification models.

2.5 Boxing Supporting System

For the boxing-related work, a Spanish start-up company VOLAVA released Fitness Boxing kit in 2020 which includes a punching bag, gloves, an exercise mat, and an IMU sensor kit [19]. The company made sensors that connect to the Volava boxing mobile app to analyze real-time data such as number of punches, punch force, calories, and heart rate to connect sensor metrics with social interaction leaderboard. Their kit, however, includes 3 IMU sensors and requires boxing pieces of equipment which may be too expensive for some people. Their system also did not recognize the type of punches which may be significant information to evaluate the punching technique when creating mobile personal trainers in the future.

Another boxing-related work is an exergame, Fitness Boxing [20] released by Nintendo Switch in 2018. They utilized Nintendo's Joy-Con motion Controllers for a player to perform punching and dodging maneuvers. In their game, players can personalize the workouts sessions by setting up their fitness goals. By making progress in the game, hit songs for background music and new personal trainers can be gradually unlocked. They can also estimate daily calories burn so that players can track their progress. However, the game only recognizes shadow-boxing punches when the controllers detected a certain motion threshold, and the type of the punch is not identified.

2.6 Remaining Problems of Existing Research

As a summary, the remaining problems of existing research are poor credibility of punch recognition accuracy, unrealistic communication method for punch recognition when applying real-world application, a solid comparison of machine learning approach and correlation-based approach for punch recognition and lack of research for validity of punch classification methods in real time. To solve these problems, our research utilized a single IMU sensor embedded in a smartwatch to achieve wireless communication and investigated if it is possible to detect and classify shadow-boxing movements and achieve high accuracy by using machine learning methods and a correlation-based method and testing person-indepenent cases with ten participants. In addition, we estimated real-time performance of the proposed classification methods.

3 Proposed Methods to Detect and Classify Punches

This section introduces the proposed methods to detect and classify punching motion using a template signal correlation approach and machine learning approach.

3.1 Overview

The end goal of this research is the development of boxing supporting system that provides useful feedbacks for users to improve boxing technique. The system configuration differs based on two different situations in boxing:

1. While sparring or in a real match
2. While practicing by oneself.

For situation 1, a boxer can wear a wearable sensor in a place where injury can be avoided, and the data collected from the sensor is sent to a web or mobile application via a Bluetooth connection. The application counts the number of punches, classifies the type of punches, and computes the punching speed or power of each punches to improve the boxing technique.

For situation 2, a boxer can wear wearable sensors to collect motion data of the boxer and provide real-time feedbacks via augmented reality (AR) or virtual reality (VR) headset as the user throw punches. As the first step to develop this system, we focused on the detection and classification of the boxing punches from the collected signal from IMUs.

3.2 Target Activities

Although there are various types of exercise done in boxing classes, shadow-boxing usually plays an important role for the class. Therefore, we focused on shadow-boxing punches first. According to Kasiri et al. [21] who recognized 6 different punches by using depth image, there are two types of boxer's stances and six basic types of shadow-boxing punches shown in Fig. 1. The stances include orthodox and southpaw. Orthodox is standing with your left foot and hand in the front and right foot and hand in the back, whereas southpaws are vice versa. The punches include straight, hook, uppercut for both lead and rear hands, respectively (the hand closest to the opponent and furthest from the opponent, respectively). In this paper, we only focused on orthodox as the stance because it is the most commonly used stance in boxing. Thus, lead hand and rear hand means left hand and right hand, respectively, in this paper. We targeted the six types of the punches thrown from orthodox stance and described them below.

1. **Lead Straight (LS)**—Lead Straight is also known as jab, and it is thrown with the lead hand from the guard position.
2. **Lead Hook (LH)**—Lead Hook is a side power punch thrown with the lead hand from the guard position.
3. **Lead Uppercut (LU)**—Lead Uppercut is a swinging upward power punch thrown with the lead hand.
4. **Rear Straight (RS)**—Rear Straight is also known as cross and it is thrown with the rear hand from the guard position.
5. **Rear Hook (RH)**— Rear Hook is a side power punch thrown with the rear hand from the guard position.
6. **Rear Uppercut (RU)**—Rear Uppercut is a swinging upward power punch thrown with the rear hand.

In this paper, we first focused on recognizing three types of rear hand punches with an IMU embedded inside a smartwatch on rear hand wrist. In addition to this, we also targeted all six types of punches performed by both lead hand and rear hand for preliminary experiment.

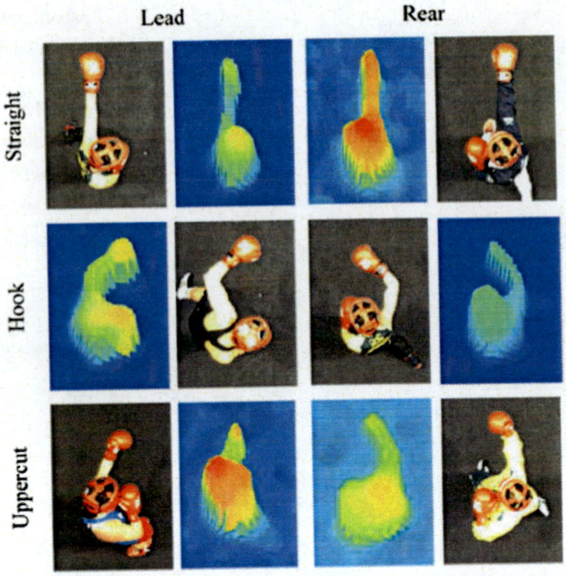

Fig. 1 Six basic boxing punches captured using overhead depth and visible cameras. This includes the straight, hook, and uppercut punches thrown from both the lead and rear hands (quoted from Kasiri et al. [21])

3.3 Activity Detection

To detect the punching activity, the process of the detection process is shown in Fig. 2. The algorithm starts with a 3D acceleration signal collected from an accelerometer. Since boxing punches contain both longitudinal and transverse motions, we calculated the synthetic acceleration, which is the norm of the 3D signal. As shown in the second plot of Fig. 2, the calculated norm contains noise. Thus, a low-pass Butterworth filter (order: 2, cut-off frequency 1hz) is applied to smooth and emphasize the rapid change of punching motion. Finally, segmentation algorithms are applied to the preprocessed data.

Two kinds of thresholds are defined for segmentation shown as the horizontal line of the third plot in Fig. 2. The lower threshold is set for detecting the starting point and ending point of an event. We set the value to 9.8 to ignore acceleration caused by gravity. The upper threshold is set to detect the rapid sensor motion. In this paper, we defined that any values above the threshold are a punch.

The segmentation algorithm starts with detecting the starting point every time preprocessed sensor value exceeds the lower threshold and saves the index of the data. After detecting the starting point, the algorithm looks for the sensor value to exceed the upper threshold. If it did exceed it, we set boolean value true, representing that upcoming sensor data is produced by a punch motion. If the boolean value is true and the preprocessed sensor value becomes lower than the lower threshold, the data point will be recognized as an endpoint of the punch, and the data between the saved starting point and endpoint is segmented as a punch. If the boolean value is false and the preprocessed sensor value becomes lower than the lower threshold, the

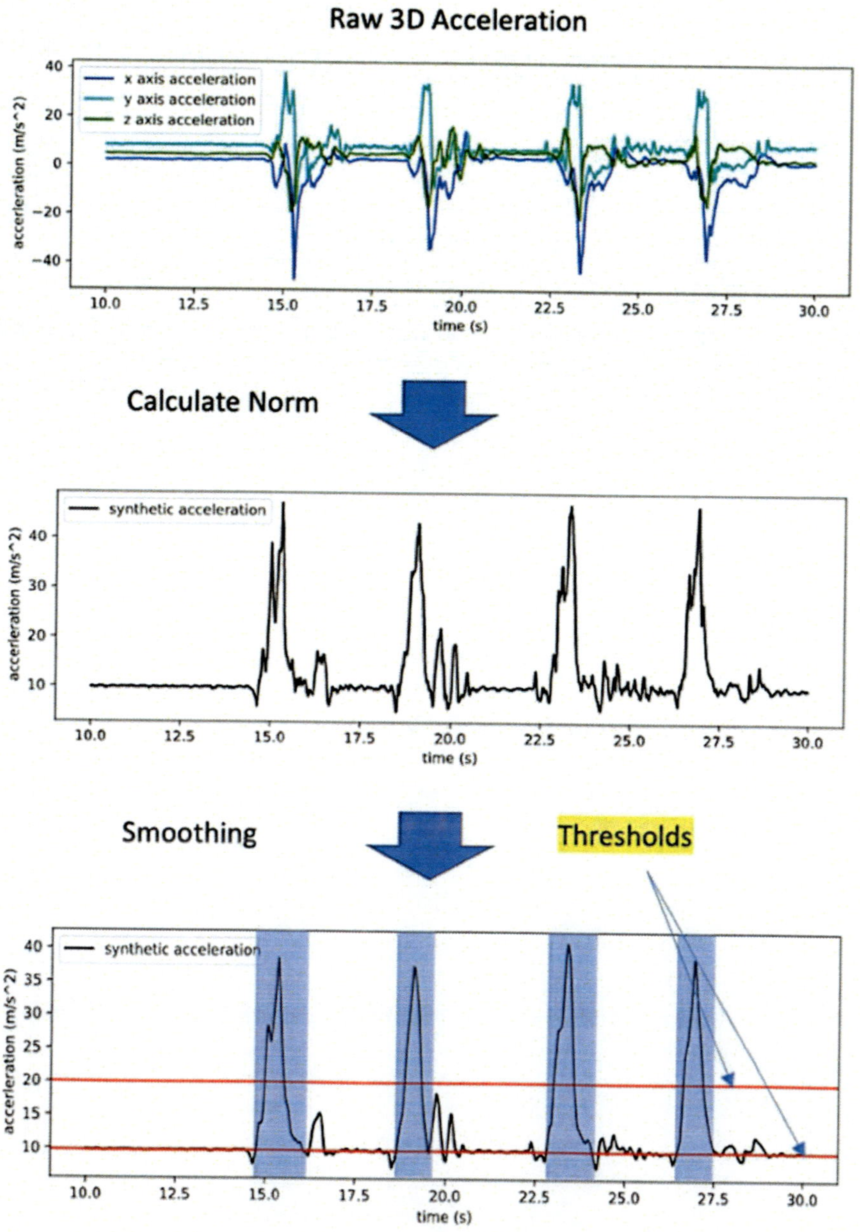

Fig. 2 Example of punch detection processing flow applied to a 3D acceleration signal gathered during the execution of four consecutive lead hooks

starting point is simply deleted from memory which implies no punching event is detected. After segmenting a punch, the saved starting point and endpoint are also deleted from memory.

3.4 Activity Classification

We chose to use machine learning methods for classification and extracted statistical features from both raw 3D acceleration and 3D angular velocity for each axis within the segment. We extracted seven features for each axis, mean, median, standard deviation, min, max, 25% percentile, and 75% percentile in a total of 42 features for each segment. We also labeled each segment as a corresponding punch type. In this work, we compared three types of classifiers, multi-class support vector machine (SVM), random forest (RF), K-nearest neighbors (KNN) from scikit-learn a machine learning library for python. We chose to set all of the parameters of machine learning models to default values of scikit-learn. Before training data with classifiers we chose, for RF and KNN classifiers which calculate distances between different points in their algorithm, we normalized extracted features between [0; 1] to maintain proportional distances.

4 Validation of Proposed Methods

Experiments for 6 punches and 2 sensor locations were done to test the proposed approach and to consider the position of sensors.

4.1 Data Collection Method

To collect data for targeted activities, we set up two different configurations of sensors as follows:

- Sensor Configuration 1
  - Sensor position: Right Wrist (RW)
  - Measuring device: Smartwatch polar m600

    Data: 3-D acceleration and 3-D angular velocity
    Sampling frequency: 100 hz
    Target activities: 3 classes (RS, RH, RU)
  - Participants: 10 people (8 male and 2 female, age 27.8 ± 12.8)

- Sensor Configuration 2
  - Sensor position: Right Wrist (RW) and Upper Back (UB)
  - Measuring device for RW: Smartwatch polar m600 [22]

    Data: 3-D acceleration
    Sampling frequency: 100 hz
    Target activities: 6 classes (LS, LH, LU, RS, RH, RU)

  - Measuring device for UB: Movesense Sensor [23]

    Data: 3-D acceleration
    Sampling frequency: 26 hz
    Target activities: 6 classes (LS, LH, LU, RS, RH, RU)

  - Participant: 1 person (age 22)

For the sensor configuration 1, we chose an IMU sensor embedded in smartwatch polar m600 [22] and developed a wear OS application. The application is used to collect acceleration and angular velocity of shadow-boxing punches from a smartwatch worn on a right-hand wrist. When a user starts the application, the user is asked to type their ID. After typing ID, the start button can be pressed whenever they are ready to start recording the sensor values. The user can press the stop button to stop recording and save sensor data as a comma-separated values format inside the device.

For the sensor configuration 2, we chose two types of IMUs for two different sensor locations as shown in Fig. 3 which are the right-hand wrist and upper back to collect 3D acceleration from the participant. There are two reasons why we chose the upper part of the back as the second sensor position. The first reason is that it is a more practical location when it comes to real boxing matches or sparring because the chance of getting hit to the upper back in boxing is low. The second reason is that we aim to compare the classification accuracy of different types of punches performed by both hands between the right wrist and upper back.

We assumed that it is more difficult to classify other hand punches from the sensor on the wrist than the sensor on the upper back. We also assumed that sensor on the wrist will score better than the upper back when it comes to classifying single hand punches because it is closer to the fist which includes more dynamic movement of the punch. For the right wrist, we used the same measuring device as configuration 1, and for the upper back, we used Movesense Sensor [23] which embeds an accelerometer 26 Hz sampling frequency. An android tablet was used to receive streaming sensor data via Bluetooth from the Movesense Sensor. We used Movesense Showcase Application [24] to collect data and converted it into comma-separated values format.

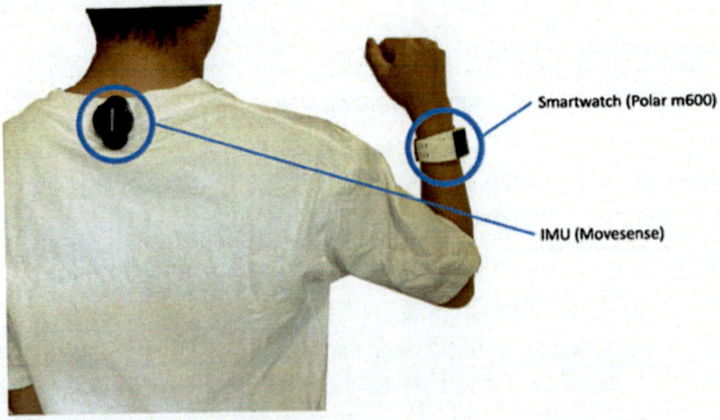

Fig. 3 Sensors used for the experiments and their positioning (An IMU on right-hand wrist and upper part of back)

4.2 Experiment

For both of the sensor configurations, the participants were instructed to punch from a static boxing orthodox stance every 4 s. Participants were asked to take breaks every 30 punches to avoid degrading the quality of the punches due to fatigue. In this experiment, we excluded boxing actions other than punches such as stepping forward or backward, slipping, and ducking by asking the participant to stay still while not performing punches.

The created dataset for sensor configuration 1 contains 924 punches with 3 types of rear hand punches (RS: 307 punches, RH: 308 punches, RU: 309 punches) performed by 10 participants. The participants' ages range from 17 to 53 years (8 male and 2 female, age 27.8 $\pm$ 12.8) and include 3 martial art experienced and 7 inexperienced persons. The ratio of created dataset for the punch classes and participants is shown in Fig. 4.

The created dataset for sensor configuration 2 contains 212 punches with 6 types of punches (LS,LU,RS,RH,RU: 35 punches, LH: 37 punches) performed by one participant who has a year of experience in boxing. The ratio of created dataset for the punch classes and participants is shown in Fig. 5.

4.3 Activity Detection Result

For sensor configuration 1, out of 924 (307 rear hand straights, 308 rear hand hooks, 309 rear hand uppercut) detected punches, 913 punches were actual punches meaning that the overall accuracy was 98.8%. We had 1 false negative (predicted that the segment is not punched but actually it is), and we had 11 false positives (predicted

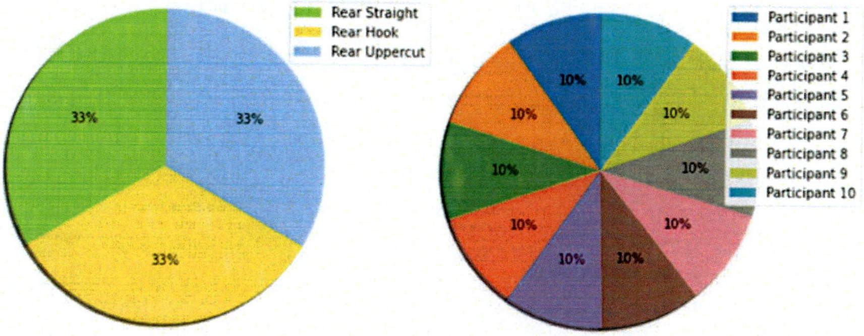

Fig. 4 Ratio of the created dataset of sensor configuration 1 for the three types of punches (left) and the participants (right)

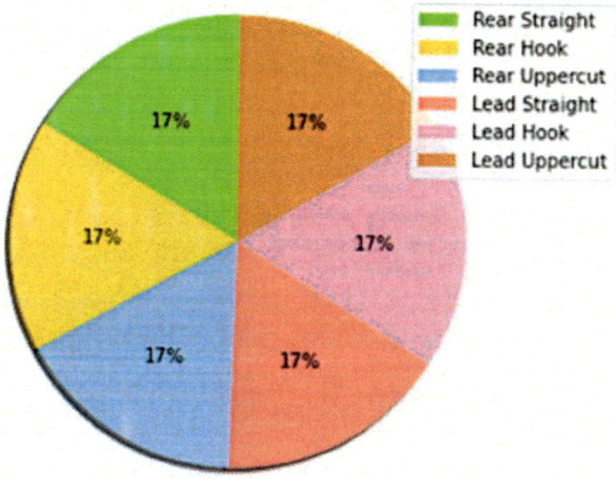

Fig. 5 Ratio of the created dataset of sensor configuration 2 for the six types of punch punches

that the segment is punch but actually it is not). Therefore, the precision of all punches detection was 98.8% and the recall of all punches was 99.9%. The accuracy, precision, and recall of each punch are shown in Table 1.

The result of detection method for sensor configuration 1 showed that it is possible to detect punches with high accuracy with the proposed method. Many of the false positives were caused by the participant's arm lowering movement when the experiment is done and they are asked to press and stop button of the data collection application. For the detection result on the right wrist of sensor configuration 2, we had 1 mistook error on LH resulting f1-score of 99.54%. For upper back as a sensor location, we had 1 mistook error on LH, LU, RS, RH resulting f1-score of 98.85%. The result of detection result on sensor configuration 2 is shown in Table 2.

Table 1 Detection result for sensor configuration 1

	RS (%)	RH (%)	RU (%)	Total punches (%)
Accuracy	99.0	98.7	98.7	98.8
Precision	100.0	100.0	98.4	98.8
Recall	99.0	99.0	99.7	99.9

Table 2 Detection result of each sensor location for sensor configuration 2 (RW = Right Wrist, UB = Upper Back)

	Precision (%)	Recall (%)	F1-score (%)
RW	100	99.1	99.5
UB	100	97.7	98.9

4.4 Activity Classification Result

For sensor configuration 1, we evaluated the three types of classifiers (SVM, KNN, RF) by two cases person-dependent case (PD) and person-independent case (PI). In the PD case, we conducted tenfold cross-validation which shuffles the data randomly in each holds. This splits 25% of the data to testing data and 75% of the data to training data. The training data is used to train classifiers, and the trained classifiers are used to predict against the testing data. This process of splitting data and predicting is repeated 10 times and average accuracy is calculated. As shown in Table 3, we achieved 97.8% of F1-score (97.8% of accuracy) with RF, 99.0% of F1-score (99.0% of accuracy) with SVM, 98.5% of F1-score (98.5% of accuracy) with KNN. Therefore, in the PD case, we confirmed the SVM is the best classifier. The confusion matrix of the best classifier is shown in Fig. 6.

In the PI case, we conducted leave-one-person-out cross-validation, wherein each fold, nine participants are used for training, and the remaining one participant was used for testing. After calculating classification accuracy for each person, the average classification accuracy of ten participants was calculated. As shown in Table 4, we achieved 85.9% F1-score (86.1% accuracy) for RF, 90.6% F1-score (91.1% accuracy) for SVM, and 85.8 F1-score (86.3% accuracy) for KNN. Therefore, in the PI case, we confirmed that the best classifier was the SVM. The confusion matrix of the best classifier is shown in Fig. 7. The confusion matrix shows that the rear hook has the least true positive rate. It also shows the most confusion occurs when the model accidentally predicted the uppercut but the true label was the rear hook.

The result of the PD case showed that it is possible to classify the three types of rear hand punches with high accuracy close to 100% in PD cases. The result of the PI case showed in table 3 that it is possible to classify the punches slightly over 90% despite a variety of the participant's age and gender.

Table 3 Classification results of each models in PD case (sensor configuration 1)

Method	Activity	Precision (%)	Recall (%)	F1-score (%)
RF	Rear straight	97.5	99.7	98.6
	Rear hook	97.7	96.4	97.1
	Rear upper	98.4	97.4	97.9
	Macro Average	97.8	97.8	97.8
KNN	Rear Straight	99.0	99.4	99.2
	Rear Hook	98.1	98.1	98.2
	Rear Upper	98.4	98.1	98.2
	Macro Average	98.5	98.5	98.5
SVM	Rear Straight	99.4	99.7	99.5
	Rear Hook	98.7	98.4	98.5
	Rear Upper	99.9	99.0	99.0
	Macro Average	99.0	99.0	99.0

Table 4 Classification results of each models in PI case (sensor configuration 1)

Method	Activity	Precision (%)	Recall (%)	F1-score (%)
RF	Rear straight	92.6	91.1	89.6
	Rear hook	84.6	81.1	79.0
	Rear upper	93.1	89.3	88.9
	Macro average	90.1	87.1	85.9
KNN	Rear straight	91.0	93.4	90.3
	Rear hook	85.6	79.0	81.6
	Rear upper	88.6	86.5	85.6
	Macro average	88.4	86.3	85.8
SVM	Rear straight	96.5	93.1	93.4
	Rear hook	91.4	84.8	85.3
	Rear upper	92.2	95.5	92.9
	Macro average	93.4	91.1	90.6

For sensor configuration 2, we evaluated the three types of classifiers (SVM, KNN, RF) by conducting fivefold cross-validation which shuffles the data randomly in each holds for both sensor position of right wrist and upper back. As a result for the right wrist, we achieved the best accuracy of 96.7% with KNN when $k = 5$ (SVM = 94.9%, RF = 95.8%). As the best result for the upper back, we achieved an accuracy of 96.3% with SVM (KNN = 95.4%, RF = 94.9%). As the best result for a combination of the right wrist and upper back, we achieved 99.0% accuracy with KNN (SVM = 98.6%, RF = 98.1%) when k = 5. To compare the results by different sensor positions, the result of classification accuracy for sensor configuration 2 is shown in Fig. 8. This figure implies that there is no much of a difference between the right wrist and upper back for classification accuracy when classifying punches

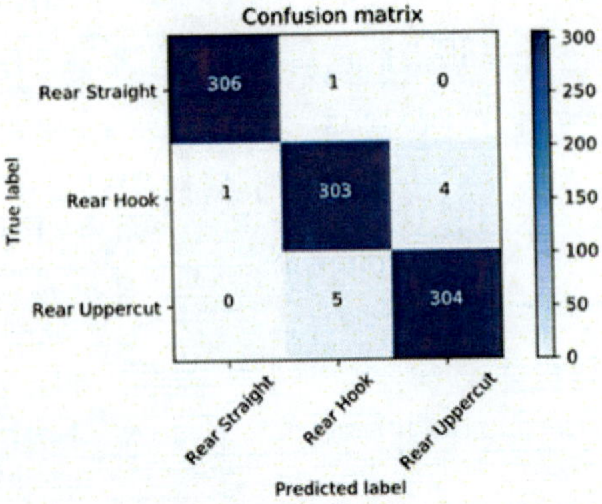

Fig. 6 Confusion matrix of the best classifier (SVM) in person-dependent case (sensor configuration 1)

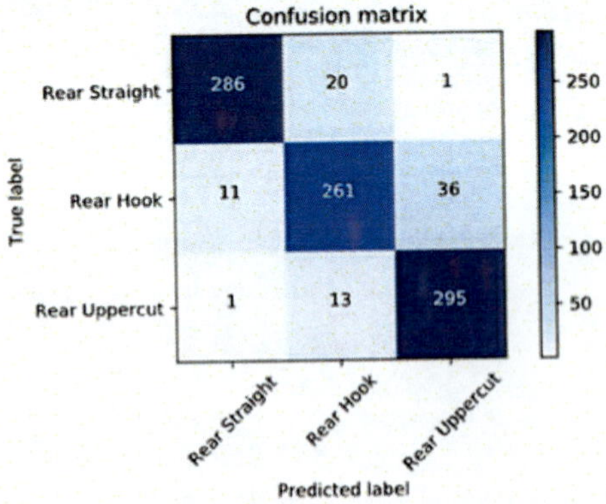

Fig. 7 Confusion matrix of the best classifier (SVM) in person-independent case (sensor configuration 1)

from both hands. The confusion matrix of the best classifier (KNN) for the six-class punch activity classification result using features from an IMU on the right wrist (RW) is shown in Fig. 9. The confusion matrix of the best classifier (SVM) for the six-class punch activity classification result using features from an IMU on the upper back (UB) is shown in Fig. 10. The numbers of miss classified punches for rear (right) hands of Figs. 9 and 10 supported our assumption that predicting single hand punches from wrist sensor score better than the sensor on the upper back. The numbers of miss classified punches for lead (left) hands of Figs. 9 and 10 supported our assumption that predicting other hand punch from the wrist sensor will be more difficult than the sensor on the upper back. Thus, it can be suggested that using an IMU on the upper back is more suited for classifying both hand punches than an IMU on the right wrist, and using the wrist are more suited for single hand punches. We will test this on more participants for our future work.

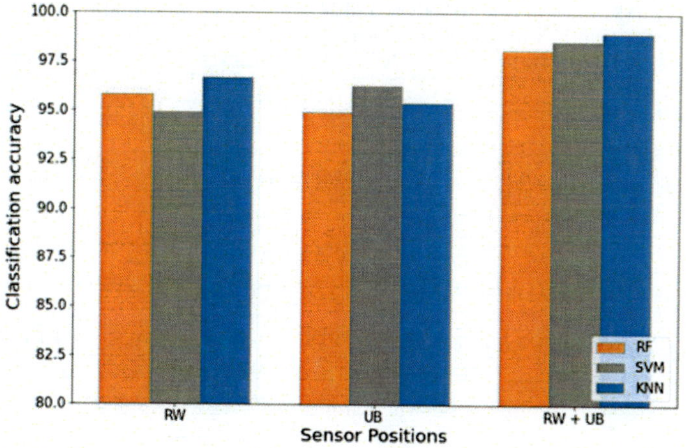

Fig. 8 Six-class punch activity classification result (sensor configuration 2) by accuracy for each IMU position and machine learning algorithm (RW = Right Wrist, UB = Upper Back)

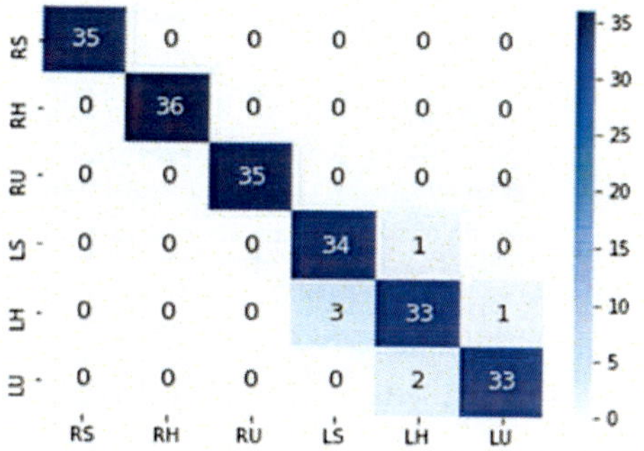

Fig. 9 Confusion matrix of the best classifier (KNN) for six-class punch activity classification result (sensor configuration 2) using features from an IMU on Right Wrist (RW)

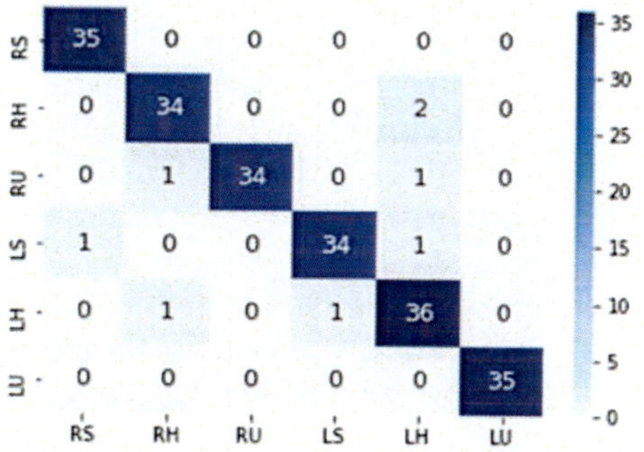

Fig. 10 Confusion matrix of the best classifier (SVM) for six-class punch activity classification result (sensor configuration 2) using features from an IMU on Upper Back (UB)

Table 5 Estimated time for real-time classification

Rank	Methods	Classification time (s)
1	SVM	0.0107
2	RF	0.0114
3	KNN	0.0120

4.4.1 Estimated Result of the Real-Time Classification Performance

Since we are assuming to provide real-time feedback when we develop boxing supporting system, we estimated the time needs to classify a single punch with each classification methods. For the estimation, we first randomly chose 31 rear straight punches performed by one participant in the experiment and classified all of the punches by using all of the classification method we proposed (RF, SVM, and KNN). Then, we calculated the average of the time required to classify a single punch for each methods. Note that in our experiment, we used a computer with an Intel(R) core(TM) i5-8250U processor running at 1.60 GHz using 8 GB of RAM, running Windows 10, and a programming language of python version 3.7.6.

As shown in Table 5, we compared the result of the estimated classification speed performed by each method that we proposed. As a result, all of the methods was able to classify a single punch in less than 0.01 s and SVM was the fastest method to classify with the record of 0.0107 s.

5 Conclusion and Future Work

In this paper, we focused on boxing and proposed punch activity detection and classification methods using acceleration and angular velocity signals obtained by an IMU. The proposed method is evaluated on 10 participants aged between 17 and 53 years old (8 male and 2 female, age 27.8 $\pm$ 12.8). As a result, we achieved 98.8% detection accuracy, 98.9% classification accuracy with SVM in-person-dependent (PD) case, and 91.1% classification accuracy with SVM in person-independent (PI) case. In addition, we conducted a preliminary experiment for classifying six different types of punches performed from both hands for two different sensor positions. Furthermore, to develop our research into a boxing personal supporting system in future work, we estimated the real-time performance of classification methods. As the result of estimation of the real-time performance of classification methods, all of our proposed classification methods could classify a single punch in less than 0.01 s and, the SVM performed the fastest speed of 0.0107 s to classify. From the result of the experiment with 10 participants, we showed that it is possible to automatically detect a single punch with high accuracy and classify three basic types of punches in high accuracy with a machine learning approach. The result of the preliminary experiment suggested that using an IMU on the upper back is more suited for classifying both hand punches than an IMU on the right wrist. We also showed that it is fast enough for all of our proposed methods to use in real-time applications.

Our aim for the future is to detect and classify boxing movements in real time to give feedback to the user through the boxing supporting system. To achieve this, we will first investigate the best position of a single sensor by extending the preliminary experiment in this paper. Then, we will build a system that can run the methods in real time on that sensor position and test their real-time validity by conducting the actual trial.

References

1. Hamer, M., Stamatakis, E., Steptoe, A.: Dose-response relationship between physical activity and mental health: the Scottish health survey. Br. J. Sports Med. **43**(14), 1111–1114 (2009)
2. Kruger, J., Blanck, H.M., Gillespie, C.: Dietary and physical activity behaviors among adults successful at weight loss maintenance. Int. J. Behav. Nutr. Phys. Act. **3**(1), 17 (2006)
3. Schutzer, K.A., Graves, B.S.: Barriers and motivations to exercise in older adults. Prev. Med. **39**(5), 1056–1061 (2004)
4. Harris, C.D., Watson, K.B., Carlson, S.A., Fulton, J.E., Dorn, J.M, Elam-Evans, L.: Adult participation in aerobic and muscle-strengthening physical activities-United States, 2011. MMWR. Morb Mort Weekly Rep 62(17), 326 (2013)
5. Antar, A.D., Ahmed, M., Ahad, M.A.R.: Sensor-Based Human Activity and Behavior Computing. pp. 147–176. Springer International Publishing, Cham (2021)
6. Ahmed, M., Antar, A.D., Ahad, A.: Static postural transition-based technique and efficient feature extraction for sensor-based activity recognition. Pattern Recogn, Lett (2021)
7. McCann, J., Bryson, D.: Smart clothes and wearable technology (2009)
8. Adidas Running. https://www.runtastic.com/
9. Kim, S., Lee, S., Han, J.: Stretcharms: promoting stretching exercise with a smartwatch. Int. J. Hum.-Comput. Interact. **34**(3), 218–225 (2018)
10. What exactly is 'Boxercise' and how can it benefit my health? https://choiceshealthclubs.com/what-exactly-is-boxercise-and-how-can-it-benefit-my-health/
11. Antón, D., Goni, A., Illarramendi, A.: Exercise recognition for kinect-based telerehabilitation. Methods Inf. Med. **54**(02), 145–155 (2015)
12. Tubez, F., Schwartz, C., Paulus, J., Croisier, J.-L., Brüls, O., Denoël, V., Forthomme, B.: Which tool for a tennis serve evaluation? a review. Int. J. Perform. Anal. Sport **17**(6), 1007–1033 (2018)
13. Ishii, S., Nkurikiyeyezu, K., Luimula, M., Yokokubo, A., Lopez, G.: Exersense: real-time physical exercise segmentation, classification, and counting algorithm using an imu sensor. In: Activity and Behavior Computing, pp. 239–255. Springer (2020)
14. Ishii, S., Yokokubo, A., Luimula, M., Lopez, G.: Exersense: physical exercise recognition and counting algorithm from wearables robust to positioning. Sensors **21**(1), 91 (2021)
15. Morris, D., Saponas, T.S., Guillory, A., Kelner, I.: RecoFit: using a wearable sensor to find, recognize, and count repetitive exercises. In: Proceedings of the SIGCHI Conference on Human Factors in Computing Systems, CHI '14, pp. 3225-3234, New York, NY, USA (2014). Association for Computing Machinery
16. Blank, P., Hoßbach, J., Schuldhaus, D., Eskofier, B.M.: Sensor-based stroke detection and stroke type classification in table tennis. In: Proceedings of the 2015 ACM International Symposium on Wearable Computers, pp. 93–100 (2015)
17. Ovalle, J.Q., Stawarz, K., Marzo, A.: Exploring the addition of audio input to wearable punch recognition. In: Proceedings of the XX International Conference on Human Computer Interaction, pp. 1–4 (2019)

18. T. Wagner, J. Jäger, V. Wolff, K. Fricke-Neuderth, A machine learning driven approach for multivariate timeseries classification of box punches using smartwatch accelerometer sensordata. In: 2019 Innovations in Intelligent Systems and Applications Conference (ASYU), pp. 1–6. IEEE
19. VOLAVA FitBoxing Kit Brings Studio Style Fitness Boxing to Home. https://www.movesense.com/news/2020/01/volava-fitboxing-kit-brings-studio-style-fitness-boxing-to-home/
20. Fitness Boxing. https://www.nintendo.com/games/detail/fitness-boxing-switch/
21. Kasiri, S., Fookes, C., Sridharan, S., Morgan, S.: Fine-grained action recognition of boxing punches from depth imagery. Comput. Vis. Image Understand. **159**, 143–153 (2017)
22. Polar m600 gps smartwatch. https://www.polar.com/blog/polar-m600-android-wear-2-0-sports-smartwatch/. Accessed on 22 July 2021
23. Movesense. https://www.movesense.com/. Accessed on 14 Jan 2021
24. Movesense showcaseapp. https://bitbucket.org/suunto/movesense-mobile-lib/downloads/. Accessed on 29 June 6 2021

FootbSense: Soccer Moves Identification Using a Single IMU

Yuki Kondo, Shun Ishii, Hikari Aoyagi, Tahera Hossain, Anna Yokokubo, and Guillaume Lopez

Abstract Although wearable technologies are commonly used for sports at elite levels, these systems are expensive, and it is still difficult to recognize detailed player movements. We introduce a soccer movements recognition system using a single wearable sensor to aid the skill improvement for amateur players. We collected 3-axis acceleration data of six soccer movements and validated the proposing system. We also compared three sensor locations to find the best accurate location. With ensemble bagged trees classification method, we achieved 78.7% classification accuracy of six basic soccer movements from the inside-ankle sensor. Moreover, our results show that it is possible to distinguish between running and dribbling, passing and shooting, even though they are similar movements in soccer. Besides, the second highest accuracy was achieved from a sensor placed on the upper part of the back, which is a safer wearing position compared to other locations. These results suggest that our approach enables a new category of wearable recognition system for amateur soccer.

Y. Kondo · S. Ishii (✉) · H. Aoyagi · T. Hossain · A. Yokokubo · G. Lopez
Aoyama Gakuin University, Kanagawa, Japan
e-mail: sishii@wil-aoyama.jp

Y. Kondo
e-mail: ykondo@wil-aoyama.jp

H. Aoyagi
e-mail: haoyagi@wil-aoyama.jp

T. Hossain
e-mail: tahera@wil-aoyama.jp

A. Yokokubo
e-mail: yokokubo@it.aoyama.ac.jp

G. Lopez
e-mail: guillaume@it.aoyama.ac.jp

M. A. R. Ahad et al. (eds.), *Sensor- and Video-Based Activity and Behavior Computing*, Smart Innovation, Systems and Technologies 291,
https://doi.org/10.1007/978-981-19-0361-8_7

1 Introduction

In recent years, an emergent area of research is analyzing human activity recognition (HAR) with body-worn inertial sensors [1–3]. In particular, accelerometers-based inertial sensors [4] are often used to collect biomechanical data in daily life and health care settings to improve people's quality of life [5, 6]. In addition, using vision-based systems for HAR is also enhancing areas of research [7]. Vision-based systems analyze three-dimensional (3-D) images from video footage and are targeted to recognize the dynamics of joint movement in part of the human body such as the shoulder, the elbow, and the knee [8–10].

Aside from the advancement of daily activity understanding, sports movement recognition technology is also advancing rapidly [11]. Soccer is one of the most popular sports in the world that uses both inertial sensors and vision-based systems to collect players' data to evaluate performance during games and training sessions [12]. In 2013, the German Football Association collaborated with SAP SE to enhance on-field performance of Germany's National Team by the software-based solutions [13]. The German national team wore vests with tiny wearable sensors connected to their backs to track their movements during training sessions. On the other hand, video recording from several cameras was analyzed to understand detailed information about the speed, distance, and heart rate of each player while they were wearing the device [14]. Coaches utilized this data to organize future training sessions and develop effective strategies for future games [15, 16].

In this way, players' bio-metrical data has become an essential component in strategizing game play in other sports too such as tennis, basketball, and volleyball, in addition to soccer [17–19]. This demonstrates how a thorough grasp of sport movement analysis aids coaches and management in evaluating players' performance. It also provides critical information to avoid injury risk, optimize training programs, and support strategic decision making [20, 21].

However, these wearable technologies are commonly used at elite levels even though these sensors are available to the general population. These devices remain expensive for amateur soccer players such as high school and university students. In addition, with the current technology, recognizing basic soccer movements such as shooting, passing, heading, and dribbling, the ball requires not only the use of a single interior sensor, but also a vision-based monitoring system, which makes it impossible for amateurs to use due to its expense and limited availability [22, 23]. The lack of availability of quality sensors to the average amateur soccer player as well as the uncertain accuracy of the readings of sensors without the addition of expensive video-monitoring systems is issues that need to be addressed to provide HAR to the everyday player.

In this study, we focus on wearable technology because it is much affordable for the general population, easy to use, and not limited location. Our goal is to provide a method that recognizes soccer movements via a single wearable sensor with an affordable system that aims to aid the soccer skills of the general population and tackle these problems. We introduce a new solution with the aim of recognizing six basic soccer movements including (shooting, passing, heading, running, dribbling the ball, and kick tricks) with a small and low-cost accelerometer worn at three body locations (inside-ankle, lower back, and upper back). We compared the effect of the sensor location and the number of soccer movements on the accuracy of various machine learning models. The collected data is classified and analyzed based on several algorithms. As a result, we achieved 79.5% accuracy for all six movements and over 83% accuracy for five of the movements except kick tricks from the right-ankle sensor. The second highest accuracy was achieved from a sensor placed on the upper part of the back, which is a safer wearing position compared to other locations. Our study proved that it is possible to distinguish between running and dribbling, passing and shooting, even though they are similar movements in soccer. Although the movement data was collected under the experimental condition and we are sure that soccer consists of various movements, it is the initial approach to recognize multiple movements of soccer by the low-cost small sensor and compare to each location. It enables us to do the following examples.

- Players can look back their movements by themselves without video.
- Coaches can analyze player's performance and manage their fatigue easily.
- Match stats are reported automatically.

2 Related Works

2.1 *Human Activity Recognition by Accelerometer*

In recent years, a variety of sizes and weights of acceleration sensors have been used during experiments to understand different types of daily activity [24, 25]. Yet, in our everyday lives, accelerometers are frequently attached in the devices we use. Smartphones are one example. Yantao et al. presented "smart jump", a study of detecting and counting human jumps by using smartphones. They first extracted three key jump features from smoothed z-axis acceleration data; (1) the peak of the taking-off phase, (2) the flat valley of the in-air phase, and (3) the peak of the landing phase by using a peak and valley detection algorithm and matching them with the derived features from the analysis of physical jumps by using an FSM for jump detection and count [26].

Another commonly used device in studies is smartwatches [27]. Gary et al. mentioned in their study that in many such studies, only the smartwatch accelerometer is used and only one physical activity, oftentimes walking, is investigated. Therefore, in their study, they used the accelerometer and gyroscope on both the smartphone and smartwatch and determined which combination of sensors performs best [28]. In addition, a similar method was performed in a free-living situation to monitor everyday life to improve our health and related habits [22, 29].

2.2 Recognition of Basic Exercise

Basic exercise such as running, walking, and jumping is key features to recognize human activity. Morris et al. developed RecoFit which is a system worn on the arm for automatically tracking repetitive exercises such as weight training and calisthenics. They show that it is possible to (1) segment exercise from intermittent non-exercise periods, (2) recognize which exercise is being performed, and (3) count repetitions [30].

Ishii et al. presented research to develop an algorithm that provides a very accurate real-time segmentation, classification, and counting of physical exercises, including both indoor and outdoor activities by only using data collected from wearable devices [31]. They collected five types of exercise data that anyone can perform anywhere which are running, walking, crotch jumps, push-ups, and sit-ups. Subjects wore four types of sensors in different body locations to develop a general-purpose algorithm that does not depend on the type of sensor or where it is worn. To classify these five different exercises, they firstly segmented raw data collected from wearable sensors into each exercise. In order to do this, the norm of 3-axis acceleration was calculated and then it was smoothed to detect the peak value. After this process, they divided the raw data to extract each action based on the peak value time and created a dataset. For the validation, they used dynamic time warping (DTW), which is a method for calculating the distance between two time series data points and calculating the correlation between runtime behavior and template data. They achieved classification accuracy of 93% for all five exercise types [31].

2.3 Recognition of Hand-Motions in Sports

Regarding specific activity recognition within the field of sports, there are several works which analyze particular movements for different sports. For example, Le et al. presented research with the purpose of monitoring basketball players with multiple inertial measurement units called BSK boards. The board contains different MEMS sensors such as accelerometer and gyroscope [32].

During the experiment, five sensors were attached to the body (top of each foot, side of each calf, and lower back) to collect basketball activity data (walking, jogging, running, sprinting, jumping, jumpshot, layup shot, and pivot). They extracted different types of features such as time and frequency domain including: range, sum, mean, standard variation, mean crossing rate, skewness, kurtosis, frequency bands, energy, and number of peaks above the threshold. They trained a model with a linear SVM classifier on range values to estimate this threshold [33]. After that, they divided moving activities into two datasets, namely step and jump activities and compared the accuracy of each activity with different subjects in the confusion matrix. The experimental results show the potential ability of the system in basketball activity recognition [32].

Sara et al. proposed a detection and classification method of three tennis strokes (serve, backhand, and forehand) via a smartwatch worn at the right-hand wrist. The collected data contained 3-D data of the accelerometer and gyroscope. The proposed approach utilized datastream alignment and signal filtering methods for data preprocessing to overcome poor smartwatch data quality. For the classification method, they used K-nearest neighbors (KNN), linear SVC, and random forest (as an ensemble method). The principal component analysis (PCA) dimension reduction method is also used to reduce dimensionality of data which consequently improves the accuracy of classification. They extracted ten time-domain features and validated them to determine which features are more effective for the classification process to achieve higher accuracy. Furthermore, 27 human actions from the provided dataset are applied to the proposed method and evaluated using their devised method to compare with existing methods. The result shows that the proposed approach has improved the overall classification accuracy by more 30% than the existing method [19].

2.4 Recognition of Foot-Works in Sports

Filip et al. presented an effective method for the recognition of fencing footwork using a single body-worn accelerometer dataset consisting of six actions. The experiment was performed by ten people and repeated ten times for each action. They proposed a segment-based SVM method for time series classification together with a set of informative features and demonstrated that the method is competitive with 1-NN DTW in terms of classification accuracy. The proposed method achieves classification accuracy slightly better than 70% on the fencing footwork dataset. In the future, they will investigate new spatio-temporal features, and another direction that will be explored is developing mechanisms for DTW to provide better generalization among different realizations of the same action [12].

The most relevant previous work for soccer movements identification is that of Omar et al., who presented research that aimed to recognize soccer movements in real time by utilizing a 3-axis accelerometer from a smartphone worn at the abdominal area with a belt. Each subject performed five soccer activities: shooting the ball, passing the ball, heading the ball, running, and dribbling. They used three different feature-based approaches which are time series forest (interval-based), fast shapelets (shapelet-based), and Bag-of-SFA symbols (dictionary-based) to train models [34–36]. They also validated that different factors might affect the accuracy and the training time, such as parameters tuning and axis elimination. Their proposed model reduces the training time by one order of magnitude achieved without sacrificing the accuracy. Furthermore, they proposed a collaborative model where they combined all three approaches in a voting mechanism using only two axes and achieved an increase in accuracy by 2–84% [37].

2.5 Issues and Our Contributions

Soccer is one of the sports that requires high ability of basic exercise such as sprinting, jogging, and jumping. Although there are many real-time applications that track human activity such as Apple Health and Google Fit, none of these applications recognize soccer moves in real time because the movements are very fast and unpredictable. These intense actions make it harder to recognize similar soccer movements such as running and dribbling or shooting and passing [37, 38]. In the most relevant previous work, Omar et al. used a smartphone worn at the abdominal area to collect data [37]. However, it is unclear whether wearing a wearable sensor at the abdominal area and using a smartphone is the best method to collect data during soccer games. Moreover, as they introduced two different types of soccer wearable sensors, the most accurate location of the wearable sensor has not been determined yet. Therefore, experimenting sensor position accuracy with small size of the sensor is needed in our research. Thus, in this study, we propose classification method of six basic soccer movements and compare with three sensor locations.

3 Proposed Method

This research aims to develop a skill improvement support system for amateur soccer players using a commercially available small wearable inertial sensor. Figure 1 shows a system overview. Players can wear a wearable sensor while playing soccer, and the data collected from the sensor is sent to the Android application via a Bluetooth connection. Through the smart devices, they can count the total number and length of each soccer movement. They can use their data to improve their soccer skills,

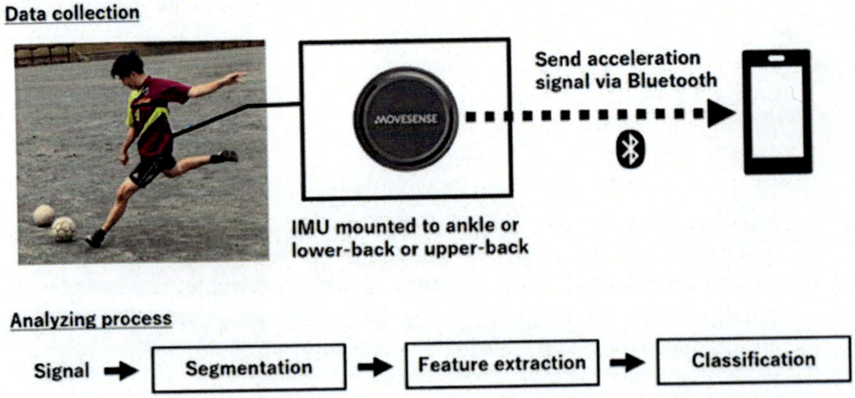

Fig. 1 System overview

manage their condition, or evaluate performance. To develop this system, we first focused on recognizing soccer movements with body-worn sensors.

The following sections provide detailed information on the data collection, definition of soccer movements, segmentation, and feature extraction.

3.1 Definition of Soccer Movements

We defined six soccer movements listed below. The definitions of each soccer movement are explained, and example pictures of six soccer movements (Fig. 2) are provided to subjects.

a. **Shooting the ball (S)**—We defined shooting as kicking the ball in a way called instep kick which uses the quadricep muscles of the thigh to provide the most powerful kick available in soccer, forcing the top of the foot to propel the soccer ball forward.
b. **Passing the ball (P)**—The passing was defined as kicking a ball with a side-foot kick which uses the inside of the foot. It is very precise and is used mostly for passing; it is not as powerful as an instep kick.
c. **Heading the ball (H)**—Subjects performed heading which hits the ball floating in the air by their head while jumping.
d. **Running (R)**—Running is defined as movement when players do not have the ball where the intensity parallels jogging in the experiment.

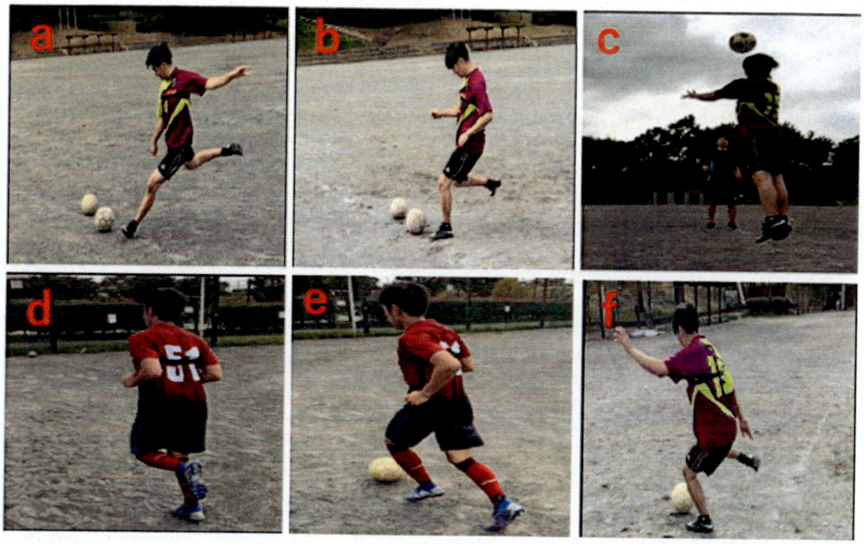

Fig. 2 Definition of soccer movements (**a** Shooting, **b** Passing, **c** Heading, **d** Running, **e** Dribbling, **f** Kick trick)

e. **Dribbling (D)**—Subjects carry the ball freely on the ground by foot.
f. **Kick trick (KT)**—Kick tricks are defined as tricks where a subject pretends to shoot the ball in front of the goal, but does not complete the shooting action. The subject swings their foot to a halfway point in the shooting motion and then stops and transitions to dribbling.

3.2 Segmentation of Individual Actions

We segmented each movement from raw data collected from each sensor. To do so, the norm was calculated from the 3-axis acceleration data, and the peak value during each movement was determined manually from video footage during the experiment. In this experiment, the range of the peak timing ±0.5 s was considered to be one action (see Fig. 3).

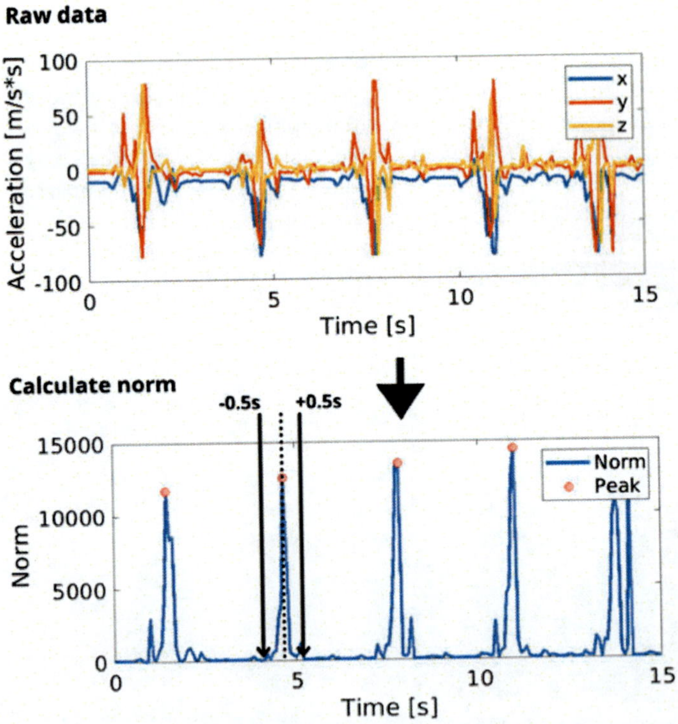

Fig. 3 Example of the processing of segmentation algorithm applied to 3-D acceleration signal collected during shooting

3.3 Feature Extraction for Classifier Building

In order to build a machine learning classification model, ten features (mean, standard deviation, maximum, minimum, median, maximum-minimum, mode, scale, skewness, and integral) were extracted from the data of one action range. The related works influenced why we selected these features. Le et al. extracted time-domain features such as sum, mean, standard variation, skewness, and number of peaks in order to train basketball motion data models [32]. Basketball and soccer are both intense sports. Therefore, we extracted similar features to train our models.

4 Validation of the Proposed Method

To validate the proposed method and considering the location of sensors, experiments have been conducted for six soccer movements and three sensor locations. Below, we have described the data collection and result analysis in details.

4.1 Data Collection

This experiment was conducted on ten right-foot subjects, aged 20–23 years old, with more than 6 years of soccer experience. We used movesense sensor [39] which embeds an accelerometer 13 Hz sampling frequency. Moto g6 [40], an Android smartphone, was used to record the data. As shown in Fig. 4, wearable sensors were attached to three locations (inside-ankle, lower back, and upper back). Although we collected data from three sensor locations at the same time, we analyzed the data separately because we aim to recognize soccer actions from one sensor.

Six soccer movements defined at Sect. 3.1 were performed 30–50 times for each participants. 3-D acceleration data was collected during the experiment, and a camera was used to simultaneously record the subject's movements. The data was sent to an Android smartphone via Bluetooth and saved as a comma-separated values (CSV) file. We used data from seven subjects excluding missing values. In the following Fig. 5, we showed the dataset which includes the collected data from sensors worn at the right ankle, lower back, and up back. This data covers all six soccer movements.

4.2 Validation Results and Discussions for All Six Actions

In our experiment, we trained models to classify data using supervised machine learning with a fivefold cross-validation on MATLAB. We performed eight classification methods, fine tree, quadratic SVM, cubic SVM, medium Gaussian SVM, fine

KNN, weighted KNN, ensemble bagged trees, and ensemble subspace KNN, which are expected high accuracy in exercise recognition.

Table 1 and Fig. 6 show the accuracy of each sensor for all actions. The highest classification accuracy was 78.7% that we achieved through the application of the ensemble bagged trees classification method to training data from the inside-ankle sensor. The highest accuracy of the lower back sensor was 67.8% when the ensemble bagged trees classification method was applied to the training data. The highest accuracy of the lower back sensor was 70.7% when it is trained on the medium Gaussian SVM. These results show that the SVM and ensemble classification methods have higher accuracy than other methods.

Besides, the data from the inside-ankle sensor was the highest accuracy, and the sensor from the upper back was the second highest accuracy among three sensors. In addition, ensemble bagged trees model was the highest accuracy on the datasets from the inside-ankle and the upper back sensor, and medium Gaussian SVM model was the highest accuracy on the datasets from the lower back.

We show a confusion matrix of all six actions (see Figs. 7, 8, and 9). We found that regardless of classification method, the accuracy for shooting (S) was the highest and that for kick tricks (KT), the lowest. Kick tricks are a soccer skill which requires the subject to dribble, and they can be done in different ways depending on the angle and play style of the subject. This leads to confusion with other movements such as pure dribbling and passing. Additionally, kick tricks are usually performed during the dribbling when playing soccer. In this experiment, kick tricks are often misclassified to dribbling for all three sensor locations as shown in Figs. 7, 8, and 9. This means that kick tricks are often included in dribbling. So that, we show the validation result excluding kick tricks in the next section.

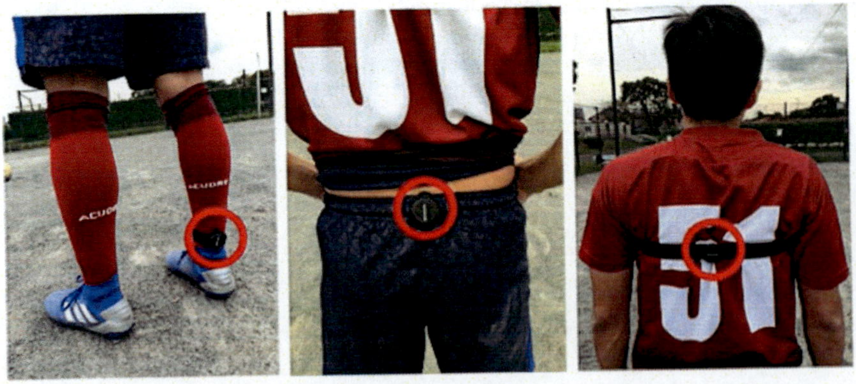

Fig. 4 Sensor locations (inside-ankle, lower back, and upper back)

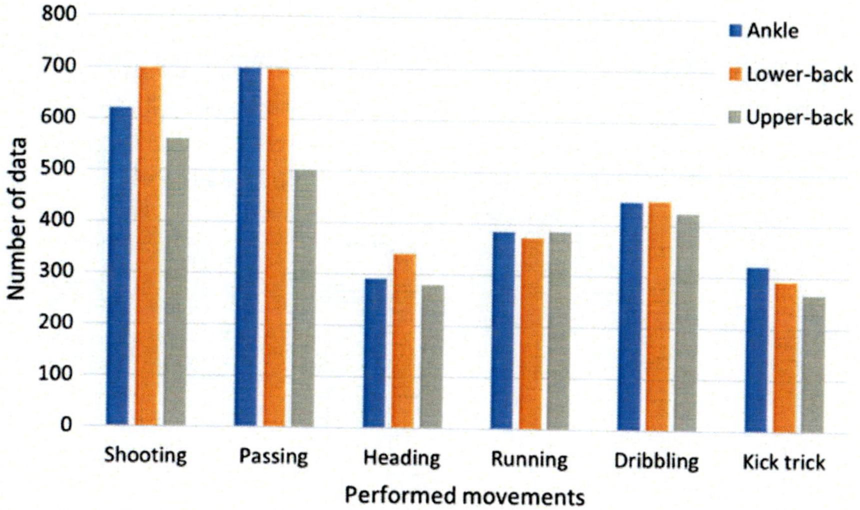

Fig. 5 Collected datasets

Table 1 Classification accuracy for all actions (shooting, passing, heading, running, dribbling, kick trick)

		Machine learning models							
		FT (%)	QS (%)	CS (%)	MGS (%)	FK (%)	WK (%)	EBT (%)	ESK (%)
Sensor locations	Inside-ankle	68.2	77.2	78.5	77.9	75.7	76.7	78.7	74.9
	Lower back	54.8	66.4	68.0	66.7	61.8	65.4	67.8	62.8
	Upper back	55.1	69.6	70.0	70.7	65.4	68.9	70.5	65.8

FT fine tree; QS quadratic SVM; CS cubic SVM; MGS medium Gaussian SVM; FK fine KNN, WK weighted KNN; EBT ensemble bagged trees; ESK ensemble subspace KNN

4.3 *Validation Results and Discussions for Selected Actions*

As mentioned at Sect. 4.2, we show the validation result excluding kick tricks because it is usually performed during the dribbling. Table 2 and Fig. 10 show the accuracy of each sensor for five of the actions excluding kick tricks. The highest classification accuracy was 83.3% which we achieved through the application of the ensemble bagged trees classification method to training data from the inside-ankle sensor. The highest accuracy of the lower-back sensor was 73.5% when the ensemble bagged trees classification method was applied to the training data. The highest accuracy of the lower-back sensor was 76.2% when the medium Gaussian SVM classification method

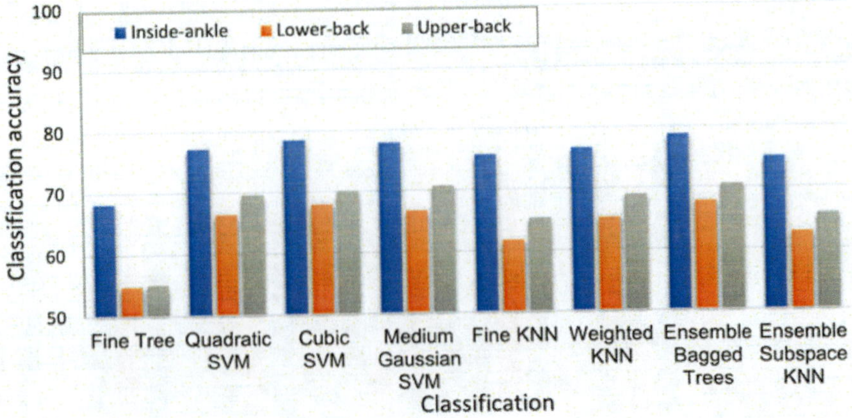

Fig. 6 Comparison of the classification accuracy of machine learning models for all actions (shooting, passing, heading, running, dribbling, kick trick)

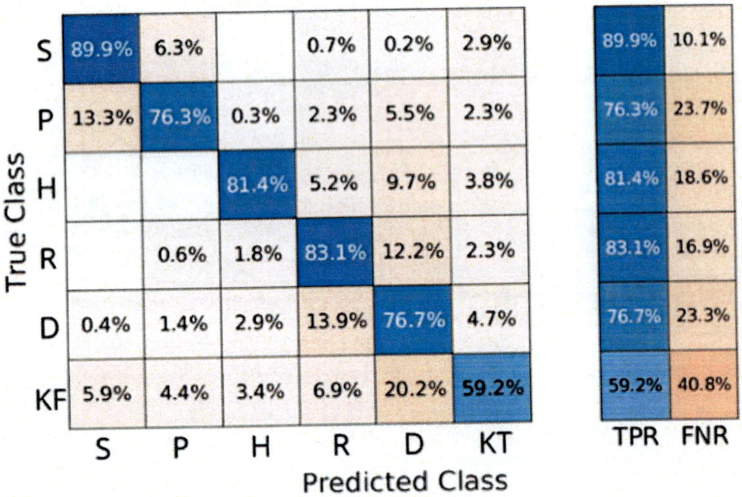

Fig. 7 Inside-ankle sensor—ensemble bagged trees (accuracy: 78.7%)

was applied to the training data. The accuracy increased when the classification method was applied to the dataset excluding dribbling in comparison with the all actions dataset.

We conducted additional validations to see effects of the combination of actions on classification accuracy. Figure 11 shows the result of the classification method accuracy with datasets as follows: (all actions), (5 actions excluding kick trick), (5 actions excluding dribbling), (shooting, passing, kick trick), (shooting, passing), and (running, dribbling). About 90.1% accuracy was achieved with shooting and passing

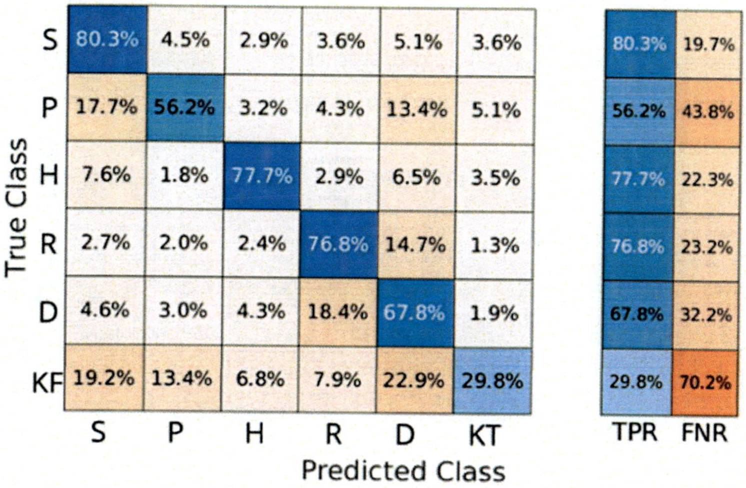

Fig. 8 Lower-back sensor—ensemble bagged trees (accuracy: 67.8%)

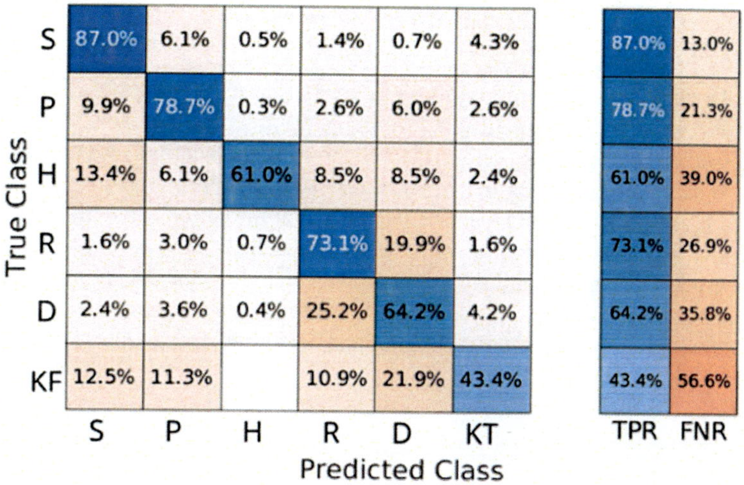

Fig. 9 Upper-back sensor—medium Gaussian SVM (accuracy: 70.7%)

dataset that we expected difficult to classify. The accuracy was almost the same for both lower- and upper-back sensors with running and dribbling datasets.

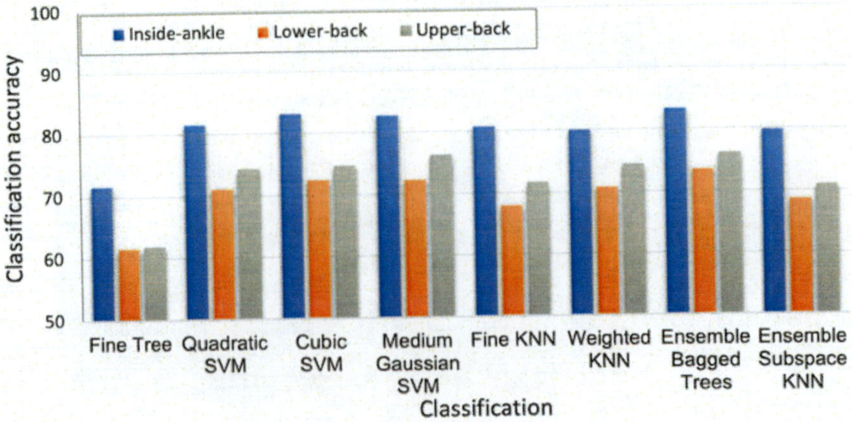

Fig. 10 Comparison of the classification accuracy of machine learning models for five actions (shooting, passing, heading, running, dribbling)

5 Conclusion and Future Work

In this paper, we proposed a peak extraction method and an identification model for shooting, passing, heading, running, dribbling, and kick tricks in soccer. We also evaluated its accuracy and compared three sensor location's accuracy which included right ankle and lower and upper back. The result shows that the accuracy was 78.7% for all six actions and over 83.3% for five of the actions from the right-ankle sensor. Our proposed method proved that it is possible to distinguish between running and dribbling, passing and shooting, even though they are similar movements in soccer. The second highest accuracy was achieved from a sensor placed on the upper part of the back, which is a safer wearing position compared to other locations.

Table 2 Classification accuracy for five actions (shooting, passing, heading, running, dribbling)

		Machine learning models							
		FT (%)	QS (%)	CS (%)	MGS (%)	FK (%)	WK (%)	EBT (%)	ESK (%)
Sensor locations	Inside-ankle	71.6	81.5	83.1	82.7	80.7	80.0	83.3	79.8
	Lower back	61.6	71.1	72.4	72.3	67.9	70.7	73.5	68.6
	Upper back	61.9	74.3	74.6	76.2	71.6	74.4	76.1	70.9

FT fine tree; *QS* quadratic SVM; *CS* cubic SVM; *MGS* medium Gaussian SVM; *FK* fine KNN; *WK* weighted KNN; *EBT* ensemble bagged trees; *ESK* ensemble subspace KNN

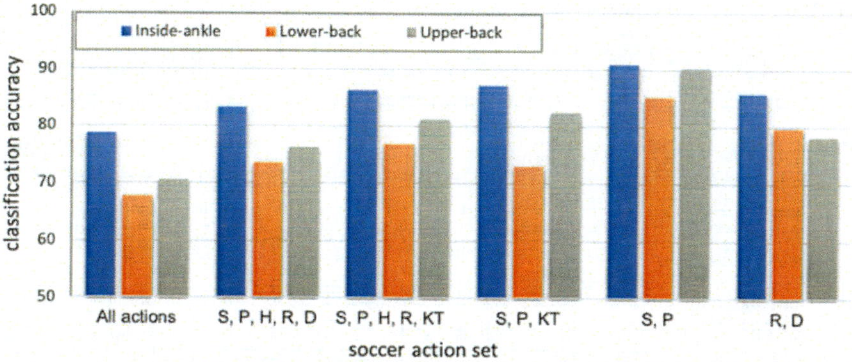

Fig. 11 Effect of the number of movements on targeted classification accuracy (S: shooting, P: passing, H: heading, R: running, D: dribbling, KT: kick trick)

We extracted features based on the manual peak detection method, which took many attempts to precisely segment each action from a video footage during the experiment. Therefore, future work would develop an automatic system to segment each soccer movement. Eventually, we would like to develop a smartphone application for skill monitoring, the aim of which would be to help improve the skills of amateur soccer players.

Acknowledgements This work was supported by Aoyama Gakuin University Research Institute grant program for creation of innovative research.

References

1. Skawinski, K., Montraveta Roca, F., Dieter Findling, R., Sigg, S.: Workout type recognition and repetition counting with CNNs from 3D acceleration sensed on the chest. In: International Work-Conference on Artificial Neural Networks, pp. 347–359. Springer, Berlin (2019)
2. Das Antar, A., Ahmed, M., Ahad, M.A.R.: Sensor-Based Human Activity and Behavior Computing, pp. 147–176. Springer International Publishing, Cham (2021)
3. Hossain, T., Islam, Md.S., Ahad, M.A.R., Inoue, S.: Human activity recognition using earable device. In: Adjunct Proceedings of the 2019 ACM International Joint Conference on Pervasive and Ubiquitous Computing and Proceedings of the 2019 ACM International Symposium on Wearable Computers, UbiComp/ISWC'19 Adjunct, pp. 81–84. Association for Computing Machinery, New York, NY, USA (2019)
4. Das Antar, A., Ahmed, M., Ahad, M.A.R.: Challenges in sensor-based human activity recognition and a comparative analysis of benchmark datasets: a review. In: 2019 Joint 8th International Conference on Informatics, Electronics Vision (ICIEV) and 2019 3rd International Conference on Imaging, Vision Pattern Recognition (icIVPR), pp. 134–139 (2019)
5. Inoue, S., Lago, P., Hossain, T., Mairittha, T., Mairittha, N.: Integrating activity recognition and nursing care records: the system, deployment, and a verification study. Proc. ACM Interact. Mob. Wearable Ubiquitous Technol. **3**(3) (2019)

6. Manjarres, J., Narvaez, P., Gasser, K., Percybrooks, W., Pardo, M.: Physical workload tracking using human activity recognition with wearable devices. Sensors **20**(1), 39 (2020)
7. Ahad, M.A.R., Das Antar, A., Shahid, O.: Vision-based action understanding for assistive healthcare: a short review. In: Proceedings of the IEEE/CVF Conference on Computer Vision and Pattern Recognition (CVPR) Workshops (2019)
8. Ahad, M.A.R., Ahmed, M., Das Antar, A., Makihara, Y., Yagi, Y.: Action recognition using kinematics posture feature on 3d skeleton joint locations. Pattern Recogn. Lett. **145**, 216–224 (2021)
9. Tong, C., Tailor, S.A., Lane, N.D.: Are accelerometers for activity recognition a dead-end? In: Proceedings of the 21st International Workshop on Mobile Computing Systems and Applications, pp. 39–44 (2020)
10. Zhang, S., Wei, Z., Nie, J., Huang, L., Wang, S., Li, Z.: A review on human activity recognition using vision-based method. J. Healthcare Eng. **2017** (2017)
11. Malawski, F., Kwolek, B.: Classification of basic footwork in fencing using accelerometer. In: 2016 Signal Processing: Algorithms, Architectures, Arrangements, and Applications (SPA), pp. 51–55. IEEE (2016)
12. Luis Felipe, J., Garcia-Unanue, J., Viejo-Romero, D., Navandar, A., Sánchez-Sánchez, J.: Validation of a video-based performance analysis system (mediacoach®) to analyze the physical demands during matches in LaLiga. Sensors **19**(19), 4113 (2019)
13. Sap and the German football association turn big data into smart decisions to improve player performance at the world cup in Brazil. https://news.sap.com/2014/06/sap-dfb-turn-big-data-smart-data-world-cup-brazil/. Accessed on 26 July 2021
14. Kim, W., Kim, M.: Sports motion analysis system using wearable sensors and video cameras. In: 2017 International Conference on Information and Communication Technology Convergence (ICTC), pp. 1089–1091. IEEE (2017)
15. Chmura, P., Andrzejewski, M., Konefał, M., Mroczek, D., Rokita, A., Chmura, J.: Analysis of motor activities of professional soccer players during the 2014 world cup in Brazil. J. Human Kinet. **56**(1), 187–195 (2017)
16. Bojanova, I.: It enhances football at world cup 2014. IT Prof. **16**(4), 12–17 (2014)
17. Metulini, R.: Players movements and team shooting performance: a data mining approach for basketball (2018). arXiv preprint arXiv:1805.02501
18. Taylor, J.B., Wright, A.A., Dischiavi, S.L., Townsend, M.A., Marmon, A.R.: Activity demands during multi-directional team sports: a systematic review. Sports Med. **47**(12), 2533–2551 (2017)
19. Taghavi, S., Davari, F., Tabatabaee Malazi, H., Ali Abin, A.: Tennis stroke detection using inertial data of a smartwatch. In: 2019 9th International Conference on Computer and Knowledge Engineering (ICCKE), pp. 466–474. IEEE (2019)
20. Pons, E., García-Calvo, T., Resta, R., Blanco, H., del Campo, R.L., Díaz García, J., José Pulido, J.: A comparison of a GPS device and a multi-camera video technology during official soccer matches: agreement between systems. Plos One **14**(8), e0220729 (2019)
21. Merton McGinnis, P.: Biomechanics of Sport and Exercise. Human Kinetics (2013)
22. Fullerton, E., Heller, B., Munoz-Organero, M.: Recognizing human activity in free-living using multiple body-worn accelerometers. IEEE Sens. J. **17**(16), 5290–5297 (2017)
23. Poppe, R.: A survey on vision-based human action recognition. Image Vis. Comput. **28**(6), 976–990 (2010)
24. Ahmed, M., Das Antar, A., Ahad, M.A.R.: An approach to classify human activities in real-time from smartphone sensor data. In: 2019 Joint 8th International Conference on Informatics, Electronics Vision (ICIEV) and 2019 3rd International Conference on Imaging, Vision Pattern Recognition (icIVPR), pp. 140–145 (2019)
25. Sayan Saha, S., Rahman, S., Ridita Haque, Z.R., Hossain, T., Inoue, S., Ahad, M.A.R.: Position independent activity recognition using shallow neural architecture and empirical modeling. In: Adjunct Proceedings of the 2019 ACM International Joint Conference on Pervasive and Ubiquitous Computing and Proceedings of the 2019 ACM International Symposium on Wearable Computers, UbiComp/ISWC'19 Adjunct, pp. 808–813. Association for Computing Machinery, New York, NY, USA (2019)

26. Li, Y., Peng, X., Zhou, G., Zhao, H.: Smartjump: a continuous jump detection framework on smartphones. IEEE Internet Comput. **24**(2), 18–26 (2020)
27. Shahmohammadi, F., Hosseini, A., King, C.E., Sarrafzadeh, M.: Smartwatch based activity recognition using active learning. In: Proceedings of the Second IEEE/ACM International Conference on Connected Health: Applications, Systems and Engineering Technologies, CHASE'17, pp. 321–329. IEEE Press (2017)
28. Weiss, G.M., Yoneda, K., Hayajneh, T.: Smartphone and smartwatch-based biometrics using activities of daily living. IEEE Access **7**, 133190–133202 (2019)
29. Sukreep, S., Elgazzar, K., Henry Chu, C., Nukoolkit, C., Mongkolnam, P.: Recognizing falls, daily activities, and health monitoring by smart devices. Sens. Mater. **31**(6), 1847–1869 (2019)
30. Morris, D., Scott Saponas, T., Guillory, A., Kelner, I.: RecoFit: using a wearable sensor to find, recognize, and count repetitive exercises. In: Proceedings of the SIGCHI Conference on Human Factors in Computing Systems, pp. 3225–3234 (2014)
31. Ishii, S., Yokokubo, A., Luimula, M., Lopez, G.: ExerSense: physical exercise recognition and counting algorithm from wearables robust to positioning. Sensors **21**(1) (2021)
32. Nguyen, L.N.N., Rodríguez-Martín, D., Català, A., Pérez-López, C., Samà, A., Cavallaro, A.: Basketball activity recognition using wearable inertial measurement units. In: Proceedings of the XVI International Conference on Human Computer Interaction, pp. 1–6 (2015)
33. Chang, C.-C., Lin, C.-J.: LIBSVM: a library for support vector machines. ACM Trans. Intell. Syst. Technol. **2**(3) (2011)
34. Deng, H., Runger, G., Tuv, E., Vladimir, M.: A time series forest for classification and feature extraction. Inf. Sci. **239**, 142–153 (2013)
35. Rakthanmanon, T., Keogh, E.: Fast shapelets: a scalable algorithm for discovering time series shapelets. In: Proceedings of the 2013 SIAM International Conference on Data Mining, pp. 668–676. SIAM (2013)
36. Schäfer, P.: The boss is concerned with time series classification in the presence of noise. Data Min. Knowl. Discov. **29**(6), 1505–1530 (2015)
37. Alobaid, O., Ramaswamy, L.: A feature-based approach for identifying soccer moves using an accelerometer sensor. In: HEALTHINF, pp. 34–44 (2020)
38. Henriksen, A., Haugen Mikalsen, M., Zebene Woldaregay, A., Muzny, M., Hartvigsen, G., Arnesdatter Hopstock, L., Grimsgaard, S.: Using fitness trackers and smartwatches to measure physical activity in research: analysis of consumer wrist-worn wearables. J. Med. Internet Res. **20**(3), e110 (2018)
39. Movesense: https://www.movesense.com/. Accessed on 26 July 2021
40. Motorola: https://www.motorola.com/us/. Accessed on 14 Jan 2021

A Data-Driven Approach for Online Pre-impact Fall Detection with Wearable Devices

Takuto Yoshida, Kazuma Kano, Keisuke Higashiura, Kohei Yamaguchi, Koki Takigami, Kenta Urano, Shunsuke Aoki, Takuro Yonezawa, and Nobuo Kawaguchi

Abstract The implementation of wearable airbags to prevent fall injuries depends on accurate pre-impact fall detection and a clear distinction between activities of daily living (ADL) and them. We propose a novel pre-impact fall detection algorithm that is robust against ambiguous falling activities. We present a data-driven approach to estimate the fall risk from acceleration and angular velocity features and use thresholding techniques to robustly detect a fall before impact. In the experiment, we collect simulated fall data from subjects wearing an inertial sensor on their waist. As a result, we succeeded in significantly improving the accuracy of fall detection from 50.00 to 96.88%, the recall from 18.75 to 93.75%, and the specificity 81.25 to 100.00% over the baseline method.

1 Introduction

It is an important issue to prevent injuries due to falls among the elderly. Falls can lead directly to death or may cause the elderly to become bedridden that may indirectly lead to death. Psychological trauma and fear of falling can cause anxiety and lack of confidence in performing daily activities, thus preventing independence. One-third to one-half of seniors aged 65 and older experience a fall [1]. About one-third of the elderly who live at home fall at least once a year. About half of the elderly living in nursing homes fall at least once a year. People who have fallen before are more likely to fall again. Of those who fall and remain lying on the floor for hours, half will be dead within half a year [2].

Many researchers have study of fall detection and its prevention. The key points of the fall detection task are to reliably detect falls and to distinguish between falls and activities of daily living (ADL). There are three main categories of fall detection meth-

T. Yoshida (✉) · K. Kano · K. Higashiura · K. Yamaguchi · K. Takigami · K. Urano · T. Yonezawa · N. Kawaguchi
Graduate School of Enginnering, Nagoya University, Nagoya, Japan
e-mail: takuto@ucl.nuee.nagoya-u.ac.jp

S. Aoki
National Institute of Informatics, Tokyo, Japan

M. A. R. Ahad et al. (eds.), *Sensor- and Video-Based Activity and Behavior Computing*, Smart Innovation, Systems and Technologies 291,
https://doi.org/10.1007/978-981-19-0361-8_8

ods: ambient device-based, vision-based, and wearable device-based [3]. Ambient device-based system is a method of recognizing human activity using video, audio, and vibrational data [4, 5]. Vision-based system detects the position and posture of a person and estimates their activity based on images from ceiling-mounted cameras [6, 7]. However, those methods are costly and not easy to set up. Additionally, it is difficult to use them for online pre-impact fall detection to prevent fall injuries. On the other hand, wearable-based systems are easy to implement and various methods have been proposed [8–16]. In most of these methods, acceleration and angular velocity are the key features for detecting falls and are applied using threshold detection algorithms. In [1, 17, 18], the approaches for online pre-impact fall detection to prevent fall injuries have been proposed. In general, the system should be able to detect a fall 0.3–0.4 s before impact, assuming that it is incorporated into a wearable airbag. Most existing methods use thresholds to perform binary classification of fall events (the timing of airbag activation) and ADL events and achieve high detection rates in experiments with some restricted activities. However, in real life, there are many ambiguous falling activities, such as ADL activities that resemble falls and fall activities that resemble ADLs, for example, sitting on a chair vigorously, jumping, falling with a defensive response, and so on. It is difficult to distinguish them by only using instantaneous acceleration and angular velocity values and thresholds. Since falls are life-threatening, there is a need for more robust fall detection algorithms.

We propose the novel pre-impact fall detection algorithm that is robust against ambiguous falling activities to prevent fall injuries. Figure 1 shows an overview of the algorithm for detecting a fall before impact based on acceleration and angular velocity. Our proposed method uses the data-driven human activity recognition (HAR) technique to improve the robustness of fall detection. First, we extract the features of acceleration and angular velocity using a sliding window and then perform feature reduction using principal component analysis (PCA) or sequential forward feature selection (SFFS). Secondly, we use a machine learning model, Bayesian decision making (BDM), the least-squares method (LSM), the k-nearest neighbor algorithm (k-NN), support vector machines (SVM), and artificial neural networks (ANN), to estimate the fall risk, which is a value that models the likelihood of a fall in the time direction. Finally, at the timing when the fall risk exceeds the threshold, the airbag activation signal is output. In our approach, we set the threshold to detect 0.3 s before the fall that is the optimal time to activate the airbag. In the experiment, we collect simulated fall data including ambiguous falling activities from subjects wearing an inertial sensor on their waist. Our contributions are as follows:

- We present a novel pre-impact fall detection algorithm that is robust against ambiguous falling activities.
- We collect simulated fall data including ambiguous falling activities from subjects wearing an inertial sensor on their waist.
- We have achieved improved robustness of fall detection against ambiguous falling activities.

The paper is structured as follows: We describe the related work in Sect. 2. We explain the detailed proposed method in Sect. 3. We conduct the experiment to search for

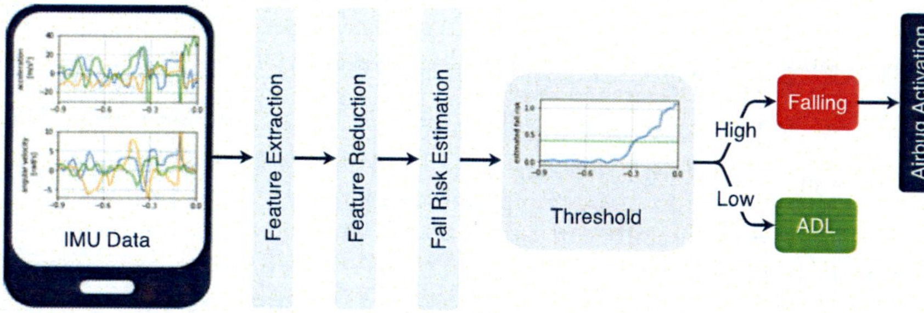

Fig. 1 Implementation flow of our pre-impact fall detection algorithm

optimal hyperparameters and regression models in Sect. 4. We evaluate the baseline and the proposed method in terms of accuracy and timing of fall detection in Sect. 5. Finally, Sect. 6 concludes the paper by discussing future directions of the research.

2 Related Work

Research on pre-impact fall detection has been conducted to prevent falls injuries in the elderly. Wu et al. in [17] have proposed that motion analysis techniques can be used to detect a fall before impact. Wu has showed that by thresholding the horizontal and vertical velocity profiles of the trunk, falls could be detected 0.3 to 0.4 s before impact. Wu et al. in [18] separated fall and ADL using a threshold detection method with the magnitude of the vertical velocity of the inertial frame as the main variable. The algorithm enables to detect all fall events at least 0.07 s before the impact. By setting the threshold for each individual subject, all falls can be detected and no false alarms occurred. Tamura et al. in [1] have developed a wearable airbag that incorporates a fall detection system. The fall detection algorithm is implemented using a thresholding technique based on accelerometers and gyroscopes. The algorithm is able to detect a signal 0.3 s before the impact. This signal triggers the airbag to inflate up to 2.4 l, preventing physical impact that could lead to injury. These methods have achieved a high fall detection rate by using raw data of acceleration and angular velocity and a threshold. Their validation data certainly includes various ADL events and fall events, but does not include data that is ambiguous about the distinction between falls and ADLs. In order to apply to real life, it is very important to validate with this ambiguous fall data and achieve a high fall detection rate.

In the field of HAR, the data-driven approach has been successfully used to improve classification accuracy and robustness. Matsuyama et al. in [19] classified dance figures based on acceleration, angular velocity, and posture extracted from images. Matsuyama has achieved high accuracy in classification by using long short-term memory (LSTM) as a classifier. Wan et al. in [20] have proposed a accelerometer-based architecture for real-time HAR. He utilizes convolutional neural network (CNN), LSTM, bidirectional LSTM (BLSTM), multilayer perceptron (MLP), and SVM models. Altun et al. in [21] have compared different techniques for HAR using small inertial and magnetic sensors attached to the body. Altun uses BDM, LSM, k-NN, DTW, SVM, and ANN as estimators and employs PCA and SFFS for feature reduction. These gave us the insight to run a general machine learning algorithm-based HAR. Furthermore, Yoshida et al. in [22] and Chen et al. in [23] have successfully applied the HAR technique to regression analysis. Yoshida has developed a method for estimating walking speed from acceleration using deep neural network (DNN). Chen has proposed a DNN framework to estimate pedestrian speed and heading from acceleration and angular velocity. In fall detection, these suggest that the fall risk over time can be estimated from acceleration and angular velocity.

3 Proposed Method

We propose a data-driven pre-impact fall detection method. In this method, we train machine learning models with feature values and fall risk that represents the potential of fall, estimate current fall risk by regression and then detect pre-impact by threshold. In this section, to begin with, we explain what features to extract and how to reduct the number of them. Next, we define fall risk to use as the target value at machine learning. Then, we train several machine learning models with sets of the feature values and fall risk calculated according to the definition. Finally, we estimate current fall risk with the trained models and detect 0.3 s before the impact by using threshold.

3.1 *Feature Extraction and Reduction*

We extract 256 features from acceleration and angular velocity for each sliding window. We apply the idea of sliding window to the model for fall-potential estimation since potential to fall at a certain time should be estimated considering the sensor data in the last certain period of time. With this model, fall potential at a time t is estimated by regressing the feature values of the window that is period from $t - W$ to t (t: time at right edge of the window, W: window size). The slide width when learning is half of the window size, and when estimation is set to 1.

As for features, 32 features are calculated from each of the eight data sets (X-axis data, Y-axis data, Z-axis data, and norm data for acceleration and angular velocity, respectively), resulting in 256 features for each single sliding window. 32 features are listed in Table 1. The 15 features in (1) are also computed in a window that took the absolute value of all the data and made into new features (1′). All features are normalized to the interval [0,1] to be used for machine learning in Sect. 3.3.

The 256 features obtained do not all have the same amount of information, and there is a potential that models cannot learn well due to their large feature dimension.

Table 1 32 features extracted from each of the eight data (X-axis data, Y-axis data, Z-axis data, and norm data for acceleration and angular velocity, respectively)

Classification	Features extracted from each Window	Data type	Number of features
(1)	Minimum value, maximum value, median value, mean value, standard deviation, total value, average of differences of neighboring elements, 0.05, 0.10, 0.25, 0.75, 0.90, 0.95 quantile, max/min value, max-min value	Original value	15
(2)	Skewness, kurtosis	Original value	2
(1′)	Same as (1)	Absolute value	15

Therefore, in order to obtain features that can calculate the fall risk more efficiently, we examine two methods: principal component analysis (PCA) for feature extraction and sequential feature forward selection (SFFS) for feature selection. PCA is a method for extracting more meaningful features by setting a new axis in the direction where the variance of the data is maximized. We use this method to reduce 256 features to 40 features with a cumulative contribution rate of about 90%. SFFS is different from PCA in that it selects features as they are. By sequentially selecting the best features, SFFS achieves feature reduction while maximizing the prediction capability of the model. The number of features to be selected is set to five because of the large computational cost.

3.2 Definition of Fall Risk

Some actions like standing or walking are classified with sufficient precision in conventional HAR research. In these general activity recognition task, the timing of recognition does not matter much. When it comes to real-time fall detection task, however, the timing of recognition needs to be carefully considered due to its time tightness. It is difficult to find the earliest time to be able to judge whether the subject is actually about to fall or not after he/she started falling. In fact, that the subject is falling does not get suddenly confirmed at some point. For example, in case a subject had stumbled on a step and eventually hit his/her hips, no one knows the exact time when that he/she was falling got confirmed. He/She might not have fallen if he/she had balanced.

Thus, we model the action of fall as its potential increases gradually, and estimate it by regression. It is expected that the index of fall potential is a value that meets the following requirements:

- Takes 0 at ADL.
- Increases gradually toward end of fall.
- Takes 1 just before end of fall.

Therefore, we introduce a new index fr (fall risk) defined by the following formula:

$$fr(t) = \begin{cases} 0 & (t < T_{\rm fs}, t > T_{\rm fe}) \\ \dfrac{t - T_{\rm fs}}{W} & (T_{\rm fs} \leq t \leq T_{\rm fs} + W) \\ 1 & (T_{\rm fs} + W < t \leq T_{\rm fe}) \end{cases}$$

fr fall risk
t time at right edge of window
$T_{\rm fs}$ fall start time
$T_{\rm fe}$ fall end time
W window size

Figure 2 shows the relationship between fr and t. We refer to period before $T_{\rm fs}$ as ADL phase and period from $T_{\rm fs}$ to $T_{\rm fe}$ as falling phase. fr is equivalent to the proportion of the area included in falling phase to the whole window. It takes 0 while the whole window is included in ADL phase. Then, it increases as the window moves and the proportion of the area included in falling phase increases. Finally, it takes 1 after the whole window gets included in falling phase.

3.3 *Training of Machine Learning Model*

We train machine learning models using the features obtained in Sect. 3.1 and fall risk calculated according to the definition in Sect. 3.2. $T_{\rm fe}$ for calculating fall risk

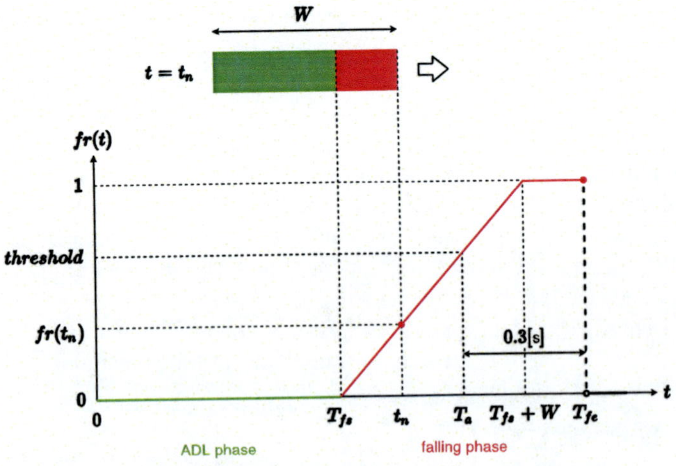

Fig. 2 Relationship between fall risk and window position

are set by labels. In our approach, we use five regression techniques : Bayesian decision making (BDM), the least-squares method (LSM), the k-nearest neighbor algorithm (k-NN), support vector machines (SVM), and artificial neural networks (ANN). The accuracy of them is evaluated by mean square error (MSE). BDM is a method of determining the most likely weights by introducing noise that follows a normal distribution to the predictions. In this case, we also added a ridge regression term to prevent overfitting. LSM is a well-known method used in linear regression analysis. It determines the plane so that the sum of the squared errors for each data and approximation plane is minimized. The k-NN and SVM are one of the most commonly used methods of regression analysis and classification. In ANN, we use a three-layer perceptron regressor. It is one of the simplest neural networks.

3.4 Estimation of Fall Risk and Fall Detection with Threshold

fr (fall risk) will be estimated by inputting the feature values of the current window to the model trained in Sect. 3.3. If estimated fr exceeds a certain threshold value, the system recognizes that the subject is falling, and outputs signal to activate the airbug which prevents him/her from getting injured. Threshold values to detect any seconds before end of fall can be given as the theoretical value of fr at that time. In this paper, we aim to detect 0.3 s before end of fall because it is generally considered that the model should be able to detect 0.3 to 0.4 s before the impact in order to activate the airbug in advance. As such, the threshold value corresponding to 0.3 s before the impact will be calculated by the following equation:

$$\text{threshold} = fr(T_a)$$

$$T_a = T_{\text{fe}} - 0.3[\text{s}] : \text{airbug activation time}$$

The relationship between the threshold value and T_a is shown in Fig. 2. The pair of parameters (T_{fs}, W) needs to satisfy following condition so that the slope of $fr(t)$ does not take 0 around $t = T_a$:

$$T_a - T_{\text{fs}} \le W \le T_{fe} - T_{\text{fs}}$$

4 Search for Hyperparameters and Regression Models

We conduct experiments to find a machine learning model that can estimate fall risk with high accuracy. Initially, we collect data from four subjects to train and evaluate the machine learning model. Then we train and cross-validate the machine learning model using the collected data to select the optimal window size, feature reduction method, and regressor.

4.1 Experimental Setup

We collect training data for the proposed method from three subjects with an average age of 21, a weight of 58.0 ± 7.0 kg, and a height of 172.0 ± 9.4 cm and test data from one subject with an age of 24, a weight of 58.2 kg, and a height of 165.5 cm. Figure 3 shows a simulated falling experiment. Three of them fall to 11 times front, 12 times back, 11 times right side, and 5 times left side and perform daily activities such as walking 39 times, a total of 78 times for training data. One of them fall to 4 times front, 4 times back, 4 times right side, and 4 times left side and perform daily activities such as walking 16 times, a total of 32 for test data. They wear the smartphones with inertial sensors (XPERIA Z5 SO-01H) that is attached to the back of the waist and the right side of the waist. The y-axis of the smartphone is aligned with the subject's foot-to-head axis, and the back of the smartphone is in close contact with the body. In other words, the z-axis of the smartphone is perpendicular to the plane of the body and points from the inside of the body to the outside. At the moment of impact, the recorder presses a button on the M5stack to record the timing of the impact of the fall. The inertial sensor data and the impact timing data are sent to the same server in real time, thus that the time is synchronized accurately.

Our data simulates real-life falls, including stumbling, losing balance, and bending the knee in defense. It is more difficult to distinguish between fall events and ADL

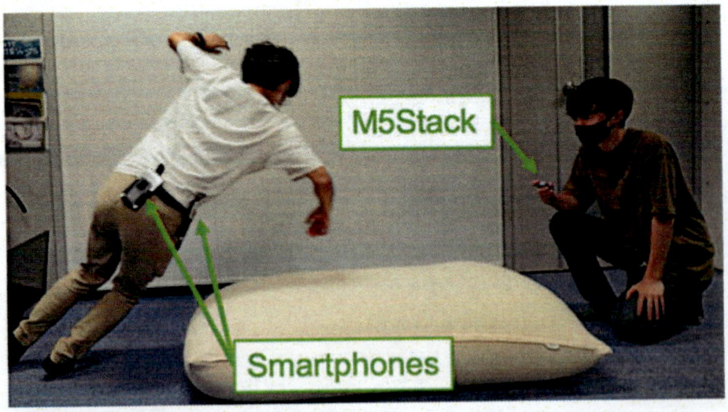

Fig. 3 A simulated falling experiment: The person wearing a smartphone on his waist falls and inertial sensor data is collected. The person holding the M5Stack presses a button at the timing of the impact of the fall and records it

Table 2 Results of cross-validation with MSE when using each window size, feature reduction, and regressor (Target fall risk when $T_{fs} = T_{fe} - 0.5$)

W	BDM		LSM		k-NN		SVM		ANN	
	PCA	SFFS	PCA	SFFS	PCA	SFFS	PCA	SFFS	PCA	SFFS
0.20	0.0157	0.0158	0.0157	0.0183	0.0133	0.0229	0.0173	0.0230	0.0183	0.0148
0.30	0.0125	0.0127	0.0120	0.0151	0.0095	0.0158	0.0142	0.0196	0.0127	0.0114
0.40	0.0096	0.0100	0.0095	0.0121	0.0064	0.0104	0.0103	0.0159	0.0104	0.0082
0.50	0.0068	0.0072	0.0067	0.0084	**0.0044**	0.0083	0.0073	0.0104	0.0078	0.0072

events in our data than in data from existing studies because there are many variations in the falling events in these data, including defensive responses. Therefore, our data set is more suitable to verify the robustness of the method against ambiguous activities.

4.2 The Result of Estimation Accuracy

Through a number of simulated fall experiments, we have found that setting T_{fs} to 0.5 s before impact is optimal for modeling fall risk well. Therefore, we search for W, reduction methods, and regressor that can estimate the fall risk with the highest accuracy when $T_{fs} = T_{fe} - 0.5$ s. Table 2 shows the results of the evaluation using mean squared error (MSE). As a result, when a window size of 0.5 s, a reduction method of PCA, and a regressor of k-NN, the MSE of fall risk is minimized. We use this setting as our method at evaluation in Sect. 5.

5 Evaluation

We evaluate the baseline and the proposed method in terms of accuracy and timing of fall detection. Firstly, we introduce the baseline method. Secondly, we define the evaluation metrics. Finally, we show the evaluation results and discuss them.

5.1 Baseline Method

We evaluate the performance of pre-impact fall detection for the proposed method and the baseline method. We select [1] as baseline. It is threshold-based pre-impact fall detection algorithm using only current acceleration and angular velocity. It assumes that the acceleration signal during the fall is similar to free fall. Additionally, it suggests that pitch angular velocity signals can also be used for fall detection. Therefore, it judges a fall when the acceleration is less than ± 3 m/s^2 and the pitch angular velocity exceeds 0.52 rad/s.

5.2 Evaluation Metrics

The results of running the fall detection algorithm on the test data can be categorized into the following four groups:

- True Positive (TP) that falls are detected in the falling phase.
- True Negative (TN) that falls are not detected in the ADL phase.
- False Positives (FP) that falls are detected in the ADL phase.
- False Negative (FN) that falls are not detected in the falling phase.

The high percentage of TP and TN indicates that the fall detection system works well to prevent falling injuries. If the percentage of FP is high that the airbag will malfunction during the ADL phase, causing inconvenience to the user. If the percentage of FN is high, the airbag will not work during the falling phase and the user will be injured by the fall. Therefore, it is ideal that FP and FN are zero. The time of airbag activation is also an important evaluation indicator to prevent fall injuries. Hence we calculate the mean and standard deviation of $T_{\text{fe}} - \hat{T}_a$. $\hat{T}_a$ denotes the estimated airbag activation time. This indicator is desirable to have a mean value of 0.3 and a standard deviation close to 0.

5.3 Evaluation Results

Table 3 shows the number of TP, TN, FP, and FN counts at each sensor position when the baseline and the proposed method detection algorithm are executed on the test data. In common with both methods, there is almost no difference in accuracy by sensor position. The results of the baseline method show that 3 for TP, 13 for TN, 3 for FP, and 13 for FN, giving an accuracy of 50.00%, a recall of 18.75% and a specificity of 81.25%. On the other hand, the results of the proposed method show that 15 for TP, 16 for TN, 0 for FP, and 1 for FN, giving an accuracy of 96.88%, a recall of 93.75%, and a specificity of 100.00%. It can be seen that the accuracy, recall, and specificity are higher in the proposed method than in the baseline. The results show that the proposed method is more accurate in detecting falls and is able to make a distinction between ADL and falling more clearly than the baseline methods.

Table 4 shows the evaluation result of airbag activation timing. The overall $T_{\text{fe}} - \hat{T}_a$ of baseline has a mean of 0.265 s and a standard deviation of 0.150 s. The overall $T_{\text{fe}} - \hat{T}_a$ of the proposed method has a mean of 0.154 and a standard deviation of 0.0965. Considering that the target $T_{\text{fe}} - \hat{T}_a$ is 0.3 s, we can see that the baseline is more accurate. On the other hand, when we focus on the standard deviation, we can see that the proposed method is more stable with less variation.

5.4 Comparison of Our Proposed with the Baseline

Table 3 shows that there is a large difference in the recall, which indicates the fall detection rate, between the proposed method (93.75%) and the baseline (18.75%). Figure 4 shows a typical example of fall detection for baseline and the proposed method when the subject has an inertial sensor attached to the right side of the waist and falls to the right side. Figure 4a shows a example of baseline. The signal is not reaching within 0.3 m/s^2 that is the threshold for acceleration. All of the test data simulated realistic falls and included behaviors such as stumbling, losing balance, and defensive reactions. There are few such data that can detect a clear free fall. As a result, the threshold-based method fails to detect it. In addition, there are some data that cannot detect a fall because the angular velocity in the free fall phase is small due to the defensive reaction of bending the knee and falling from the knee that is also mentioned in the discussion of [1]. This experiment has shown that it is difficult to implement a threshold-based system that works reliably in real-world fall accidents and does not cause the airbag to malfunction during the ADL phase.

Table 3 Number of TP, FP, and FN counts when the proposed method and the baseline fall detection algorithm are executed on the test data

	Sensor position	TP	TN	FP	FN
Baseline	Right	1	7	1	7
	Back	2	6	2	6
	Overall	3	13	3	13
Proposal	Right	8	8	0	0
	Back	7	8	0	1
	Overall	15	16	0	1

Table 4 Mean and standard deviation of $T_{fe} - \hat{T}_a$ s that is time difference between falling impact and the airbag activation

	Sensor position	$T_{fe} - \hat{T}_a$	
		Mean	Std
Baseline	Right	0.334	–
	Back	0.231	0.174
	Overall	0.265	0.150
Proposal	Right	0.168	0.097
	Back	0.137	0.094
	Overall	0.154	0.097

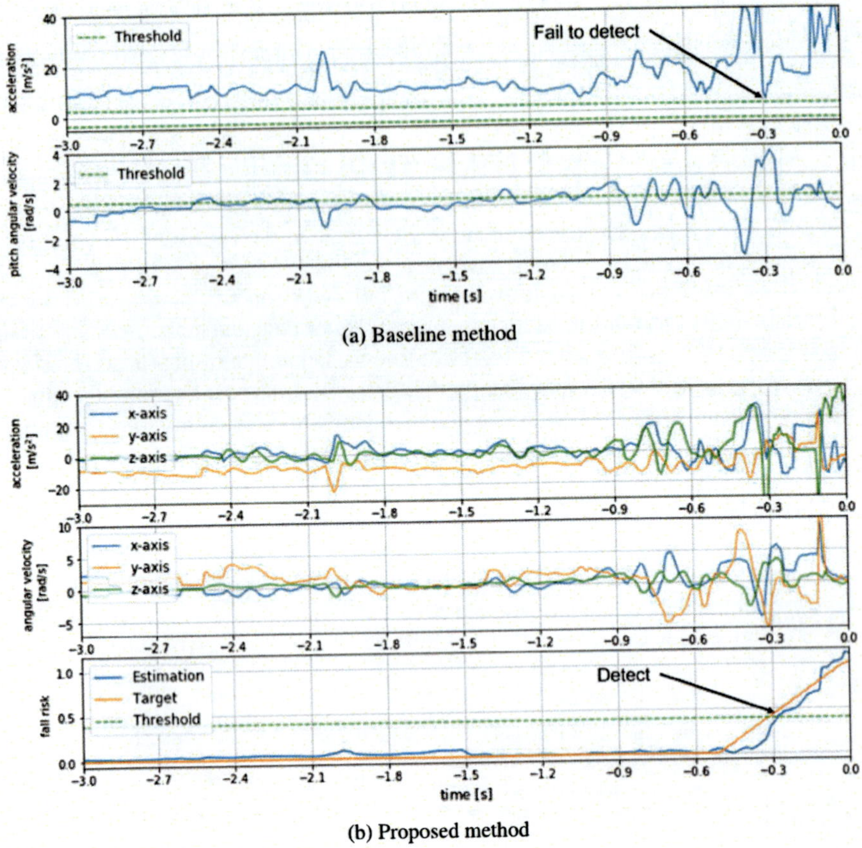

Fig. 4 Example of fall detection for baseline and proposed methods

Figure 4b shows the results of pre-impact fall detection based on proposed method that uses a threshold and fall risk estimation with a window size of 0.5 s, a reduction method of PCA, and a regressor of k-NN. k-NN has successfully estimated the fall risk we defined in the Sect. 3 from the acceleration and angular velocity. This result supports the validity of our assumed fall risk model.

We can see that we have succeeded in detecting the fall 0.3 s before the impact from the time of the crossing point between a threshold of 0.4 and the fall risk. This result shows that improving the accuracy of fall risk estimation contributes to improving the accuracy and robustness of pre-impact fall detection and reducing the number of false fall detections. In other words, we only need to focus on improving the accuracy of fall risk to improve the performance of pre-impact fall detection.

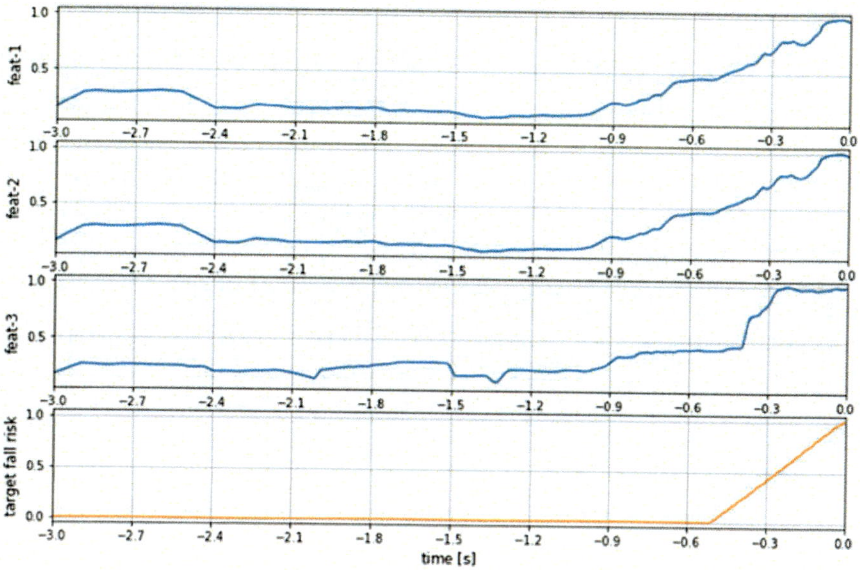

Fig. 5 Example of three features that are important for estimating fall risk in k-NN that is selected by SFFS

5.5 *The Importance of Features*

We use the SFFS results to discuss the features that are important in estimating the fall risk. We have found three features that are important for estimating fall risk in k-NN in the process of feature extraction by SFFS. The features are the 0.05 quantile of y-axis acceleration (feat-1) and the kurtosis of y-axis acceleration (feat-2) and average of the differences of neighboring elements in absolute value of z-axis acceleration (feat-3). Figure 5 shows an example of these features and the target fall risk. Each features are shown as feat-1, feat-2, and feat-3 in order. It can be seen from Fig. 5 that there is a strong correlation between target fall risk and these features. The values of feat-1 and feat-2 rise faster than the target fall risk; however, the values from -0.9 to -0.6 s are close to the values around -2.7 s, and therefore, it is difficult to use them as a basis for activating the fall risk. However, after -0.6 s, the value of feat-1,2 exceeds 0.5, and after -0.4, the value of feat-3 increases significantly that determines the increase in falling risk.

5.6 *Evaluation of Airbag Activation Time*

The $T_{\text{fe}} - \hat{T}_a$ of the proposed method, 0.15, is smaller than the target of 0.3. This means that the time to activate the airbag is shortened that needs to be improved.

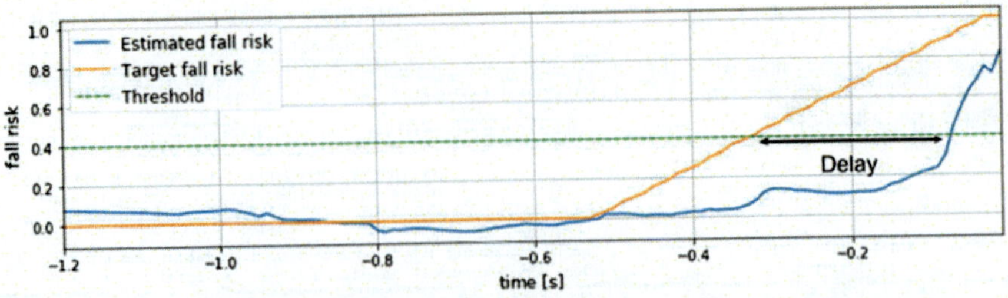

Fig. 6 Example of the delay in the rise of the fall risk estimated by our proposed method

The reason is the delay in the rise of the fall risk estimated by the proposed method. Figure 6 shows an example of the delay in the rise of the fall risk. To solve this problem, we can increase the number of training data or improve the learning model. These are future issues.

6 Conclusion

We have developed an online pre-impact fall detection algorithm for airbags to prevent fall injuries. Our algorithm uses a data-driven approach to calculate the risk of falling based on acceleration and angular velocity features and uses a thresholding technique to robustly detect a fall before impact. As a result of evaluating the algorithm on data simulating real-life falls, we succeeded in significantly improving the accuracy of fall detection from 50.00 to 96.88% and the recall from 18.75 to 93.75% over the baseline method. However, the fall detection time of the proposed method is on average 0.15 s before the impact that is shorter than 0.3 s that is enough time to activate the airbag. As a solution, we consider a method to increase the training data to improve the accuracy of fall risk estimation and reduce the delay of airbag activation. In addition, the current evaluation data set does not have enough variation and quantity in terms of age, gender, etc., and therefore these need to be increased.

Acknowledgements This work is supported by JSPS KAKENHI Grant Number JP17H01762, JST CREST, and NICT.

References

1. Tamura, T., Yoshimura, T., Sekine, M., Uchida, M., Tanaka, O.: A wearable airbag to prevent fall injuries. IEEE Trans. Inf. Technol. Biomed. **13**(6), 910–914 (2009)
2. Mulley, G.: Falls in older people. J. Royal Soc. Med. **94**(4), 202–202 (2001). PMC1281399[pmcid]
3. Mubashir, M., Shao, L., Seed, L.: A survey on fall detection: principles and approaches. Neurocomputing **100**, 144–152 (2013). Special issue: Behaviours in video

4. Zhuang, X., Huang, J., Potamianos, G., Hasegawa-Johnson, M.: Acoustic fall detection using gaussian mixture models and gmm supervectors. In: 2009 IEEE International Conference on Acoustics, Speech and Signal Processing, pp. 69–72
5. Alwan, M., Rajendran, P.J., Kell, S., Mack, D., Dalal, S., Wolfe, M., Felder, R.: A smart and passive floor-vibration based fall detector for elderly. In: 2006 2nd International Conference on Information Communication Technologies, vol. 1, pp. 1003–1007 (2006)
6. Nait-Charif, H., McKenna, S.J.: Activity summarisation and fall detection in a supportive home environment. In: Proceedings of the 17th International Conference on Pattern Recognition, 2004. ICPR 2004., vol. 4, pp. 323–326 (2004)
7. Lee, T., Mihailidis, A.: An intelligent emergency response system: preliminary development and testing of automated fall detection. J. Telemed. Telecare **11**, 194–198 (2005)
8. Hwang, J.Y., Kang, J.M., Jang, Y.W., Kim, H.C.: Development of novel algorithm and real-time monitoring ambulatory system using bluetooth module for fall detection in the elderly. In: The 26th Annual International Conference of the IEEE Engineering in Medicine and Biology Society, vol. 1, pp. 2204–2207
9. Diaz, A., Prado, M., Roa, L.M., Reina-Tosina, J., Sanchez, G.: Preliminary evaluation of a full-time falling monitor for the elderly. In: The 26th Annual International Conference of the IEEE Engineering in Medicine and Biology Society, vol. 1, pp. 2180–2183
10. Bourke, A., O'Brien, J.V., ÓLaighin, G.: Evaluation of threshold-based tri-axial accelerometer fall detection algorithm. Gait Posture, **26**, 194–199 (2007)
11. Bourke, A.K., Lyons, G.M.: A threshold-based fall-detection algorithm using a bi-axial gyroscope sensor. Med. Eng. Phys. **30**(1), 84–90 (2008)
12. Bagalà, F., Becker, C., Cappello, A., Chiari, L., Aminian, K., Hausdorff, J.M., Zijlstra, W., Klenk, J.: Evaluation of accelerometer-based fall detection algorithms on real-world falls. PLOS ONE **7**, 1–9 (2012)
13. Habib, M.A., Mohktar, M.S., Kamaruzzaman, S.B., Lim, K.S., Pin, T.M., Ibrahim, F.: Smartphone-based solutions for fall detection and prevention: challenges and open issues. Sensors **14**(4), 7181–7208 (2014)
14. Wang, J., Zhang, Z., Li, B., Lee, S., Sherratt, R.S.: An enhanced fall detection system for elderly person monitoring using consumer home networks. IEEE Trans Consumer. Electron. **60**(1), 23–29 (2014)
15. Najafi, B., Aminian, K., Loew, F., Blanc, Y., Prince, R.: Measurement of stand-sit and sit-stand transitions using a miniature gyroscope and its application in fall risk evaluation in the elderly. IEEE Trans. Bio-med. Eng. **49**, 843–51 (2002)
16. Zhang, T., Wang, J., Xu, L., Liu, P.: Using wearable sensor and nmf algorithm to realize ambulatory fall detection. In: Jiao, L., Wang, L., Gao, X., Liu, J., Wu, F. (eds.) Advances in natural computation, pp. 488–491, Berlin, Heidelberg (2006). Springer Berlin Heidelberg
17. Wu, G.: Distinguishing fall activities from normal activities by velocity characteristics. J. Biomech. **33**(11), 1497–1500 (2000)
18. Ge, W., Xue, S.: Portable preimpact fall detector with inertial sensors. IEEE Trans. Neu. Syst. Rehabil. Eng. **16**(2), 178–183 (2008)
19. Matsuyama, H., Aoki, S., Yonezawa, T., Hiroi, K., Kaji, K., Kawaguchi, N.: Deep learning for ballroom dance: a performance classification model with three-dimensional body joints and wearable sensor. IEEE Sens. J. 1–1 (2021)
20. Wan, S., Qi, L., Xiaolong, X., Tong, C., Zonghua, G.: Deep learning models for real-time human activity recognition with smartphones. Mob. Netw. Appl. **25**(2), 743–755 (2020)
21. Altun, K., Barshan, B.: Human activity recognition using inertial/magnetic sensor units **6219**, 38–51 (2010)
22. Yoshida, T., Nozaki, J., Urano, K., Hiroi, K., Yonezawa, T., Kawaguchi, N.: Gait dependency of smartphone walking speed estimation using deep learning 641–642 (2019)
23. Chen, C., Lu, X., Markham, A., Trigoni, N.: Ionet: learning to cure the curse of drift in inertial odometry (2018)

Modelling Reminder System for Dementia by Reinforcement Learning

Muhammad Fikry, Nattaya Mairittha, and Sozo Inoue

Abstract Prospective memory refers to preparing, remembering and recalling plans that have been conceived in an intended manner. Various busyness and distractions can make people forget the activities that must be done the next time, especially for people with cognitive memory problems such as dementia. In this paper, we propose a reminder system with the idea of taking time and response into consideration to assist in remembering activities. Using the reinforcement learning method, this idea predicts the right time to remind users through notifications on smartphones. The notification delivery time will be adjusted to the user's response history, which becomes feedback at any available time. Thus, users will get notifications based on the ideal time for each individual either, either with repetition or without repetition, so as not to miss the planned activity. By evaluating the dataset, the results show that our proposed modelling is able to optimize the time to send notifications. The eight alternative times to send notifications can be optimized to get the best time to notify the user with dementia. This implies that our algorithm propose can adjust to individual personality characteristics, which might be a stumbling block in dementia patient care, and solve multi-routine plan problems. Our propose can be useful for users with dementia because we can remind very well that the execution time of notifications is right on target, so it can prevent users with dementia from stressing out over a lot of notifications, but those who miss notifications can receive them back at a later time step, with the result that information on activities to be completed is still available.

M. Fikry · N. Mairittha · S. Inoue
Kyushu Institute of Technology, Kitakyushu, Fukuoka, Japan
e-mail: sozo@brain.kyutech.ac.jp

M. Fikry (✉)
Universitas Malikussaleh, Aceh Utara, Aceh, Indonesia
e-mail: muh.fikry@unimal.ac.id

M. A. R. Ahad et al. (eds.), *Sensor- and Video-Based Activity and Behavior Computing*, Smart Innovation, Systems and Technologies 291,
https://doi.org/10.1007/978-981-19-0361-8_9

1 Introduction

Using a mobile phone as an assistant while carrying out the regular activity is commonplace for some people. This is due to many activities for humans, which might cause them to miss planned activities, particularly for persons with memory issues. Stress or depression can make it difficult for people to receive information and concentrate, causing frequent forgetting. The people may have to reschedule their plans because they forgot to have previous commitments. Even people who live an organized life can forget promises over time. The ability to recall to do something in future is referred to as prospective memory [21], time-based prospective memory refers to remembering to do something at a specific time. Prospective memory can impact anyone, but it is most common in people with dementia because prospective memory affects various cognitive functions. Therefore, assistive technology to remind activities based on an existing schedule needs to be developed.

Reminder is a system that can help everyone remember something and record essential things so that the people are not forgotten. Through reminders, it can make it easier for users to remember various important information. Some reminder systems only notify predefined time-based events and then send notifications based on that plan. Normal people can set the reminder system themselves according to their wishes because they can know the best time for them. They can set the time of reminder on schedule, some hours or minutes before the schedule, make one, two, or more notifications. However, it will be very difficult for people with memory function disorders; they can forget their mobile phones, so they do not see reminders or be through forgetting the activity again even though the system has previously reminded them. Even for people with dementia who also have the effects like abnormal motor activity, anxiety, irritability, depression, apathy, disinhibition, delusions and hallucinations, the reminder system will be complicated to do set by manually because the best time to remind for today is not necessarily to be an excellent time to remind for the next day, one or two notifications may not be enough for them; on the other hand, too many notifications might be a harmful impact for them because people with dementia can have unstable emotions.

To solve this problem, we aim to leverage the reinforcement learning method [32] to estimate the time it will take to remind the user to perform an activity. The goal is to remind the user before the schedule at the right time with or without repetition that does not distract the user from the notification and does not hallucinate the schedule of activities; for example, the user has an activity at 09:00 a.m., then the system will remind the user before 09:00 a.m. The agent in reinforcement learning is learning based on the experience, the reminder technology with this method is considered suitable for people with memory problems like dementia to overcome difficulties in setting fixed rules for each individual because of the variety of symptoms and life changes they face [12]. We introduce a new model in the initial definition using the q-learning algorithm [36] to evaluate the time, taking into account the user's response. So that users will get effective time feedback to remind the activity that will occur, the time for sending notifications and repeating reminders may vary for each user according to the response given. We have eight-time options (see details in Table 2) to remind the users, we will start from the longest time to the nearest time before the scheduled time. The reminder system with our proposed model is capable of being dynamic, meaning that if the user can respond to notifications appropriately, the time will be optimized, and the number of notifications sent can be minimized. This solves a number of issues that dementia patients have, including forgetting things, ignoring notifications, multi-routine plans and difficulties in establishing permanent rules for each individual.

2 Related Work

2.1 *Assistive Technology*

Dementia is an illness marked by a variety of cognitive impairments that vary depending on the disease that causes it. Memory loss is the most frequent cognitive sign. Short-term memory impairment is the initial complaint of patients who have trouble acquiring new material. After that, the problem of remembering substantial memory comes up [33]. Assistive technology for dementia sufferers is still being researched and developed, because people with temporal and memory impairments require reminders of upcoming and previous activities and events [34]. For elderly with moderate dementia, HYCARE introduced a hybrid context-aware reminding architecture that can handle both synchronous time-based and asynchronous event-based reminders [10]. ehcoBUTLER designed a program that uses the Internet to link multiple users to provide health care to the elderly, including features of diagnostic, treatment and amusement [5]. The COGKNOW project's application provides activity assistance, reminders, a visual dialing system, alerts and a GPS service to assist individuals with dementia in locating their home [25]. The ROBADOM project designed a robot that provides verbal and nonverbal conversations and feedback to help older individuals with moderate dementia with their everyday activities [37]. eHealth system proposed a medication reminder system that uses smartphone alerts, home voice and video notifications in the context of a smart home environment [30]. The MultiMemoHome project provides an overview of the many electronic reminder delivery modes accessible in the house [22].

2.2 *Reminder System*

A reminder system is used to aid memories. Various reminder strategies are used by people to support in daily life, such as calendars, diaries, sticky notes or smartphones [2]. Reminders have good in many aspects of life, for example, taking medication, exercising, or meeting. Many studies related to reminder systems have been carried out with various technologies to help humans. Using RFID technology to detect objects when the user leaves the house, this system compares the object in his pocket with the thing with a list of items so that the user can retrieve the forgotten object [17]. Automatic reminder system for medical orders from the doctor's office to the smart box in the nurse's room, accompanied by text messages from doctors to nurse [35]. Using the accelerometer and camera sensors, the system provides reminders for coupling activities, such as having to close an opened bottle [7]. A reminder system using a smartphone was developed to support patient self-medication management [13] because it can improve medication adherence through short messages from mobile phones [20]. Technologies for reminder systems can be used separately or in combination to achieve the goals of context-aware reminder systems.

Reminder systems help people to improve cognitive disabilities, such as instructional prompts and scheduling assistance [29]. In smartphones, information to be delivered to users is one of them through notifications [23, 24, 26, 28]. Notifications become visual cues, auditory signals or haptic alerts generated by the application to convey information to the user [15]. However, with the increasing number of notifications that demand the attention of smartphone users, often notifications appear at inopportune times or carry irrelevant content. Notifications at inappropriate times can cause annoyance; previous research has shown that notifications at inappropriate times can increase anxiety [28], and interfere with task completion time [9, 16], people find it difficult to refocus on their previous task after being distracted by calls or instant messages [16] let alone if the task demands cognitive work, it will certainly have a more pronounced effect [19].

Because the notification on the smartphone plays an essential role in communicating information to the user about the event or action to be done, it is critical to verify the appropriate time to remind the user. In self-medication management of patients, forty-six per cent (41.1%) forget or are late to take their medicine more than two hours from schedule [13], to monitor dementia patients taking medicine or monitoring glucose, 38.4% of caregivers require a reminder feature on their smartphones [6] because dementia patient often forget to take their medication and even forget their personal belongings [18]. This issue makes researchers develop various assistive technologies to remind individuals with dementia [3, 4, 11] that have impaired cognitive function. Dementia that is mostly experienced by older people, they require the special requirements for reminders [1, 11] even previous research carried out a combination of human and artificial intelligence to design reminder systems [8, 31].

To optimize the time when sending notifications, one method that can be used is reinforcement learning. Bo-Jhang Ho et al. [14] explored the use of reinforcement learning by modelling the problem as a Markov decision process and the advantage actor–critic algorithm to identify interruptible moments, to schedule microtasks while minimizing user distraction, by setting sensor data as state, notify and stay silent as an action. James Obert and Angie Shia [27] analysed dynamic time optimization with reinforcement learning to reduce time and resources in manufacturing ASICI/VLSI chips. Reinforcement learning is an algorithm that can make agents work automatically to determine the ideal behaviour in order to improve the performance of the algorithm. From experimental tests and feedback, reinforcement learning learns effective strategies for an agent; an agent is able to actively adapt with the environment to optimize time by maximizing future rewards. Our work differs from these works in the application of reinforcement learning techniques. These works remind the user according to a predetermined schedule. In contrast, we remind the user before the schedule with several alternative times available to get reminders more than once. Our system will learn the best time to send notifications before the schedule to address problems of users with dementia so that they can prepare activity needs and not miss activities due to ignoring information or forgetting something.

3 Method

In this section, we present our approach to modelling the exact timing of sending notifications to users ahead of schedule. In the reminder system that we propose, the user can set the scheduled time according to their needs, but the system will remind the user before the scheduled time, not the time that has been set by the user. We set a reminder time starting from the furthest distance to the time that is closest to the schedule. The system will choose an action to be applied to the user; if the action is silent, then the user response will automatically be ignored, but if the action is notify, then the user is asked to respond by selecting the option that appears on the notification, such as accept or dismiss. Accept response means that the user likes the time and considers the information is sufficient to send notification of time schedule. Dismiss response means that the user does not like the time or needs the information the next time. If the user does not select that option within fifteen minutes due to forgetting or something else, then our system decides that the user choice was ignored at that point. After we get the user's response, we optimize the time for the next notify based on the response for each user. In Fig. 1,we provide an overview of the relationship between an agent and the environment.

In our framework, the agent is our system, and the environment is the smartphone. The agent observes the user context to take the action of sending a notification or

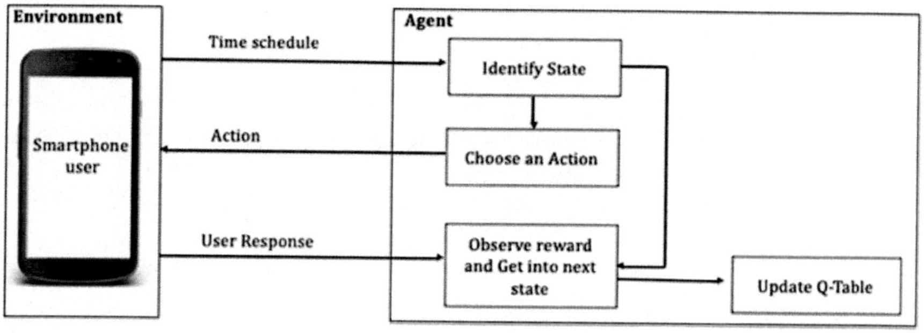

Fig. 1 Reinforcement learning setup

remaining silent. From the notification that appears, it allows the user to make a response that will be input for the agent to assign the reward. The possible response for the user is to accept, dismiss, or ignore the notification.

The relationship between agent and environment is that the agent makes observations to get a representation of the environment called state, then takes action based on its policies. Based on the action taken, the environment moves from the state to the next state and returns the reward. The agent will maximize the amount of the accumulated future reward discount. We use q-learning as a reinforcement learning algorithm. We show the processing flow of the method proposed in Algorithm 1, and Table 1 summarizes the definitions of the mathematical expressions used in the algorithm.

Algorithm 1 Proposed reminder system using reinforcement learning

Initial definition:
T = {120, 105, 90, 75, 60, 45, 30, 15}
A = {notify, silent}
R = {+1, -1, 0}
X = {accept, dismiss, ignore}
S = T × X
S = {S1, S2, S2, ..., S24}
r: S × A → R
δ: S × A → S
π(s) = a

1. Initialize, for all $S_t \in$ S; $A_t \in$ A;
t = 0.
2. Start with S_0
3. At time step t, choose action $A_t = argmax_{(a \in A)}$ Q(S_t,a), ϵ-greedy is applied
4. Apply action A_t
5. Observe reward $R^{(t+1)}$ and get into the next state $S^{(t+1)}$
6. Update the Q-value function:
Q(S_t,A_t)← Q(S_t,A_t)+α($R_{(t+1)}$+$\gamma max_{(a \in A)}$ Q($S_{(t+1)}$,a)-Q(S_t,A_t))
7. Set t=t+1 and repeat from step 3

In the reinforcement learning algorithm we use, time step t is the time to send a notification if the action chosen by an agent is notify; state is the product of time and input. The selection of actions will be applied using the epsilon greedy method. After applying the action, an agent will observe the reward and go to the next state based on the user's response, the reward function shows how the agent benefits from action A at time t in state S at time t, while the next state is determined from the transition state S at time t after taking action A at time t; after that, the agent will calculate the q-value to be updated into the q-table.

The furthest time is two hours before the schedule, and the shortest time is fifteen minutes before the schedule. From two hours will move to schedule time every fifteen minutes, so we have eight times to remind the user. Table 2 shows the time features of our approach.

Table 1 Nomenclature reference

Symbol	Summary
α	The learning rate
γ	The discount factor
s	State
a	Action
r	Reward
t	Time step
n	Final time step
S	Set of all states (the product of time and input)
A	Set of action possible in state s
R	Set of possible rewards
T	Time
St	State at t
At	Action at t
Rt	Reward at t
π	Policy, decision making rule
X	Input
δ(s, a)	The state transition

Table 2 Feature of time

Time (T)	Description
120	2 h before time schedule
105	1 h 45 min before time schedule
90	1 h 30 min before time schedule
75	1 h 15 min before time schedule
60	1 h before time schedule
45	45 min before time schedule
30	30 min before time schedule
15	15 min before time schedule)

In our method focus on the time before the schedule, so we propose that state is the product of time and input. For each time, it has the same possible response from the user shown in Table 3 so that each time has three states because we have eight times to remind the user, then the number of states we have is twenty-four. Table 4 shows the relationship between time and inputs that make up the state of our method.

Table 3 Feature of input

Input (X)	Description
Accept	User response: accept
Dismiss	User response: dismiss
Ignore	User response: not answer

Table 4 Feature of state

State (S)	Description	State (S)	Description
S1	(120, accept)	S13	(60, accept)
S2	(120, ignore)	S14	(60, ignore)
S3	(120, dismiss)	S15	(60, dismiss)
S4	(105, accept)	S16	(45, accept)
S5	(105, ignore)	S17	(45, ignore)
S6	(105, dismiss)	S18	(45, dismiss)
S7	(90, accept)	S19	(30, accept)
S8	(90, ignore)	S20	(30, ignore)
S9	(90, dismiss)	S21	(30, dismiss)
S10	(75, accept)	S22	(15, accept)
S11	(75, ignore)	S23	(15, ignore)
S12	(75, dismiss)	S24	(15, dismiss)

4 Experimental Evaluation

To evaluate our proposed model, we conducted several experiments to see if the system worked as intended. To calculate the estimated time of each activity, the agent needs to get initial feedback from the user when the notification appears to remind the user based on the existing schedule and optimize it with reinforcement learning, then conduct tests the next time based on the response carried out before for each activity.

4.1 Data Description

The dataset that we use in the experiment is the EngagementService dataset [14] and synthetically generated data as a proof-of-concept study. The EngagementService dataset contains some information such as CreationTime, AssignmentStatus, AcceptTime, SubmitTime, Input.content, and Answer.sentiment. However, in this case, we only use Answer sentiment information as a user response that we will test on our system; there are 100 user responses that will be used in our experiment. As

Table 5 An example of synthetically generated data

Activity ID	User ID	Time schedule	Action	Time action	Time response	User response
1	1	9:00	Notify	7:00		
1	1	9:00	Notify	7:15		
1	1	9:00	Notify	7:30	07:34	Dismiss
1	1	9:00	Notify	7:45	07:48	Accept

for synthetically generated data, we have 124 actions of notify and 126 actions of silent, we create a synthetic dataset by giving random user responses. When sending notifications, we have 30.65% of responses are accepted, 31.45% of responses are dismissed and 37.9% did not answer. In this process, the system will call the available user responses directly, agents learn by trial and error while interacting with the environment and get rewards for their actions. An example of synthetically generated data is shown in Table 5.

We also generate data that is resulted from the system to simulate an agent learn from the environment, from the experiments we conducted we got 1324 actions is notify, and 1426 actions are silent. To choose an action, the agent does random exploration occasionally with probability ϵ and takes the optimal action most of the time with probability 1-ϵ.

4.2 Evaluation Method

To evaluate our proposed method, we performed a synthetic simulation in which the human responses are collected in the wild and approximated from two datasets: (1) Engagement service dataset and (2) Synthetically generated data to show the advantage of repeatedly and systematically iterating over our proposed algorithms. Three performance measures are defined in this paper: number of notifications, user response rate and time optimization. The number of notifications is number of the alert that are sent to remind users of the activities they will be doing. Next, we count the number of users who responded to the notification divided by the number of notifications sent. This is a critical metric for determining the algorithm's performance. Time optimization relates to the status of the q-table, and it is an essential measure for the next action, whether to send a notification or remain silent. It is defined as the ratio of updated entries in the q-table of our proposed algorithm.

5 Result

As explained in Sect. 3, we have eight alternative times to notify the user. For people with dementia, eight times are certainly better than one or two timestamps, as the algorithm is able to achieve higher response rates over time. Because each time

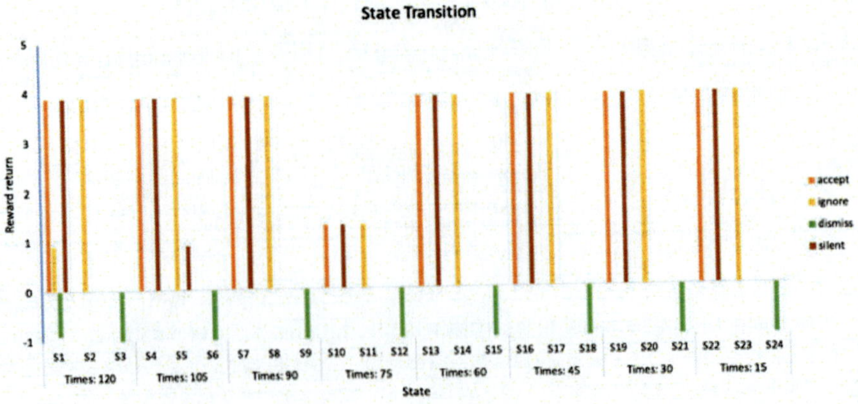

Fig. 2 State transition

has three possible responses that result in three states for each time, we conducted an experiment to see the state transition by assuming the user's response is always accept, dismiss, ignore and the action is always silent. The results show the transition can occur from the time to the next time, not the transition from the state to the next state at the same time as shown in Fig. 2.

In the next experiment, we use the dataset from EngagementService, we take the existing user responses, in this dataset, all the answers are filled in, so we assume that the action that occurs is notify, then we experiment on our system assuming that the activity occurs at one time and the notification sent before the scheduled activity. The result is shown in Fig. 3 that all silent values in our q-table are zero, and the transition of state to the next state occurs based on the response from the user. Then we perform simulations to see the agent work automatically to determine the ideal behaviour to maximize the performance of the algorithm because the goal of reinforcement learning is to choose the most appropriate action in each particular state. To prevent overfitting, we balance exploration and exploitation by applying an epsilon greedy action selection, we choose a random action with probability ϵ and otherwise the max q-value. If the action is notify, then the user response will be retrieved from the EngagementService dataset. The number of rounds performed is until the agent gets the last response from the user in the dataset. The result shows that 53.5% reminder system sends a notification to notify the user and 46.5% reminder system stays silent as shown in Fig. 4. From this result, we can see that an agent can work well by learning from the environment based on user feedback. In other words, the system can decide the right time to send notifications to users, which means we do not send notifications every time so as not to disturb the user.

Irrelevant time to context can cause distraction and make the information that the reminder system wants to convey can be unacceptable to users, especially people with dementia who often forget and have unstable emotions. Therefore, before we apply this system to humans who have a lot of notifications that will appear in

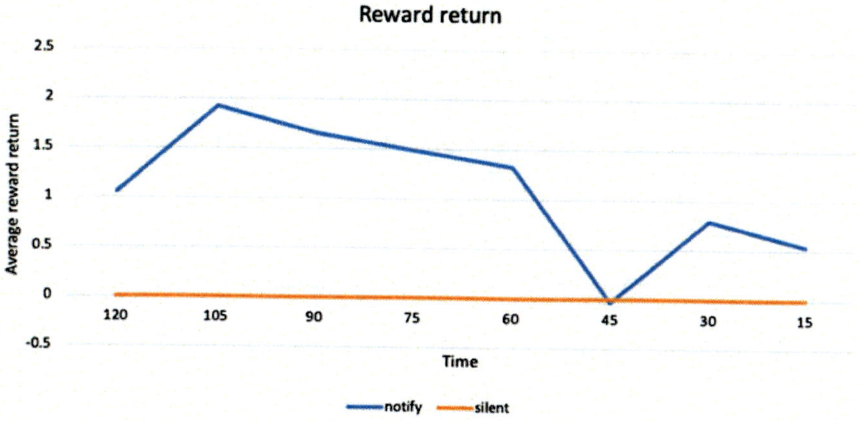

Fig. 3 Reward return with EngagementService dataset

Fig. 4 Percentage of actions with user responses from the EngagementService dataset

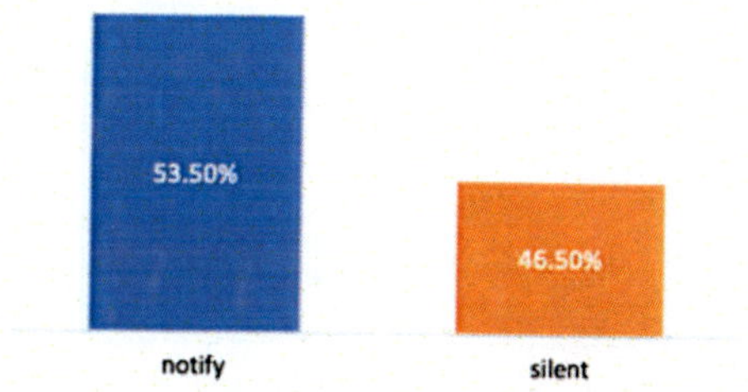

their smartphones, we carried out the next experiment using synthetically generated data. The synthetics data we generated manually and then input it into the system. The system takes the input and calculates it to get a q-table, then we reprocess reinforcement learning by applying random user responses that generate new data. We show the number of notifications in Fig. 5a for synthetically generated data in the wild and Fig. 5b for synthetically generated data with iterating by our proposed algorithms, for the user response rate we show in Fig. 6 (see details for each user in Fig. 7). From this process, it can be seen that when the first process is done, the agent can calculate properly and set the state correctly, but the agent does not learn directly from the environment, while during the second process, the agent learns more from the environment so that the reminder system gets the best time to send notifications to users.

The result of this process is the accept rate of user responses processed using our proposed algorithm is better (see details in Table 8), as our proposed algorithm is able to send notifications at the right time, this depends on the preferred time of each user, near or far from the schedule; some users with dementia might be like reminders that are far from the schedule because they have time to prepare some items, other people may like near time schedule, so they can immediately do activities. The more often users choose to dismiss or ignore, the more notifications they receive; we show

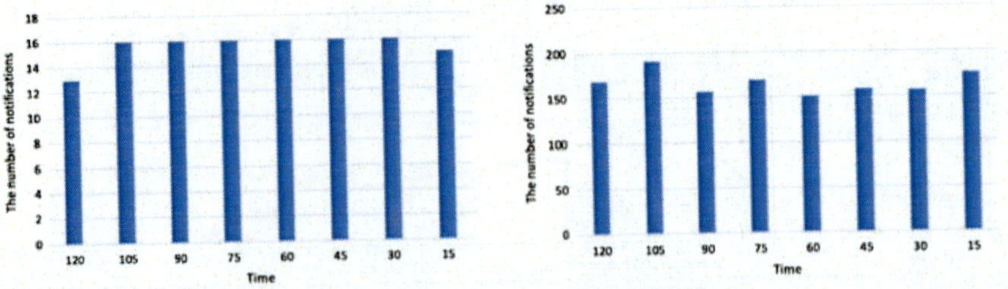

(a) Synthetically generated data (in the wild) (b) Synthetically generated data (iterating by our proposed algorithms)

Fig. 5 Number of notifications

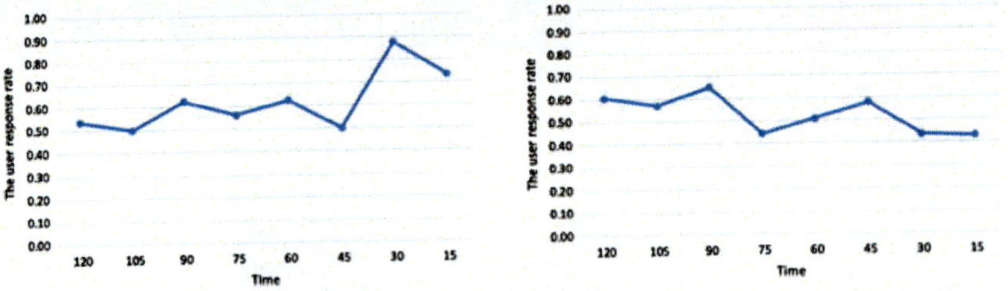

(a) Synthetically generated data (in the wild) (b) Synthetically generated data (iterating by our proposed algorithms)

Fig. 6 User response rate

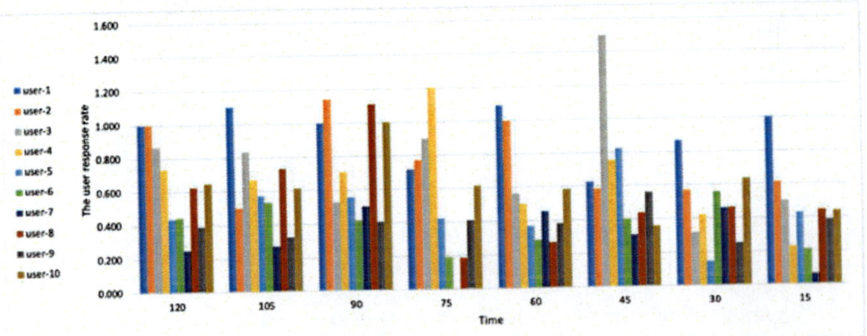

Fig. 7 Response rate comparison for each user

Table 6 Average number of notification for each user

User	The average number of notification
1	0.084
2	0.085
3	0.090
4	0.088
5	0.099
6	0.089
7	0.091
8	0.088
9	0.194
10	0.093

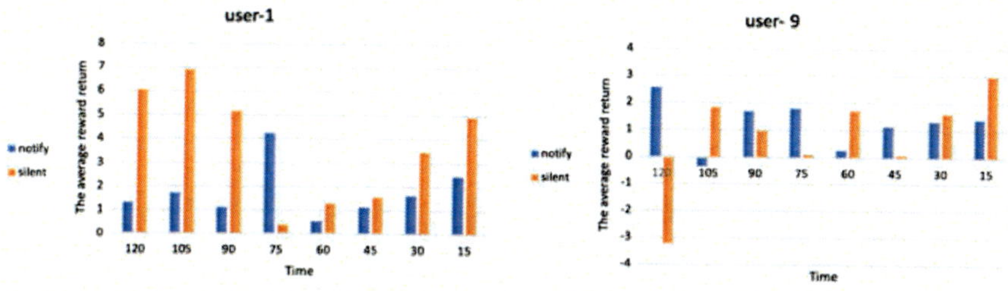

(a) The highest user response rate

(b) The lowest user response rate

Fig. 8 Average reward return

the average number of notifications for each user in Table 6, the average reward return per user for each action in Table 7, and we show in Fig. 8 the comparison of response rates for each user. Timing optimization is based on the response of each user, the user with the highest response rate may only need one notification for the time, the user with the lowest response rate in this experiment will still have to be reminded four times for the next time; indeed, optimize time-consuming to remind users in this experiment is not an absolute requirement at that time, as changes in notification delivery timings may vary again based on subsequent responses. This implies that our algorithm can adjust to individual personality characteristics, which might be a stumbling block in the care of dementia patients. Our propose can work for people with dementia because we can remind very well, the high accept rate proves the execution time of notifications is right on target, so it can prevent users with dementia from stressing out over a lot of notifications, but for those who missed notifications can receive them back at a later time step, with the result that information on activities to be carried out is still available.

Table 7 Average reward return per user for each action based on times

Times	A1	A2	A1	A2	A1	A2	A1	A2	A1	A2	A1	A2	A1	A2	A1	A2	A1	A2	A1	A2
120	1.3	6.1	1.7	5.5	0.0	3.3	−7.0	6.9	0.5	0.6	0.6	2.1	0.1	2.1	1.2	0.4	2.6	−3.2	1.4	0.1
105	1.7	6.9	2.3	−1.6	3.0	0.8	0.3	2.9	1.7	0.0	5.0	−0.8	3.6	−0.5	−1.4	2.3	−0.3	1.8	2.0	5.0
90	1.1	5.2	0.0	3.8	4.6	0.3	0.4	4.3	2.2	−0.6	0.7	1.5	6.4	1.7	−0.9	2.1	1.7	1.0	0.7	4.2
75	4.2	0.4	1.4	3.1	3.3	4.1	4.5	19.3	0.9	3.8	0.1	0.6	6.5	5.5	−0.8	1.4	1.8	0.1	−2.3	10.7
60	0.5	1.3	−1.5	10.0	1.9	11.3	1.0	23.6	2.0	0.5	0.9	0.4	0.2	1.8	0.2	1.8	0.2	1.7	−6.1	8.4
45	1.2	1.6	−8.1	9.3	−9.2	10.5	2.9	33.5	0.9	0.0	0.3	1.2	−1.5	5.3	1.7	1.6	1.1	0.1	1.5	6.7
30	1.6	3.5	−1.8	14.9	2.7	1.8	9.9	1.5	0.8	1.0	0.0	0.8	1.1	3.9	−1.0	−0.2	1.3	1.6	−1.2	6.5
15	2.5	4.9	5.3	9.3	1.4	1.0	−15	87.0	−1.7	0.8	0.9	0.7	−2.4	3.2	0.6	0.3	1.4	3.0	0.8	3.9

A1: The action is notify; A2: The action is silent

Table 8 Comparison of synthetically generated data

Time	In the wild		Iterating by our proposed algorithms	
	Accept rate	Dismiss rate	Accept rate	Dismiss rate
120	0.31	0.23	0.32	0.28
105	0.13	0.38	0.36	0.21
90	0.38	0.25	0.42	0.23
75	0.38	0.19	0.26	0.18
60	0.38	0.25	0.26	0.25
45	0.19	0.31	0.31	0.27
30	0.44	0.44	0.27	0.21
15	0.27	0.47	0.28	0.15

6 Discussion and Future Work

By evaluating with dataset and conducting various experiments, the results reflect that our proposed model using the reinforcement learning method can optimize the time to send notifications. The eight alternative times to send notifications can be optimized to get the best time to alert the user. We set eight alternatives of times because in this case we have users with dementia, which means if healthy people do not need a system with time optimization. After all, they can set the times of reminder manually as they wish unless they are also having problems with memory such as dementia symptoms, then this system might be able to help them. Although this model allows us to optimize time effectively, there are some limitations that we would like to address.

In this work, we do not claim that the data can represent the actual user data, so the dynamic time only occurs in eight parts. If the data has been obtained from humans, we can make the eight parts of the time more flexible based on the response time of the user, which can make the notification delivery time even more precise.

We also do not know how many notifications the user receives on their phone because interruptions from notifications can cause people to turn off notifications or make them ignore notifications more often. Examining the number of notifications that appear at any given time may give better results for increasing user engagement.

We cannot tell if the user is doing the activity as scheduled or not after being reminded. In future, we are interested in identifying user activities because it could be that the user accepts the notification on the reminder system but does not carry out activities according to schedule, or otherwise, the user directly carries out their activities after responding to the notification.

We believe that real-world application and testing are critical to developing practical solutions for people with dementia. We hope that our proposed method and the results of our trial will ease the burden on caregivers and families for the issues commonly handled by persons with dementia. The reminder system with our proposed model has notifications at every available time step and is capable of being dynamic so that if the user can respond to notifications correctly, the time will be optimized, and the number of notifications sent can be minimized. This is overcome several problems of users with dementia such as forgetting something (eating, taking medication, events) including forgetting newly learned information, improper execution time that makes them forget about the activity they are doing, ignoring notifications with various influencing factors (e.g. they are far from the location of the phone), stress remembering the activities to be carried out, multi-routine plans and difficulty in setting fixed rules for each individual. However, we acknowledge that the reminder system for dementia users has a number of additional problems that must be addressed, such as dementia-friendly design (simple, flexible, recognizable), information related to activities to be completed, and external support for setting the reminder.

7 Conclusions

In this paper, the reminder will notify each time step available before the scheduled time so that people with prospective memory failure that directly impacts daily life, such as dementia, do not forget the activities they will do or ask their caregivers or family repeatedly. Because one notification on the schedule may not be enough for them, on the contrary, too many notifications can have the effect of being a nuisance. It is also used so that people with dementia do not experience stress to remember the activities they will do and overcome difficulties in setting fixed rules for each individual because they have varied life behaviours. Furthermore, the timing of our idea is dynamic, meaning that if the user responds appropriately to notification, the system will optimize the time such that the number of notifications issued is decreased.

The main contribution of this research is that we have a different initial definition of the reinforcement learning process generally for time optimization. Here we make the state as a combination of the time and the possible response of the user so that the system can remind the user before the time scheduled about the activities to be carried out and prepare the required items. The purpose of modelling using reinforcement learning is to get the best time and number of notifications to notify the users. With this model, we can observe the user's response from time to time and estimate the time and future actions. Reinforcement learning can work well to optimize the time for each user response by balancing exploration and exploitation.

In our experiment, we randomly generated user responses because the user's response might be unpredictable, especially for people with dementia. In addition, we show user responses based on dataset from existing research, and it can be seen that the optimal timing is easy to obtain if the user response is constant but different if the user response is very random. Other than that, more experiments carried out will make the agent learn more so that the choice of action to send notifications or remain silent, and optimization of time to send notifications can be better.

References

1. Abdul Razak, F.H., Sulo, R., Wan Adnan, W.A.: Elderly mental model of reminder system. In: Proceedings of the 10th Asia Pacific Conference on Computer Human Interaction, pp. 193–200 (2012)
2. Ahmed, Q., Mujib, S.: Activity recognition using smartphone accelerometer and gyroscope sensors supporting context-based reminder systems. In: Context Aware Reminder System, Faculty of Computing at Blekinge Institute of Technology (2014)
3. Alharbi, S., Altamimi, A., Al-Qahtani, F., Aljofi, B., Alsmadi, M., Alshabanah, M., Alrajhi, D., Almarashdeh, I.: Analyzing and implementing a mobile reminder system for alzheimer's patients. In: Alharbi, S., Altamimi, A., Al-Qahtani, F., Aljofi, B., Alsmadi, MK, Alshabanah, M., Alrajhi, D., Almarashdeh, I., pp. 444–454 (2019)
4. Asghar, I., Cang, S., Yu, H.: A systematic mapping study on assitive technologies for people with dementia. In: 2015 9th International Conference on Software, Knowledge, Information Management and Applications (SKIMA), pp. 1–8. IEEE (2015)
5. Botella, C., Etchemendy, E., Castilla, D., Baños, R.M., García-Palacios, A., Quero, S., Alcaniz, M., Lozano, J.A.: An e-health system for the elderly (butler project): a pilot study on acceptance and satisfaction. CyberPsychology Behav. **12**(3), 255–262 (2009)
6. Brown, E.L., Ruggiano, N., Li, J., Clarke, P.J., Kay, E.S., Hristidis, V.: Smartphone-based health technologies for dementia care: opportunities, challenges, and current practices. J. Appl. Gerontol. **38**(1), 73–91 (2019)
7. Chaminda, H.T., Klyuev, V., Naruse, K.: A smart reminder system for complex human activities. In: 2012 14th international conference on advanced communication technology (ICACT), pp. 235–240. IEEE (2012)
8. Chen, H., Soh, Y.C.: A cooking assistance system for patients with alzheimers disease using reinforcement learning. Int. J. Inf. Technol. **23**(2) (2017)
9. Czerwinski, M., Cutrell, E., Horvitz, E.: Instant messaging and interruption: Influence of task type on performance. In: OZCHI 2000 Conference Proceedings, vol. 356, pp. 361–367. Citeseer (2000)
10. Du, K., Zhang, D., Zhou, X., Mokhtari, M., Hariz, M., Qin, W.: Hycare: A hybrid context-aware reminding framework for elders with mild dementia. In: International Conference On Smart homes and health Telematics, pp. 9–17. Springer (2008)
11. Fikry, M.: Requirements analysis for reminder system in daily activity recognition dementia: Phd forum abstract. In: Proceedings of the 18th Conference on Embedded Networked Sensor Systems, pp. 815–816 (2020)
12. Fikry, M., Hamdhana, D., Lago, P., Inoue, S.: Activity recognition for assisting people with dementia. Contactless Hum. Act. Anal. **200**, 271 (2021)
13. Hayakawa, M., Uchimura, Y., Omae, K., Waki, K., Fujita, H., Ohe, K.: A smartphone-based medication self-management system with real-time medication monitoring. Appl. Clin. Inf. **4**(01), 37–52 (2013)
14. Ho, B.J., Balaji, B., Koseoglu, M., Sandha, S., Pei, S., Srivastava, M.: Quick question: interrupting users for microtasks with reinforcement learning. arXiv preprint arXiv:2007.09515 (2020)
15. Horvitz, E., Apacible, J., Subramani, M.: Balancing awareness and interruption: investigation of notification deferral policies. In: International Conference on User Modeling, pp. 433–437. Springer (2005)
16. Horvitz, E.C.M.C.E.: Notification, disruption, and memory: effects of messaging interruptions on memory and performance. In: Human-Computer Interaction: INTERACT, vol. 1, p. 263 (2001)
17. Hsu, H.H., Lee, C.N., Chen, Y.F.: An rfid-based reminder system for smart home. In: 2011 IEEE International Conference on Advanced Information Networking and Applications, pp. 264–269. IEEE (2011)

18. Koumakis, L., Chatzaki, C., Kazantzaki, E., Maniadi, E., Tsiknakis, M.: Dementia care frameworks and assistive technologies for their implementation: a review. IEEE Rev. Biomed. Eng. **12**, 4–18 (2019)
19. Leiva, L., Böhmer, M., Gehring, S., Krüger, A.: Back to the app: the costs of mobile application interruptions. In: Proceedings of the 14th International Conference on Human-computer Interaction with Mobile Devices and Services, pp. 291–294 (2012)
20. Lester, R.T., Ritvo, P., Mills, E.J., Kariri, A., Karanja, S., Chung, M.H., Jack, W., Habyarimana, J., Sadatsafavi, M., Najafzadeh, M., et al.: Effects of a mobile phone short message service on antiretroviral treatment adherence in Kenya (Weltel Kenya1): a randomised trial. The Lancet **376**(9755), 1838–1845 (2010)
21. McDaniel, M.A., Einstein, G.O.: The neuropsychology of prospective memory in normal aging: a componential approach. Neuropsychologia **49**(8), 2147–2155 (2011)
22. McGee-Lennon, M.R., Brewster, S.: Reminders that make sense: designing multimodal notifications for the home. In: 2011 5th International Conference on Pervasive Computing Technologies for Healthcare (PervasiveHealth) and Workshops, pp. 495–501. IEEE (2011)
23. Mehrotra, A., Hendley, R., Musolesi, M.: Notifymehere: Intelligent notification delivery in multi-device environments. In: Proceedings of the 2019 Conference on Human Information Interaction and Retrieval, pp. 103–111 (2019)
24. Mehrotra, A., Musolesi, M., Hendley, R., Pejovic, V.: Designing content-driven intelligent notification mechanisms for mobile applications. In: Proceedings of the 2015 ACM International Joint Conference on Pervasive and Ubiquitous Computing, pp. 813–824 (2015)
25. Meiland, F.J., Reinersmann, A., Sävenstedt, S., Bergvall-Kåreborn, B., Hettinga, M., Craig, D., Andersson, A.L., Dröes, R.M.: User-participatory development of assistive technology for people with dementia-from needs to functional requirements. first results of the cogknow project. Dementia, pp. 71–91 (2012)
26. Morrison, L.G., Hargood, C., Pejovic, V., Geraghty, A.W., Lloyd, S., Goodman, N., Michaelides, D.T., Weston, A., Musolesi, M., Weal, M.J., et al.: The effect of timing and frequency of push notifications on usage of a smartphone-based stress management intervention: an exploratory trial. PloS one **12**(1), e0169162 (2017)
27. Obert, J., Shia, A.: Optimizing dynamic timing analysis with reinforcement learning. Tech. rep., Sandia National Lab.(SNL-NM), Albuquerque, NM (United States) (2019)
28. Pielot, M., Church, K., De Oliveira, R.: An in-situ study of mobile phone notifications. In: Proceedings of the 16th International Conference on Human-Computer Interaction with Mobile Devices and Services, pp. 233–242 (2014)
29. Pollack, M.E., Brown, L., Colbry, D., McCarthy, C.E., Orosz, C., Peintner, B., Ramakrishnan, S., Tsamardinos, I.: Autominder: an intelligent cognitive orthotic system for people with memory impairment. Robot. Auton. Syst. **44**(3–4), 273–282 (2003)
30. Ramljak, M.: Smart home medication reminder system. In: 2017 25th International Conference on Software, Telecommunications and Computer Networks (SoftCOM), pp. 1–5. IEEE (2017)
31. Sanchez, V.G., Pfeiffer, C.F., Skeie, N.O.: A review of smart house analysis methods for assisting older people living alone. J. Sens. Actuator Netw. **6**(3), 11 (2017)
32. Sutton, R.S., Barto, A.G.: Reinforcement learning: an introduction. MIT press (2018)
33. Tarawneh, R., Holtzman, D.M.: The clinical problem of symptomatic Alzheimer disease and mild cognitive impairment. Cold Spring Harb. Perspect. Med. **2**(5), a006148 (2012)
34. Vogt, J., Luyten, K., Van den Bergh, J., Coninx, K., Meier, A.: Putting dementia into context. In: International Conference on Human-Centred Software Engineering, pp. 181–198. Springer (2012)
35. Wang, H.J., Shi, Y., Zhao, D., Liu, A., Yang, C.: Automatic reminder system of medical orders based on bluetooth. In: 2011 7th International Conference on Wireless Communications, Networking and Mobile Computing, pp. 1–4. IEEE (2011)
36. Watkins, C.J., Dayan, P.: Q-learning. Mach. Learn. **8**(3–4), 279–292 (1992)
37. Wu, Y.H., Wrobel, J., Cristancho-Lacroix, V., Kamali, L., Chetouani, M., Duhaut, D., Le Pévédic, B., Jost, C., Dupourque, V., Ghrissi, M., et al.: Designing an assistive robot for older adults: the ROBADOM project. Irbm **34**(2), 119–123 (2013)

Can Ensemble of Classifiers Provide Better Recognition Results in Packaging Activity?

A. H. M. Nazmus Sakib, Promit Basak, Syed Doha Uddin, Shahamat Mustavi Tasin, and Md Atiqur Rahman Ahad

Abstract Skeleton-based motion capture (MoCap) systems have been widely used in the game and film industry for mimicking complex human actions for a long time. MoCap data has also proved its effectiveness in human activity recognition tasks. However, it is a quite challenging task for smaller datasets. The lack of such data for industrial activities further adds to the difficulties. In this work, we have proposed an ensemble-based machine learning methodology that is targeted to work better on MoCap datasets. The experiments have been performed on the MoCap data given in the Bento Packaging Activity Recognition Challenge 2021. *Bento* is a Japanese word that resembles *lunch-box*. Upon processing the raw MoCap data at first, we have achieved an astonishing accuracy of 98% on tenfold cross-Validation and 82% on leave-one-out cross-validation by using the proposed ensemble model.

1 Introduction

Human activity recognition has been one of the major concentrations for researchers for over a decade. Previously, human activity recognition tasks only used data from geospatial sensors such as accelerometers, gyroscopes, GPS sensors [1]. But in the last few years, skeleton-based human action recognition (SHAR) became quite popular because of its better performance and accuracy [2–5]. In SHAR, the human skeleton is typically represented by a set of body markers which are tracked by several specialized cameras. In such work, computer vision or sensor data can also be used. In the case of sensor data, the use of motion capture, kinematic sensors, etc. are prominent [6]. Although skeleton-based data is already being used widely in many cases, such applications are quite rare in fields such as packaging, cooking [7], nurse care [8]. Among these fields, packaging activity recognition can be very effective in

A. H. M. Nazmus Sakib · P. Basak · S. Doha Uddin · S. Mustavi Tasin
Electrical and Electronic Engineering, University of Dhaka, Dhaka, Bangladesh

M. A. R. Ahad (✉)
University of East London, London, UK
e-mail: atiqahad@du.ac.bd; atiqahad@yahoo.com

M. A. R. Ahad et al. (eds.), *Sensor- and Video-Based Activity and Behavior Computing*, Smart Innovation, Systems and Technologies 291,
https://doi.org/10.1007/978-981-19-0361-8_10

the industrial arena and can solve multi-modal problems like industrial automation, quality assessment, and reducing errors.

Packaging activity recognition is a relatively newer field of SHAR. Hence, scarcity of data and lack of previous examples are some of the main problems of this task. Usually, in such tasks, items are put on a conveyor belt and packaged by a subject. The items to be put on the conveyor belt are dictated by the company. Hence, the location of the item on the belt is also important as it produces new scenarios for different positions. The size of the dataset to perform such experiments is another important factor because small datasets often limit the scope of work. In this paper, our team *Nirban* proposes an approach to solve these issues and detect such activities in the Bento Packaging Activity Recognition Challenge 2021 [9, 10].

The dataset used in this work is based on Bento box packaging activities. Bento is a single-serving lunch-box originated in Japan. The dataset contains motion capture data with 13 body markers with no previous preprocessing. The raw motion capture data is first preprocessed, and then a total of 2400 features are extracted. Furthermore, feature selection is used to select the best 396 features based on "mean decrease in impurity" and chi-square score. Then, the processed data is trained on several classical machine learning models, and their performances are evaluated using tenfold cross-validation (CV) and leave-one-out cross-validation (LOOCV). Lastly, an ensemble of the best five models is done to generate predictions on the test data. Deep learning (DL) methods were also considered, in which case raw data was fed to one-dimensional CNN, LSTM, and bidirectional LSTM. The results of all the approaches and models are included in this paper.

The rest of the paper is organized as follows: Sect. 2 describes the previous works that are relevant to the approach described here. Section 3 provides a detailed description of the dataset, including its settings and challenges. Section 4 entails the detailed methodology used in this work. Section 5 describes the results and analysis of the results, including the approach, as well as the future scopes of this work. Finally, the conclusion is drawn in Sect. 6.

2 Related Work

Several pieces of research regarding SHAR have been carried out where the dataset had motion capture data. Picard et al. [11] used motion capture data to recognize cooking activities. The method achieved a score of 95% on cross-validation of the training set. In this work, a subject has been visualized as a stickman using the MoCap data. For temporal information to be taken into consideration, an HMM model was used in post-processing to get a better result. It should be noted that the dataset had few wrong labels, which were manually labeled here, and data was shuffled which was also ordered before training. It helped them reach such a high accuracy. For different classes, two specialized classifiers were used, and their results were merged.

Image-based approaches have been also observed in the industrial packing process of range hood (meaning kitchen chimney) [12]. In this case, local image-directed graph neural network (LI-DGNN) is used on a set of different types of data. The dataset includes RGB videos, 3D skeleton data extracted by pose estimation algorithm AlphaPose, local images, and bounding-box data of accessories. However, since it uses local images from video frames, it is subjected to object occlusion and viewpoint changes if used solely. Also, as the items are needed to be tracked continuously, it causes a bottleneck in using local images. As a result, a combination of local images and other sensor data is required.

An important observation regarding SHAR works is the size of the datasets. In most cases, the dataset is large enough to experiment with deep learning approaches. Deep learning methods are expected to outperform classical machine learning models with hand-crafted features [13]. In this case, a large dataset is advantageous for a data-driven method. However, such an approach is not expected to work well on smaller datasets as given in the Bento Packaging Activity Recognition Challenge 2021.

3 Dataset

3.1 Data Collection Setup

In any activity recognition challenge, the environment in which data is collected is very crucial. For the Bento Packaging Activity Recognition Challenge 2021, data is collected in the Smart Life Care Unit of the Kyushu Institute of Technology in Japan. Motion Analysis Company [14] has provided the necessary instruments to collect motion capture data. The setup consists of 29 different body markers, 20 infrared cameras to track those markers, and a conveyor belt, where the Bento boxes are passed. Though there were 29 different body markers initially, data for only 13 markers of the upper body is provided for this challenge. The marker positions are shown in Fig. 1.

The data is collected from 4 subjects aged from 20 to 40. While collecting data, empty Bento boxes are passed to the subject using a conveyor belt, and the subject has to put three kinds of foods in the box. The data collection setup is given in Fig. 2, where a subject is taking food and putting it in the Bento box. The face is covered with a white rectangular mask to protect privacy.

3.2 Dataset Description

The dataset for the Bento Packaging Activity Recognition Challenge 2021 consists of activities from five different scenarios necessary for packaging a Bento box. For

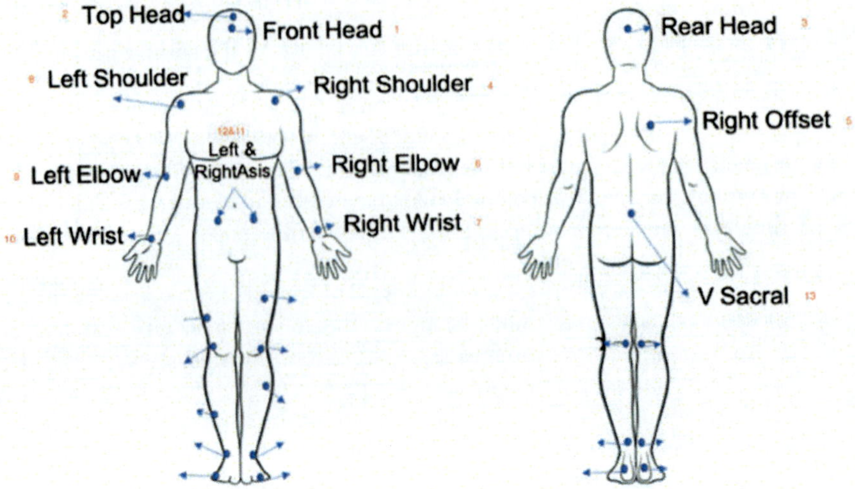

Fig. 1 Position of the markers (*Source* https://abc-research.github.io/bento2021/data/)

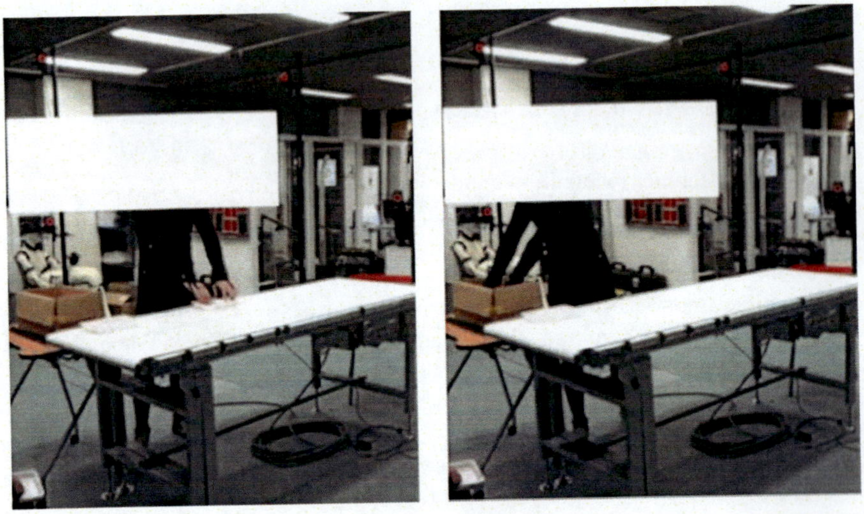

Fig. 2 Data collection setup. A subject is putting items in a Bento box, which is on the white conveyer belt in the middle. At left-mid, the rectangular box is used to cover the subject's face to retain privacy (*Source* https://youtu.be/mQgCaCjC7fI)

each scenario, the activity is done in two different patterns which are inward and outward. The name and label for each activity are listed in Table 1.

The provided data contains three-dimensional coordinates for each of the body markers sampled at a frequency 100 Hz. Each subject has performed each activity approximately five times, and the duration of each activity is between 50 and 70 s. There are a total of 151 training files and 50 test files where each file represents a single activity. From the subject-wise data distributions shown in Fig. 3, it is evident that the dataset is well balanced and each of the subjects has done almost an equal number of different activities.

Table 1 Activity names and corresponding labels

Activity name	Label
Normal (inward)	1
Normal (outward)	2
Forgot to put ingredients (inward)	3
Forgot to put ingredients (outward)	4
Failed to put ingredients (inward)	5
Failed to put ingredients (outward)	6
Turn over bento box (inward)	7
Turn over Bento box (outward)	8
Fix/rearranging ingredients (inward)	9
Fix/rearranging ingredients (outward)	10

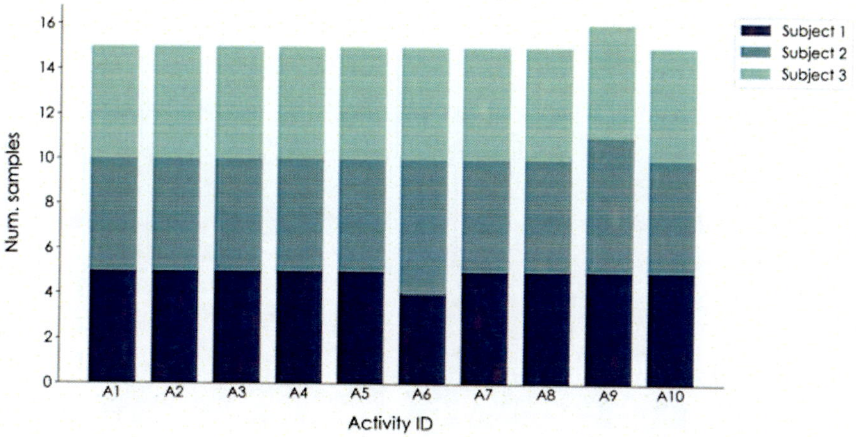

Fig. 3 Distribution of samples for every class (A1~A10). Data of three subjects (as per the training set) is shown

3.3 Dataset Challenges

In most cases, a real-life data collection setup has some inevitable inconsistencies, which make it challenging to work on. The dataset given in this challenge is not free from this issue too. The biggest challenge of this dataset is the small amount of data. There is only a total of 151 instances in the training set which is extremely low considering the complexity of each activity. This problem makes it very hard to use deep learning models that require large datasets to perform well [15]. Another difficulty of the dataset is shown in Fig. 4, which compares the average execution time of each activity for different subjects. It is obvious that different subjects have done the activities differently. Subject 2 has taken a significantly longer period to execute the activities in comparison with Subjects 1 and 3. This problem is more evident for Activities 7, 8, and 9. As the test set contains actions from a different subject who is not present in the training set, this cross-subject inconsistency is likely to take a toll on the overall performance of the model.

However, there are some other problems in the dataset. The data is provided in raw *.csv files rather than any conventional motion capture data format such as *.bvh, *.htr *.c3d, *.asf [16]. The base positions of the body joints are not provided too. As a result, many important features can not be extracted properly from the files. The setting of data collection is very complex which caused incorrect marker labeling, missing data, and unwanted noises which offered further challenges. Of the 29 markers, data from only 13 markers of the upper body was given. Some of the activities are easily separable if lower body marker data is provided. We have addressed almost every issue in our work, which will be covered in the next sections.

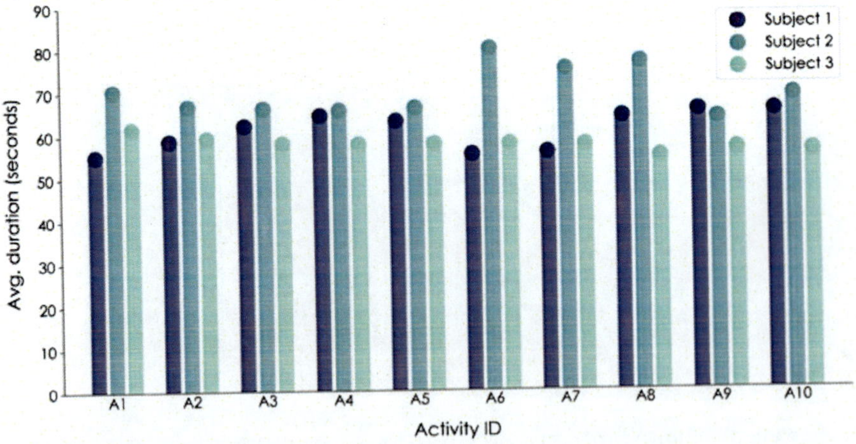

Fig. 4 Subject-wise average activity distribution for three subjects. Distribution for test subject is unknown

4 Methodology

4.1 Preprocessing

fs The most prominent challenge of this dataset is the low number of instances in the training data. To minimize the problem of data scarcity, we have divided each data into multiple overlapped segments of 20–40 s. Smaller segments increase the number of instances sacrificing the global trend, while larger segments decrease the number of instances retaining the global trend. Hence, we have treated the segment size as one of the hyperparameters and have tuned it to the perfect value. A similar approach is taken on the overlapping rate of two consecutive segments. After completing the preprocessing, we were able to increase the number of instances to a range of 300–600 for different combinations of segment size and overlapping rate.

Also, there are some missing values in the dataset. We have interpolated them linearly instead of imputation as the dataset has been resampled at a constant frequency. We have extracted features for each segment which will be described in the following subsection.

4.2 Stream and Feature Extraction

In this dataset, only the cartesian coordinates of 13 upper body joints are given (Fig. 5). So, for each activity, there is a sequence of positions in three axes for all 13 markers. For describing purposes, we will call each of the temporal sequences a stream. This position stream is not enough to describe each activity. So, we have

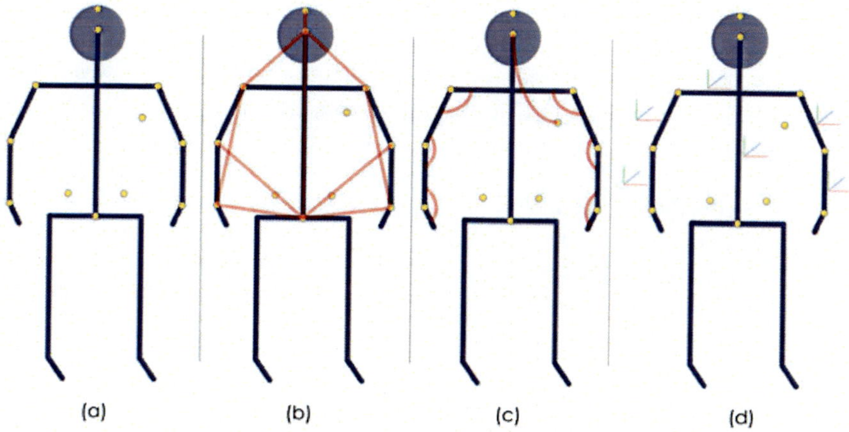

Fig. 5 Stream extraction steps: **a** Skeleton model, **b** Extraction of distance streams, **c** Extraction of joint angle streams, and **d** Extraction of planer angle streams

differentiated it repeatedly to get the speed, acceleration, and jerk streams. In Fig. 5, stream extraction steps are mentioned.

In real life, we move our certain limbs to execute any action, and the distances between certain body joints, d, are crucial for detecting any action [2]. From this point of view, we have calculated distances between selected body joints (i.e., the distance between wrist and shoulder, between v-sacral and elbow, between front head and elbows, between the wrists) to create the distance stream. Each distance signifies a separate concept. For example, the distance between the v-sacral and front head helps to determine if the person has bent his/her head or not. The distance is defined as,

$$d = \sqrt{x^2 + y^2 + z^2} \tag{1}$$

For different activities, the angle between three consecutive joints, θ, and the orientation of the selected bones (i.e., forehand, hand) should be very important. Hence, we have extracted selected joint angle streams and planar angles for bone streams too. In both cases, we have differentiated each stream to get the angular speed streams, according to the following expression,

$$\theta = \arccos\left(\frac{\mathbf{v_1}}{\|v_1\|} \cdot \frac{\mathbf{v_2}}{\|v_2\|}\right) \tag{2}$$

We have synthesized a total of 218 streams after the stream extraction process. The next process is different for RNN-based models and traditional machine learning models. RNN-based deep learning models like LSTM can take each stream directly as the input of the network as well-crafted deep learning networks can learn features from data on their own. Hand-crafted feature extraction is unnecessary for these models. But, the number of streams is too much for the dataset size. For this reason, we have selected the most important 40 streams for LSTM to train on.

We have observed that the deep learning models performed very poorly because the dataset was so small. So, we have constructed a separate feature extraction pipeline for traditional machine learning models. From each of the selected streams, we have extracted the basic frequency-domain features (i.e., median, skew, kurtosis, energy) apart from some statistical features (i.e., median, min, max, standard deviation).

After the execution of the feature extraction pipeline, the feature set became quite large compared to the dataset. So, we had to remove a considerable portion of the feature set to prevent overfitting. We have used the mean decrease in impurity [17] and chi-square techniques [15] to select the most significant 496 features for the later workflow.

4.3 Model Selection and Post-processing

Even after taking a much smaller set of features through the feature selection methods, the number of features remains quite high compared to the dataset size. After preprocessing, the highest number of instances we have produced is less than 600, where the number of features is already as many as 496. This data-to-feature ratio will highly likely lead to overfitting. So, we have proposed a model ensembling system to solve this problem (Fig. 6).

First, we have divided the feature set into 13 overlapped feature subsets each of which contained approximately 150–250 features. For each model, we have trained on different feature subsets and evaluated its result on both tenfold CV and LOOCV. We have selected the top five models based on both the evaluation scores and added a majority voting layer on top of each of the models' predictions. The intuition behind the proposed ensemble system is that the reduced feature set will make the models less prone to overfitting, and majority voting will combine all predictions and give us a final prediction that considers the full feature set [18].

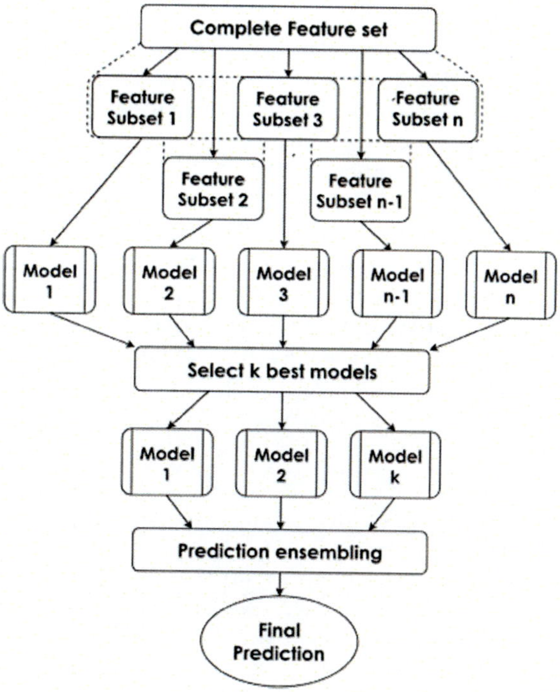

Fig. 6 Our propesed ensemble-based framework

5 Results and Analysis

We have used different tuned models and evaluated them based on tenfold CV and LOOCV. We have found the extra trees classifier to perform best on our framework. The detailed results are portrayed in Table 2. The confusion matrices of the best model found after LOOCV and tenfold CV are depicted in Fig. 7.

The highest accuracy we have achieved in this work is 98% for tenfold CV and 82% for LOOCV. Though the result we obtained is not perfect, this is a very competitive result considering the dataset challenges. There are several reasons behind it. As we can see from Table 2, the evaluation on LOOCV is pretty much less than that of the tenfold CV score. The reason behind it is the lower number of samples for each activity. Each subject has only five samples for each activity which is too low for generalizing on another subject, and this leads to a significantly lower score on LOOCV.

Also from Table 2, we can see that some models have done significantly poorer than other models. LSTM has performed the worst because of the small dataset size. Deep learning models generally need a lot of data to obtain a generalized performance on data. In this case, the dataset size is so small that LSTM has performed even lower than the baseline model, which is the naive Bayes classifier. Gradient boosting models, XGBoost, and LightGBM also suffered a lot from this problem and do not perform very well.

If we look at the confusion matrix for LOOCV in Fig. 7a, we can notice that the model can not differentiate between Classes 2 and 3, 7 and 8, and 6 and 10. It is because different subjects carried out the activities differently to some extent. This problem is also evident in Fig. 4, which depicts the average activity execution time for different subjects. For example, for Activity 6, Subject 1 and Subject 3 took 60 s on average to perform, but Subject 2 took more than 80 s to perform the same task. This problem is reflected in the confusion matrix as we can see that the model was severely confused between Activity 6 and Activity 10. Also, Activities 2 and 3 are typically distinguishable, but there are some confusions observed in the confusion

Table 2 Accuracy of different models

Model	Tenfold CV accuracy	LOOCV accuracy
Naive Bayes	0.84	0.64
Support vector machine (SVM)	0.92	0.73
Random forest classifier (RFC)	0.96	0.77
Extra trees classifier (ETC)	0.96	0.78
LightGBM	0.94	0.74
XGBoost	0.88	0.67
Long short-term memory (LSTM)	0.61	0.37
Ensemble of four RFC models and one ETC model	0.98	0.82

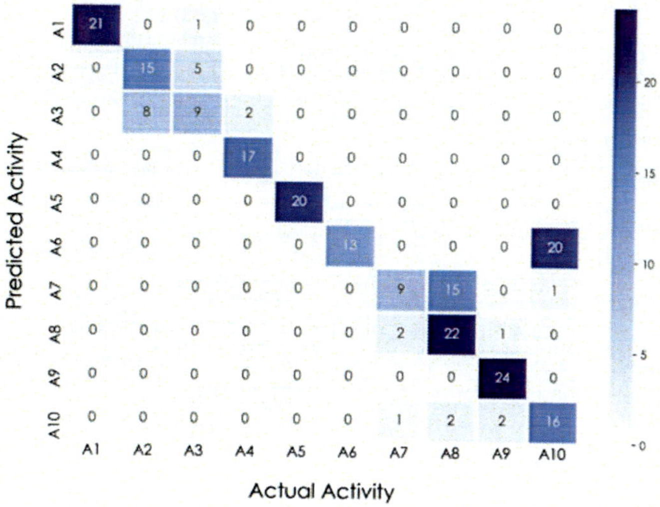

(a) Confusion matrix for the best model after LOOCV.

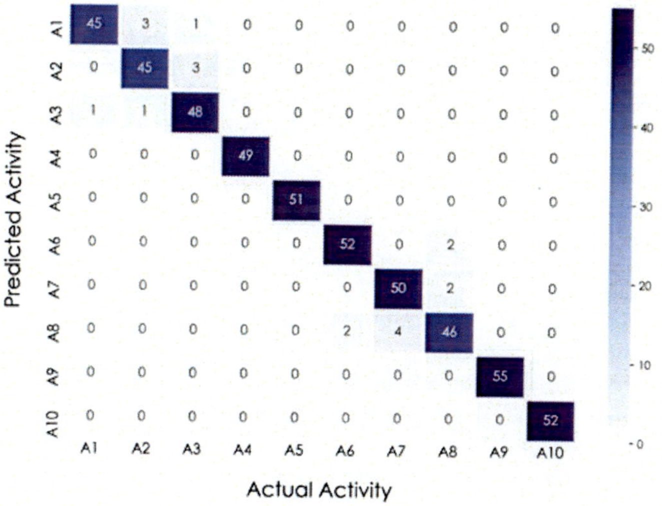

(b) Confusion matrix for the best model after 10-fold CV.

Fig. 7 Confusion matrices

matrix for LOOCV. On the other hand, Activities 7 and 8 are similar, but confusions are observed in this case too. Video data of these activities might help to solve these issues in the future. Despite different challenges and complications of the dataset, our proposed procedure has managed to achieve a quite promising result.

6 Conclusion

In this paper, we have provided a method to tackle the challenges of activity recognition in an industrial setting. Though human activity recognition is a very popular field and a wide variety of work has been done, our work still manages to provide a solution in a less explored arena of this field. After comparing various methods used in previous works by applying them to our dataset, we have decided to use a hand-crafted feature-based solution for our final approach. We have calculated various streams such as speed, joint angle, marker distance from the given data. Furthermore, we have used segmentation with overlap to increase the amount of the data. After that, we have extracted statistical features from each stream. The features are then used to train different machine learning models. After tuning the models and evaluating them using LOOCV and tenfold CV methods, five best-performing models (four random forest classifiers and one extra tree classifier) were selected. The models are used to make predictions on different segments generated from the files of the test dataset, and a majority voting system among the models generates the final predictions.

Our method provides a good amount of precision, but further improvement is still possible. We have experimented with quaternion data generated from provided three-dimensional coordinates but it could not manage to obtain significant improvement through its use. Finding a system to incorporate this data might provide better accuracy. We have also explored different deep learning methods (i.e., temporal convolutional network, LSTM-based encoder-decoder, bidirectional LSTM-based network), but they perform poorly. We believe that the reason for this is the small size of the dataset. Deep learning approaches have the potential to perform better than machine learning approaches, provided that more data is collected. It will also be able to provide end-to-end solutions in contrast to our hand-crafted feature-based solution, which will streamline its integration in the industry. Thus, the collection of more data and exploring deep learning approaches on the data should be strongly considered for future works.

Appendix

See Table 3.

Table 3 Miscellanious information

Information heading	Description
Used sensor modalities	Motion capture (MoCap)
Features used	As described in Sect. 4.2
Programming language	Python 3.8
Packages used	Pandas, NumPy, SciPy, Scikit-learn, XGBoost, TensorFlow, Keras
Machine specifications	Intel(R) Core(TM) i5-7200U CPU @ 2.50GHz, 8 GB RAM
Training and testing time	Time to process and train on full training data—12 min Time to predict on full test data—3 min

References

1. Óscar D. Lara, Labrador, M.A.: A survey on human activity recognition using wearable sensors. IEEE Commun. Surveys Tutorials **15**, 1192–1209 (2013). https://doi.org/10.1109/SURV.2012.110112.00192
2. Cippitelli, E., Gasparrini, S., Gambi, E., Spinsante, S.: A human activity recognition system using skeleton data from rgbd sensors. Comput. Intell. Neurosc. **2016** (2016). https://doi.org/10.1155/2016/4351435
3. Núñez, J.C., Cabido, R., Pantrigo, J.J., Montemayor, A.S., Vélez, J.F.: Convolutional neural networks and long short-term memory for skeleton-based human activity and hand gesture recognition. Pattern Recogn. **76**, 80–94 (2018). https://doi.org/10.1016/J.PATCOG.2017.10.033
4. Sarker, S., Rahman, S., Hossain, T., Ahmed, S.F., Jamal, L., Ahad, M.A.R.: Skeleton-Based Activity Recognition: Preprocessing and Approaches, pp. 43–81. Springer International Publishing (2021). https://doi.org/10.1007/978-3-030-68590-4_2
5. Zhu, W., Lan, C., Xing, J., Zeng, W., Li, Y., Shen, L., Xie, X.: Co-occurrence feature learning for skeleton based action recognition using regularized deep lstm networks. In: Proceedings of the AAAI Conference on Artificial Intelligence **30** (2016). https://ojs.aaai.org/index.php/AAAI/article/view/10451
6. Ahad, M.A.R., Ahmed, M., Antar, A.D., Makihara, Y., Yagi, Y.: Action recognition using kinematics posture feature on 3d skeleton joint locations. Pattern Recogn. Lett. **145**, 216–224 (2021). https://doi.org/10.1016/J.PATREC.2021.02.013
7. Cooking activity recognition challenge. https://abc-research.github.io/cook2020/ (2020). Accessed: 21 Aug 2021
8. Basak, P., Tasin, S.M., Tapotee, M.I., Sheikh, M.M., Sakib, A.H., Baray, S.B., Ahad, M.A.: Complex nurse care activity recognition using statistical features. In: UbiComp/ISWC 2020 Adjunct—Proceedings of the 2020 ACM International Joint Conference on Pervasive and Ubiquitous Computing and Proceedings of the 2020 ACM International Symposium on Wearable Computers, pp. 384–389 (2020). https://doi.org/10.1145/3410530.3414338
9. Adachi, K., Alia, S.S., Nahid, N., Kaneko, H., Lago, P., Inoue, S.: Summary of the bento packaging activity recognition challenge. In: The 3rd International Conference on Activity and Behavior Computing (ABC2021) (2021)
10. Alia, S.S., Adachi, K., Nahid, N., Kaneko, H., Lago, P., Inoue, S.: Bento packaging activity recognition challenge (2021). https://doi.org/10.21227/cwhs-t440
11. Picard, C., Janko, V., Reščič, N., Gjoreski, M., Luštrek, M.: Identification of cooking preparation using motion capture data: A submission to the cooking activity recognition challenge.

Smart Innovation, Syst. Technol. **199**, 103–113 (2021). https://doi.org/10.1007/978-981-15-8269-1_9
12. Chen, Z., Hu, H., Li, Z., Qi, X., Zhang, H., Hu, H., Chang, V.: Skeleton-based action recognition for industrial packing process. In: IoTBDS 2020—Proceedings of the 5th International Conference on Internet of Things, Big Data and Security pp. 36–45 (2020). https://doi.org/10.5220/0009340800360045
13. Hossain, T., Sarker, S., Rahman, S., Ahad, M.A.R.: Skeleton-based human action recognition on large-scale datasets. Intell. Syst. Ref. Libr. **207**, 125–146 (2021). https://doi.org/10.1007/978-3-030-75490-7_5
14. Motion capture analysis software. https://motionanalysis.com/movement-analysis/ (2021). Accessed: 21 Aug 2021
15. Suto, J., Oniga, S., Sitar, P.P.: Comparison of wrapper and filter feature selection algorithms on human activity recognition. In: 2016 6th International Conference on Computers Communications and Control, ICCCC 2016 pp. 124–129 (2016). https://doi.org/10.1109/ICCCC.2016.7496749
16. Meredith, M., Maddock, S.: Motion capture file formats explained. Production (2001)
17. Nguyen, T.T., Huang, J.Z., Nguyen, T.T.: Unbiased feature selection in learning random forests for high-dimensional data. Scientific World J. **2015** (2015). https://doi.org/10.1155/2015/471371
18. Bayat, A., Pomplun, M., Tran, D.A.: A study on human activity recognition using accelerometer data from smartphones. Proced. Comput. Sci. **34**, 450–457 (2014). https://doi.org/10.1016/J.PROCS.2014.07.009

Identification of Food Packaging Activity Using MoCap Sensor Data

Adrita Anwar, Malisha Islam Tapotee, Purnata Saha, and Md Atiqur Rahman Ahad

Abstract The automation system has brought a revolutionary change in our lives. Food packaging activity recognition can add a new dimension to industrial automation systems. However, it is challenging to identify the packaging activities using only skeleton data of the upper body due to the similarities between the activities and subject-dependent results. Bento Packaging Activity Recognition Challenge 2021 provides us with a dataset of ten different activities performed during *Bento* box packaging in a laboratory using MoCap (motion capture) sensors. Bento box is a single-serving packed meal that is very popular in Japanese cuisine. In this paper, we develop methods using the classical machine learning approach, as the given dataset is small compared to other skeleton datasets. After preprocessing, we extract different hand-crafted features and train different models like extremely randomized trees, random forest, and XGBoost classifiers and select the best model based on cross-validation score. Then, we explore different combinations of features and use the best combination of features for prediction. By applying our methodology, we achieve 64% accuracy and 53.66% average accuracy in tenfold cross-validation and leave-one-subject-out cross-validation, respectively.

1 Introduction

Human activity recognition (HAR) has been a very useful and significant topic in the research field over the last decade [1]. This study has two mainstream methods, sensor-based activity recognition [2] and vision-based activity recognition [3, 4]. With the increasing availability of sensors and devices, such as the Microsoft Kinect [5] and MoCap sensor [6], data collection using sensors has been more convenient, and sensor-based activity recognition has improved a lot. This kind of sensor

A. Anwar · M. Islam Tapotee · P. Saha
Electrical and Electronic Engineering, University of Dhaka, Dhaka, Bangladesh

M. A. R. Ahad (✉)
University of East London, London, UK
e-mail: atiqahad@du.ac.bd; atiqahad@yahoo.com

M. A. R. Ahad et al. (eds.), *Sensor- and Video-Based Activity and Behavior Computing*, Smart Innovation, Systems and Technologies 291,
https://doi.org/10.1007/978-981-19-0361-8_11

basically provides the skeleton data points. Skeleton-based methods have contributed substantially and achieved good performance in recent studies [7, 8]. In addition, the acceleration data has also been very crucial and effective in activity recognition [9].

HAR also plays an important role in human-robot collaborative work, which has become very popular now in industries and the health care sector [10]. The use of robots in nursing and monitoring patients has been introduced to make their lives easier [11]. Such robots decrease nurses' workload efficiently. In industrial works, human-assisting robots have also been familiar. A large number of robots have been deployed in industries for assisting humans to perform different manufacturing tasks [12].

HAR is used in monitoring many complex activities like cooking activity recognition [13] and nurse care activity recognition [14]. In cooking activity recognition, both motion capture and accelerometer sensor data have been used to classify various cooking steps [15]. On the other hand, nurse care activity recognition focuses on the recognition of activities conducted by the nurses in both the laboratory and real-life settings using accelerometer data [16]. By keeping these studies in mind, Bento Packaging Activity Recognition Challenge 2021 has been arranged. Human-robot collaboration in packaging Bento boxes can be a great solution for the betterment of our lifestyle. In this modern era, getting a large workforce for packaging Bento boxes with lower wages is very tough. Robots can be an alternative to human workers in this field if they are trained efficiently to recognize the activities performed while packing the boxes [17].

Bento Packaging Activity Recognition Challenge 2021 [17] offers a dataset where MoCap sensor data for 13 markers is available to classify 10 different tasks. The key challenge in this dataset has been similarities in the activities. In this paper, we have proposed a classical machine learning approach for recognizing the activities comprising preprocessing, feature extraction, and classification.

This paper is outlined as follows: After giving an overview in Sect. 1, the description of the challenge dataset is presented in Sect. 2. In Sect. 3, we have described the necessary steps of our method, and in Sects. 4 and 5, the outcome of our results and difficulties in the dataset are described. Finally, we have concluded the paper in Sect. 6, discussing future developments and possibilities of our work.

2 Dataset Description

The main motive of Bento Packaging Activity Recognition Challenge 2021 is to replace the human workforce with robots in Bento box packaging tasks. If we want robots to be an alternative to humans, first, it is required to understand how humans are performing the task. To implement this plan, Bento Packaging Activity Recognition Challenge 2021 data has been collected. The dataset [17] contains Bento box packaging data collected from MoCap sensors. The whole data collection process has been conducted in the Smart Life Care Unit of the Kyushu Institute of Technology, Japan. The Bento box packaging activities were performed by four subjects (men).

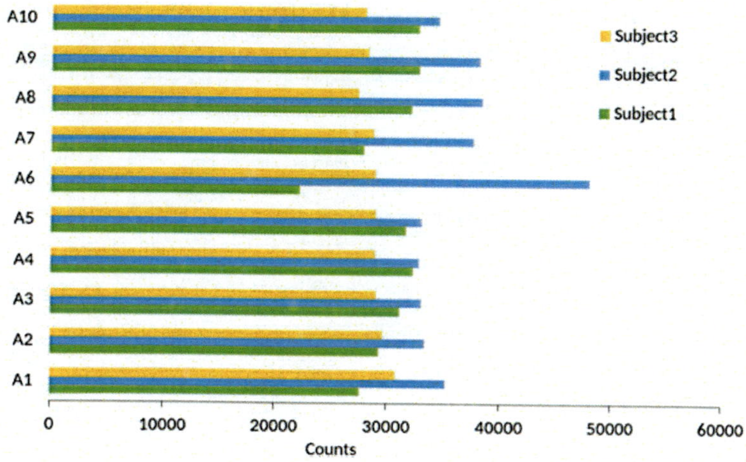

Fig. 1 Number of samples for each activity performed by three subjects

The organizers have kept the data of three subjects in the training set and the fourth subject's data in the test set. There are missing entries in both the train and test sets.

In the train set, there are 0.47%, 4.74%, and 0.039% null values in Subject 1, Subject 2, and Subject 3, respectively. On the contrary, 42% null values are present in the test set which is really a huge amount.

Figure 1 represents the number of samples for each activity performed by three subjects in the training set. According to this figure, the subjects were instructed to perform ten different tasks of packaging, namely normal, forgot to put ingredients, failed to put ingredients, turn over Bento box, and fix/rearranging ingredients, each inward and outward, which are represented as A1–A10.

While data collection, 29 body markers were used, but they made 13 body markers data available. Participants repeated each work 5 times, and 20 infrared cameras were used to track the markers. The three-dimensional position of each marker is recorded with a frequency 100 Hz.

3 Methodology

In this section, our proposed method for Bento Packaging Activity Recognition Challenge 2021 has been illustrated. We have followed the classical machine learning approach and put an emphasis on data preprocessing and feature engineering so that the learning algorithm can classify the activities easily using the best combination of features. The block diagram of our process is represented in Fig. 2.

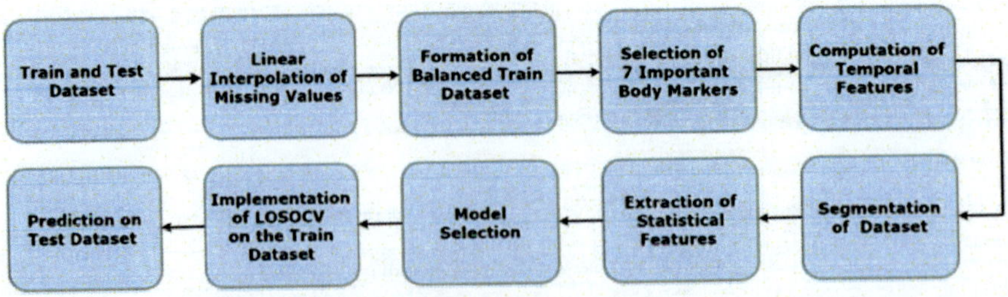

Fig. 2 Block diagram of our proposed methodology

3.1 *Preprocessing*

3.1.1 Handling Missing Values and Class Imbalance

The motion capture data obtained from the 13 body markers contains several missing values. We have used linear interpolation to handle the missing values. After that, the data of three train subjects containing ten different activities has been merged in order to form a complete dataset. In the dataset, the number of samples for each activity has turned out to be unequal. Activity 2 named normal (outward) has the least number of samples (92,218), and Activity 6 named failed to put ingredients (inward) has the highest number of samples (98,929).

Machine learning models perform better when the number of samples for each class is equal [18]. To deal with the class imbalance, we have used the undersampling method which removes samples from the majority class to even out the class distribution [19]. We have taken the sample size of Activity 2 which is the least encountered in the dataset and made other activities of the same size by deleting several data points.

3.1.2 Marker Selection

The contribution of different body markers in detecting different activities has been studied by plotting the 3-D position of individual markers for every activity and experimentally training machine learning models with different combinations of these markers. Out of the 13 given body markers, we have only used 7 markers to train our final model. Each marker has three space coordinates, and not all space coordinates are equally important as they do not change significantly while performing the activities. The selected seven markers are shown in Fig. 3.

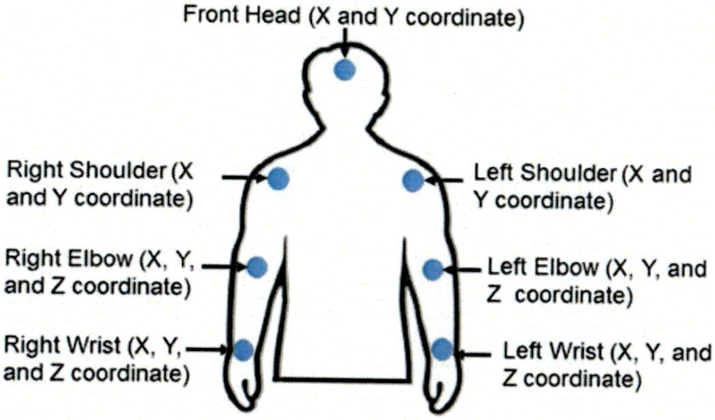

Fig. 3 Selected seven body markers

3.2 *Feature Engineering*

Using the motion capture data, temporal features like velocity, acceleration, and jerk have been extracted. Joint-to-joint distance [20], joint-to-joint orientation, the angle between selected body parts, verticality [21], horizontality, and few other hand-crafted features have also been determined.

However, only the motion capture data, velocity, acceleration, and jerk have been used for the final model training as these features have given comparatively better results than the others. Combining all the temporal features, we have divided the data into smaller segments using a sliding window of 5 s and 20% overlap. The window size and overlap rate have been determined empirically. From each segment, statistical features such as mean, median, standard deviation, skew, kurtosis, maximum value, and minimum value have been obtained. After empirically experimenting with these statistical features, we have found that mean, standard deviation, maximum value and minimum value perform well for the dataset, and thus, we have selected these features for the final model training.

For preprocessing and feature extraction of the test data, a similar procedure has been used except with a minor change. In one of the files in the test dataset, no data for Marker 6 (right elbow) was provided. We have filled it with the value of Marker 7 (right wrist) as we have observed that Markers 6 and 7 have similar plots for most of the activities.

Finally, a skeleton normalization [22] process has been implemented to make the 3-D position data from the motion capture subject size invariant. However, this process requires a user's torso length, and from the given data, it is difficult to measure the length as it varies while performing the activities. Therefore, the normalization process has not performed as expected, and we could not use it to reduce subject dependency of the data.

3.3 Classification

After the statistical feature extraction, we have used different machine learning (ML) models to train the data and compared the results for the final model selection. The use of ML algorithms such as SVM, *k*-NN, random forest, and LightGBM is observed for cooking activity recognition [23]. We have mainly used extremely randomized trees [24], random forest [25], and XGBoost classifiers [26] for model training.

Based on our result, extremely randomized trees classifier has outperformed the other classifiers. Extremely randomized trees classifier is an ensemble of decision trees that selects the split point of a tree randomly and fits each decision tree on the whole dataset. The randomness makes the decision trees less correlated. It has helped to subdue the noise in the dataset. As a result, we have obtained better results using this classifier. We have tuned the number of trees of the selected classifier and found that 1000 trees give the best accuracy. Finally, we have used this tuned classifier to generate predictions for the test set.

Tenfold cross-validation, along with leave-one-subject-out cross-validation, has been employed to evaluate model performance. Leave-one-subject-out cross-validation has been performed three times, keeping one subject as the validation set and the other two as train set. This cross-validation method has helped us to measure the robustness of our model as each time the prediction was performed using unseen data.

4 Results

In this section, results from the two different cross-validation methods are presented. Table 1 shows the tenfold cross-validation accuracy of extremely randomized trees classifier (EXT), random forest classifier (RF), and XGBoost classifier (XGB). Although the accuracy from extremely randomized trees classifier and random forest classifier is nearly the same, extremely randomized trees classifier shows higher accuracy when leave-one-subject-out cross-validation is performed.

The leave-one-subject-out cross-validation accuracy using extremely randomized trees classifier is shown in Table 2. It is seen that the accuracy is at most 59% and at least 44% when the valid subject is 1 and 2, respectively. The reason for poor

Table 1 Tenfold cross-validation accuracy of selected models

Model	Accuracy (%)
Extremely randomized trees	64
Random forest	63
XGBoost	59

Table 2 Leave-one-subject-out cross-validation accuracy

Valid subject	Train subject	Accuracy (%)
1	2, 3	59
2	1, 3	44
3	1, 2	58

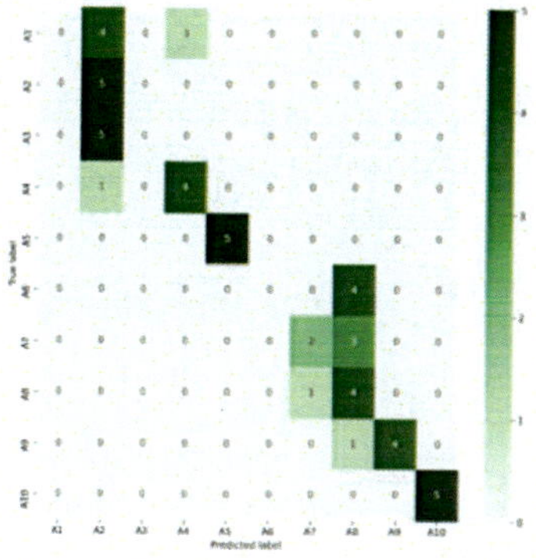

(a) Confusion matrix for subject 1

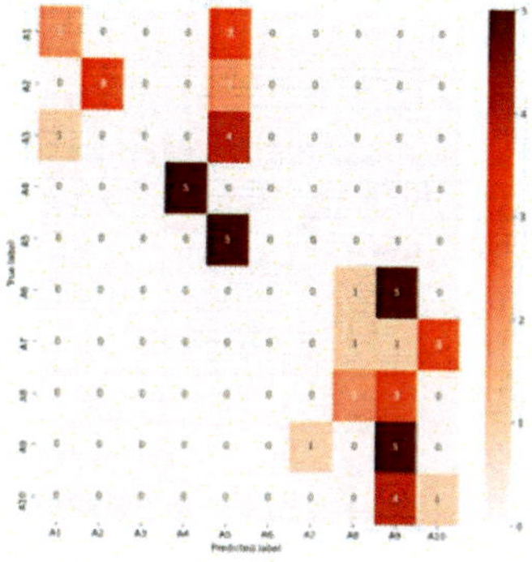

(b) Confusion matrix for subject 2

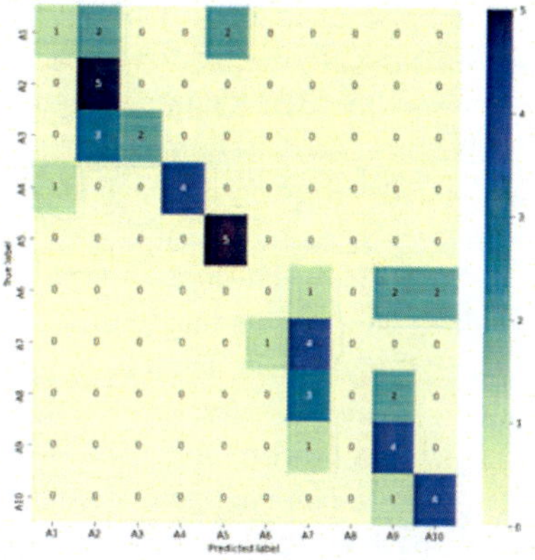

(c) Confusion matrix for subject 1

Fig. 4 Confusion matrix of leave-one-subject-out cross-validation

performance on Valid subject 2 is that it contains the most missing values (17,244), whereas Subjects 1 and 3 contain 1416 and 114 missing values, respectively.

Figure 4 shows the confusion matrix plot when Subjects 1–3 are held out as validation sets, respectively. From the confusion matrix, it is seen that Activities 4, 5, and 9 are predicted correctly for all subjects. These activities are expected to be predicted correctly for the test subject. However, Activities 6, 8, and 10 often get misclassified as Activity 9.

Activities 2, 7, and 10 are distinguishable for some subjects but not for all. Activities 1, 3, and 6 are the hardest to classify, with Activity 6 not being correctly predicted for any subject. Activity 6 is mostly misclassified as Activity 8 or 9. That means the model is confusing failing to put ingredients (inward) with turning over the Bento box (outward) and fixing/rearranging ingredients (inward). The features and window size we used may not be good enough to distinguish these three activities. The model struggles to identify some activities due to their similar nature and variation added to the activities by how they were performed by the individual subjects. The easily separable activities such as forgot to put ingredients (outward), failed to put ingredients (inward), and fix/rearranging ingredients (inward) common in all subjects get correctly classified by the model.

5 Discussion

The challenge dataset only provides body markers for upper body parts, contains several missing values, and can be considered as a small dataset in human activity recognition literature [27]. Deep learning models are more popular and effective for skeleton-based human activity recognition on large datasets [28]. As the dataset has a small number of samples containing data of only three subjects, we have used traditional machine learning algorithms for the activity recognition.

The similarity between the Bento box packaging activities makes the classification task really challenging. As class imbalance is present in the dataset, some data has been discarded in order to make it a balanced dataset. It is also observed that the three subjects perform the same activities differently, which adds more complexity. Features like the angle between selected body parts, joint-to-joint distance, and orientation have yielded poor results due to this problem. Merging these features to the dataset has dropped the accuracy. Therefore, we have only explored the temporal features (e.g., motion capture, velocity, acceleration, and jerk) and extracted statistical features from them to train our model. Moreover, we have only used 3-D MoCap sensor data to identify these complex activities. If the video data of the experiment was provided, it could have given us some insight on how to design features in order to perfectly classify the confusing activities.

6 Conclusion

In this paper, we have come up with a straightforward method to distinguish Bento box packaging tasks using motion capture data. We have interpolated the missing values and dealt with the class imbalance, extracted many hand-crafted features, carefully selected the body markers, experimented with the sliding window size and overlapping rate, tried different machine learning algorithms, and tuned the hyperparameters of the models. We also tried incorporating a skeleton normalization process to make the data subject independent, which we could not use due to some limitations mentioned earlier. However, the dataset is really challenging and small, and more data should be collected in order to achieve better results. The recognition results for the testing dataset will be presented in the summary paper of the challenge [29]. In our future work, we want to use more advanced methods for skeleton data normalization. Also, we would like to introduce smarter feature sets than what we have explored in this paper, increase the sliding window size, and implement other models for improving our results. If possible, a larger dataset can be created.

Appendix

See Table 3.

Table 3 The summary of the resources used

Items	Details
Sensor modalities	MoCap sensor
Features used	Section 3.2
Window size	5s
Post processing	NA
Programming language and library	Python: Scikit-learn, Numpy, Pandas, Matplotlib
Training and testing time	<1 min
Machine specification	RAM: 25 GB, CPU: Intel Xeon @2.20 GHz, Cores: 2

References

1. Kim, E., Helal, S., Cook, D.: Human activity recognition and pattern discovery. IEEE Pervasive Comput. **9**, 48–53 (2009)
2. Chen, L., Hoey, J., Nugent, C., Cook, D., Yu, Z.: Sensor-based activity recognition. IEEE Trans. Syst. Man Cybern. Part C (Appl. Rev.) **42**, 790–808 (2012)
3. Bodor, R., Jackson, B., Papanikolopoulos, N.: Vision-based human tracking and activity recognition. In: Proceedings of the 11th Mediterranean Conference on Control and Automation, vol. 1 (2003)
4. Bux, A., Angelov, P., Habib, Z.: Vision based human activity recognition: a review. In: Advances In Computational Intelligence Systems, pp. 341–371 (2017)
5. Zhang, Z.: Microsoft kinect sensor and its effect. IEEE Multimedia **19**, 4–10 (2012)
6. Mitobe, K., Kaiga, T., Yukawa, T., Miura, T., Tamamoto, H., Rodgers, A., Yoshimura, N.: Development of a motion capture system for a hand using a magnetic three dimensional position sensor. In: ACM SIGGRAPH 2006 Research Posters, pp. 102-es (2006)
7. Sarker, S., Rahman, S., Hossain, T., Ahmed, S., Jamal, L., Ahad, M.A.R.: Skeleton-based activity recognition: preprocessing and approaches. Contactless Human Act. Anal. **200**, 43 (2021)
8. Hbali, Y., Hbali, S., Ballihi, L., Sadgal, M.: Skeleton-based human activity recognition for elderly monitoring systems. IET Comput. Vis. **12**, 16–26 (2018)
9. Slim, S., Atia, A., Elfattah, M., Mostafa, M.: Survey on human activity recognition based on acceleration data. Intl. J. Adv. Comput. Sci. Appl. **10**, 84–98 (2019)
10. Maurtua, I., Ibarguren, A., Kildal, J., Susperregi, L., Sierra, B.: Human-robot collaboration in industrial applications: safety, interaction and trust. Int. J. Adv. Robot. Syst. **14**, 1729881417716010 (2017)
11. Mesquita, A., Zamarioli, C., Carvalho, E.: The use of robots in nursing care practices: an exploratory descriptive study. Online Braz. J. Nurs. **15**, 404–413 (2016)
12. Hentout, A., Aouache, M., Maoudj, A., Akli, I.: Human-robot interaction in industrial collaborative robotics: a literature review of the decade 2008–2017. Adv. Robot. **33**, 764–799 (2019)
13. Alia, S., Lago, P., Takeda, S., Adachi, K., Benaissa, B., Ahad, M.A.R., Inoue, S.: Summary of the cooking activity recognition challenge. In: Human Activity Recognition Challenge, pp. 1–13 (2021)
14. Lago, P., Alia, S., Takeda, S., Mairittha, T., Mairittha, N., Faiz, F., Nishimura, Y., Adachi, K., Okita, T., Charpillet, F., et al.: Nurse care activity recognition challenge: summary and results. In: Adjunct Proceedings of the 2019 ACM International Joint Conference on Pervasive and Ubiquitous Computing and Proceedings of the 2019 ACM International Symposium on Wearable Computers, pp. 746–751 (2019)
15. Siraj, M., Shahid, O., Ahad, M.A.R.: Cooking activity recognition with varying sampling rates using deep convolutional GRU framework. In: Human Activity Recognition Challenge, pp. 115–126 (2021)
16. Basak, P., Tasin, S., Tapotee, M., Sheikh, M., Sakib, A., Baray, S., Ahad, M.A.R.: Complex nurse care activity recognition using statistical features. In: Adjunct Proceedings of the 2020 ACM International Joint Conference on Pervasive and Ubiquitous Computing and Proceedings of the 2020 ACM International Symposium on Wearable Computers, pp. 384–389 (2020). https://doi.org/10.1145/3410530.3414338
17. Alia, S.S., Adachi, K., Nahid, N., Kaneko, H., Lago, P., Bento, S.I.: Packaging Activity Recognition Challenge. IEEE DataPort (2021). https://doi.org/10.21227/cwhs-t440
18. Brownlee, J.: A gentle introduction to imbalanced classification. Mach. Learn. Mastery **22** (2019)
19. Bach, M., Werner, A., Palt, M.: The proposal of under sampling method for learning from imbalanced datasets. Procedia Comput. Sci. **159**, 125–134 (2019)

20. Kadir, M., Akash, P., Sharmin, S., Ali, A., Shoyaib, M.: Can a simple approach identify complex nurse care activity? In: Adjunct Proceedings of the 2019 ACM International Joint Conference on Pervasive and Ubiquitous Computing and Proceedings of the 2019 ACM International Symposium on Wearable Computers, pp. 736–740 (2019)
21. Tits, M.: Expert gesture analysis through motion capture using statistical modeling and machine learning. Ph.D. Dissertation (2018)
22. Sie, M., Cheng, Y., Chiang, C.: Key motion spotting in continuous motion sequences using motion sensing devices. In: 2014 IEEE International Conference on Signal Processing, Communications and Computing (ICSPCC), pp. 326–331 (2014)
23. Ahad, M.A.R., Lago, P., Inoue, S.: Human Activity Recognition Challenge. Springer, Berlin (2021)
24. Geurts, P., Ernst, D., Wehenkel, L.: Extremely randomized trees. Mach. Learn. **63**, 3–42 (2006)
25. Oshiro, T., Perez, P., Baranauskas, J.: How many trees in a random forest? In: International Workshop on Machine Learning and Data Mining in Pattern Recognition, pp. 154–168 (2012)
26. Chen, T., Guestrin, C., et al.: XGBoost: a scalable tree boosting system. In: Proceedings of the 22nd ACM SIGKDD International Conference on Knowledge Discovery and Data Mining (KDD'16), pp. 785–794 (2016)
27. Yu, B., Liu, Y., Chan, K.: Effective human activity recognition based on small datasets (2020). ArXiv Preprint ArXiv:2004.13977
28. Hossain, T., Sarker, S., Rahman, S., Ahad, M.A.R.: Skeleton-based human action recognition on large-scale datasets. In: Vision, Sensing and Analytics: Integrative Approaches, pp. 125–146 (2021)
29. Adachi, K., Alia, S.S., Nahid, N., Kaneko, H., Lago, P., Inoue, S.: Summary of the Bento packaging activity recognition challenge. In: The 3rd International Conference on Activity and Behavior Computing (ABC2021)

Lunch-Box Preparation Activity Understanding from Motion Capture Data Using Handcrafted Features

Yeasin Arafat Pritom, Md. Sohanur Rahman, Hasib Ryan Rahman, M. Ashikuzzaman Kowshik, and Md Atiqur Rahman Ahad

Abstract Japanese packed-meal or *Bento* preparation or packaging automated by a robot is a recent challenge. It is one of the latest cementations in human activity recognition systems. It shows contingency on physical gesture recognition techniques using some sensor-based datasets, especially some motion capture data or skeleton data. To get a firm grip on the recognition, we (Team Boson Kona) implement a method dealing with some handcrafted features gained from the filtered data. We employ several pre-processing steps to handle any inconsistency of the dataset: after cleaning the data, we use filtering and windowing techniques to process the raw data. Then we figure out multiple statistical and geometrical features from joints-based handcrafted features. After considering the most significant features for model training, we try out support vector machine classifier, random forest classifier and extra tree classifier. After applying all these methodologies, we obtain maximum accuracy of 64.6% using the extra tree classifier.

1 Introduction

The human body can carry out innumerable compound movements owing to its complicated joint positions, muscle functioning and hybrid peripheral nervous system.

Y. A. Pritom (✉) · Md. S. Rahman · H. R. Rahman · M. A. Kowshik
University of Dhaka, Dhaka, Bangladesh
e-mail: yeasinarafat-2018726167@eee.du.ac.bd

Md. S. Rahman
e-mail: mdsohanur-2018226199@eee.du.ac.bd

H. R. Rahman
e-mail: hasibryan-2018326152@eee.du.ac.bd

M. A. Kowshik
e-mail: mashikuzzaman-2018926183@eee.du.ac.bd

M. A. R. Ahad
University of East London, London, UK
e-mail: atiqahad@du.ac.bd; atiqahad@yahoo.com

M. A. R. Ahad et al. (eds.), *Sensor- and Video-Based Activity and Behavior Computing*, Smart Innovation, Systems and Technologies 291,
https://doi.org/10.1007/978-981-19-0361-8_12

Standing up, sitting down, bending, walking, jogging, etc., are quotidian actions by the human body. Human actions got to be recognized through some sensor data for observing those complex activities and implementing them artificially [1]. Thereupon, in human–computer alliance, food manufacturing, video surveillance, virtual reality (VR), medical recovery and other fields, human activity recognition (HAR) is a time-honoured major theme.

Optical human action recognition and wearable human action recognition are two major wings for HAR in the prevailing sectors. For as much as wireless sensor mechanics has evolved moderately, wearable human motion projection has flourished swiftly during past years [2]. Owing to the easy accessibility and budget-friendliness of numerous sensors, they can now be integrated into smart appliances (smartwatches, smartphones, and so on) [3].

Accelerometers, motion capture sensors at different body joints, heart rate belt sensor [4], magnetometer [5], gyroscope [6] are some frequently used sensor modules in HAR implementations [7]. Among them, in 'Bento Packaging Activity Recognition Challenge', motion capture sensors stand out in the crowd. Because motion capture systems provide substantial accuracy compared to other sensors, these sensors are attached in such an orientation to resemble a skeleton structure. Hence, it produces data that can effortlessly identify any certain sophisticated activity. The skeleton data is extremely effective in sketching accurate models which can predict activities like walking, jogging and jumping. Over the years, many researchers have been developing deep learning neural network models to predict such activities with extreme precision. However, skeleton-based activity recognition demands for deep learning-based methods—specifically for large datasets [8]. However, machine learning and deep learning models have hardly been implemented for any packing purposes. Such a unique initiation is at the cutting edge of sensor-based motion capture data.

The paper is organized as follows: after a short description in Sect. 1, some related works have been demonstrated in Sect. 2 and dataset has been presented in Sect. 3. Overall methodology has been illustrated in Sect. 4. Results and a short discussion have been described in Sect. 5. Finally, the paper has been concluded in Sect. 6 with our purposes, contributions and future guidelines.

2 Backgrounds

Sensor data and signals originated from the attached sensors are predominantly used to track human movements. Skeleton data has been a very prevalent practice to researchers and organizers over the past decades in human activity recognition. Many different techniques and methods have been brought to light as the need arises. Reference [9] has elaborated various representation strategies, pre-processing steps, feature extraction methods and so on. Many approaches have been tabled like self-attention-based neural network model, universal spatial modelling technique perpendicular to recurrent neural network (RNN) model, multi-layer LSTM framework, etc., to handle skeleton data or mocap data.

A spatial–temporal graph convolutional network (ST-GCN) has been introduced by Cao et al. [10] to process 3D motion capture data. In [2], a two-level hierarchical framework based on a 3D skeleton dataset has been proposed where support vector machine (SVM) and the hidden Markov model were used to classify all categories. This resulted in an average accuracy of 91.41%. A prototype-based approach was initiated by [11], which represented an action as a sequence of prototypes in extended video sequences. The method finally resulted in a recognition rate of 90% to 96%. Hierarchy theory can be brought into play for the efficient projection of knotty hierarchical relationships of human movements. A two-level hierarchical projection framework has been built by the authors of [12].

A legion of encouraging research has been derived, resulting in state-of-the-art performance by manipulating multi-layer geometrical features. For example, the authors of [13] have provided a unique and straightforward universal spatial modelling technique perpendicular to the recurrent neural network (RNN) model. They fed each type of geometrical feature to a three-layer LSTM framework. Also, in [14, 15], some geometrical features based on different body joints have been proposed to verify the activities based on skeleton data. In [16], it is claimed that extracting handcrafted features and employing simple classifiers makes it possible to get up to mark performance.

3 Data Description

The provided datasets were meticulously collected from a motion capture system attached to the 29 body joints of 4 subjects. During the data extraction, they put three types of food items in the bento box at the Smart Life Care Unit of the Kyushu Institute of Technology in Japan. Data of 13 body markers have been provided for the recognition purpose. The three-axis positional data of each marker have been supplied for the training purpose.

We were provided with subjects 1, 2, 3 as training data and left with subject four as test data. The data were sampled with 100 Hz frequency. Each subject performed every activity repeatedly five times in two different-pattern (inward and outward). All the ten activities are presented accordingly in Table 1. The provided pie chart (Fig. 1)

Table 1 Activity list

Activity name	Label	Activity name	Label
Normal (inward)	1	Failed to put ingredients (outward)	6
Normal (outward)	2	Turn over bento box (inward)	7
Forgot to put ingredients (inward)	3	Turn over bento box (outward)	8
Forgot to put ingredients (outward)	4	Fix/rearranging ingredients (inward)	9
Failed to put ingredients (inward)	5	Fix/rearranging ingredients (outward)	10

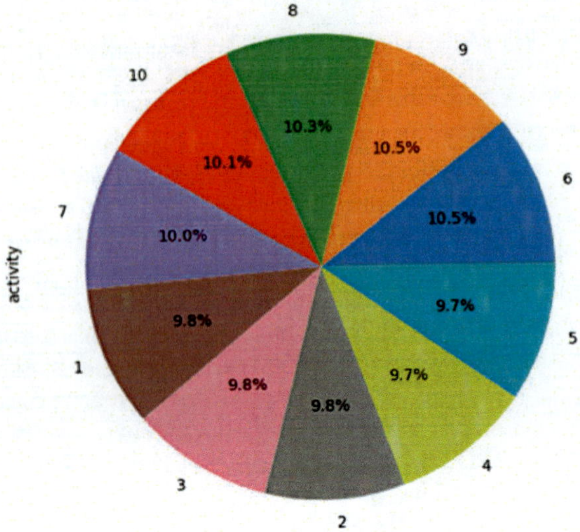

Fig. 1 Here is a pie chart that illustrates the distribution of different activities. It also shows us that all the activities are almost similarly distributed

has demonstrated a crystal clear depiction of uniformly distributed data against each activity. Every single activity cuts nearly equal share from the pie chart. Activity 6 and activity 9 hold a percentage of 10.5% each from the provided data, whereas activity 4 and activity 5 have a share of 9.7% each [17].

4 Methodology

Human gesture fluctuates from plain to complex, from simple to advanced, with a climbing degree of intricacy and noise. That is to say, there is a labyrinthine hierarchy in locomotion actions. In this section, we have outlined and elaborately explained the procedure we have tried out in this research. The whole process can be distinguished into four significant steps, which are as follows: data pre-processing, feature extraction, feature selection and model selection. Data cleaning, filtering and windowing have been elaborately explained in the pre-processing section. Similar kinds of steps have been followed for both train dataset and test dataset. In Fig. 2, we have visualized the whole methodology through a flowchart.

4.1 Data Pre-processing

Data processing consists of the following steps: data cleaning, filtering and windowing. The provided dataset has been carefully checked for any not a number (NaN) values. The NaN values in each column have been interpolated up to 100 successive

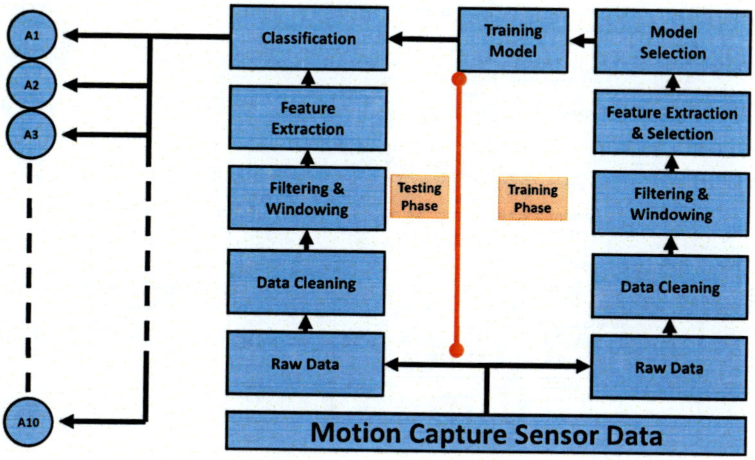

Fig. 2 Flowchart illustrates the overview of our whole method

Fig. 3 Graph demonstrates the difference between the filtered and the unfiltered data of one of the sensors of activity 1

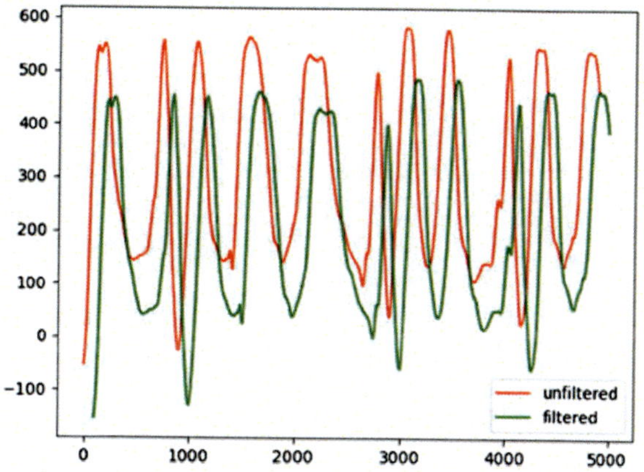

rows, and then the rest of the NaN values have been removed [3]. Any motion sensor has an additional bias towards gravity, which triggers the human motion mechanism towards the vertex. Usually, this bias affects the Z-axis data of the dataset as it directly opposes the gravity comparing the other two axes (Fig. 3).

A high-pass Butterworth filter has been applied with a cut-off frequency of 0.5 Hz to avoid such gravitational effects from the dataset. Different sizes of windows were used, and large windows provided the most stable information. Datasets have been windowed for every 20 s with 95% overlapping with the successive windows. Each window has been mapped after a single activity [18].

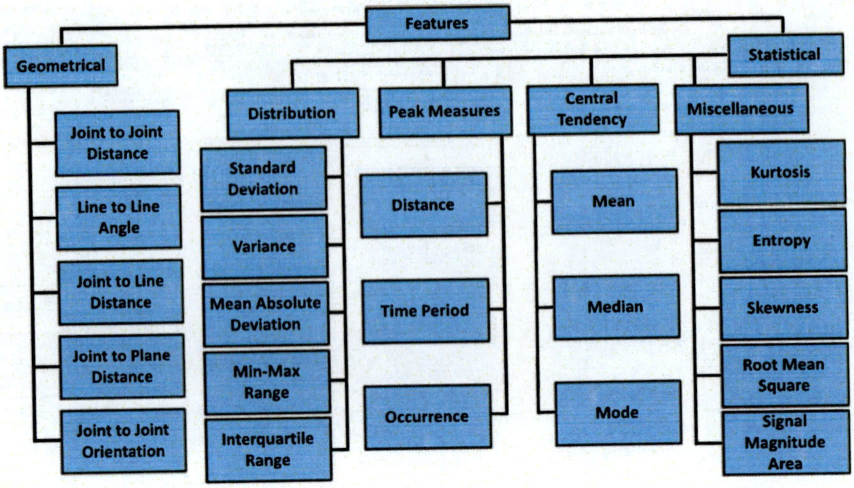

Fig. 4 Handcrafted statistical and geometrical characteristics have been extracted for improved recognition

4.2 Feature Extraction

In the case of motion capture sensors, the sensor's data positioned in different joints of the body can be utilized to identify any specific activity. Both handcrafted statistical and geometrical features have been pulled out for better recognition. In order to identify and study the versatile movements such as a wide range of hand movements while packaging food items in the bento box by the test subjects, we have extracted some geometrical features (Fig. 4).

The most common of those features are as follows, joint-to-joint distance, line-to-line angle, etc. We have introduced some distribution features to determine the repetition of a particular activity of the test subjects. It sheds some light on the point that how often the data differs within a certain interval. Apart from that there is another feature section, which deals with the central tendency of the provided data. The purpose of this feature is to visualize the intermediate state of the given data. Finally, we have also filtered out some miscellaneous features. Some notable mentions are kurtosis, entropy, skewness.

4.2.1 Statistical Features

From the windowed data, some handcrafted statistical features have been extracted from each window. To understand the frequency and occurrence interval of a specific activity, some features like peak-to-peak distance, peak-to-peak period, upper and lower peak number and so on have been measured. We have also determined mean, rms, maximum, minimum, variance, interquartile range, etc., to understand the central tendency of the data. The skewness of the data has been determined to analyse whether the data is symmetrical or not. Another crucial feature, kurtosis, has been found to know the degree of the presence of outliers in the distribution. The determination of entropy has figured out the average level of information innated in the dataset. Signal magnitude area (SMA) has been calculated using the curve under the three axis's magnitude.

4.2.2 Geometrical Features

For geometrical features, the rms value of each window has been calculated, and after that, numerous geometrical features have been pulled out. Figure 5 demonstrates the body marker orientation of a subject and depicts the movement of marker position for different activities. Depending on them, we have extracted our geometrical features.

1. **Joint Coordinates**: Joint coordinates are nothing but the 3D coordinate of each joint of the body, such as (X_m, Y_m, Z_m), representing coordinates and a joint's three-dimensional position. From the joint coordinates, positions of each joint can easily be identified.
2. **Joint to Joint Distance**: Joint-to-joint distance between (X_n, Y_n, Z_n) and (X_m, Y_m, Z_m) is nothing but the magnitude of joint-to-joint vector. Joint coordinates have been subtracted to determine the joint-to-joint vector. Distances between body joints (JJ_D in Fig. 5b) have been calculated using the mathematical equation:

$$J_{mn} = \sqrt{(X_m - X_n)^2 + (Y_m - Y_n)^2 + (Z_m - Z_n)^2} \tag{1}$$

3. **Joint to Line Distance**: A perpendicular was drawn from a joint to opposite line vector. The line equation can be stated as:

$$\frac{X - a}{f} = \frac{Y - b}{g} = \frac{Z - c}{h} \tag{2}$$

Here, directing vector of this line is: $s = \{f, g, h\}$, coordinate of a point on this line: $M_1 = \{a, b, c\}$, and joint coordination is $M_2 = \{X_m, Y_m, Z_m\}$. So, distance of the joint from that line (JL_D in Fig. 5b) will be:

$$d = \frac{M_2 M_1 \times s}{s} \tag{3}$$

where M_2M_1 refers the distance vector from M_2 to M_1. So, $M_2M_1 = M_2 - M_1$.
4. **Joint to Joint orientation:** It represents the unit vectors along the line vectors [19]. By subtracting one joint coordinate from another, line vectors have been calculated. Dividing line vectors by their magnitudes has given the joint-to-joint orientation (JJ_O in Fig. 5b) the following equation:

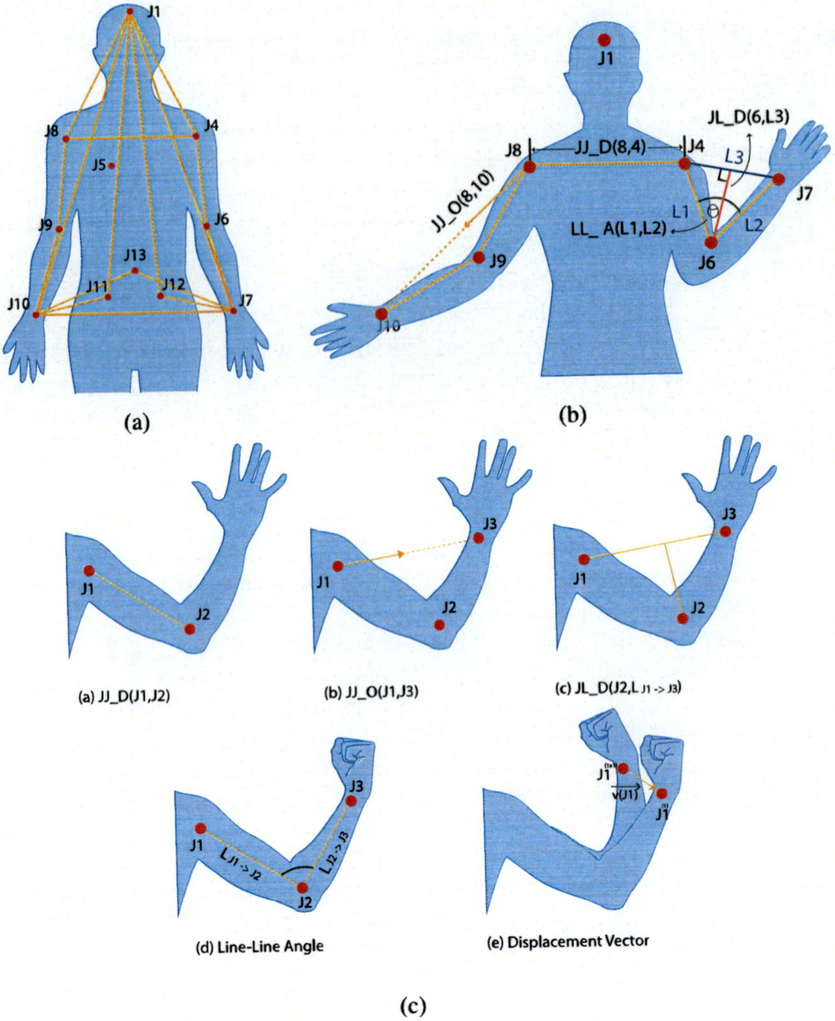

Fig. 5 Geometrical Feature extraction: **a** Body markers, **b** Joint movements and **c** Hand movements

$$J_m to J_n = \frac{(X_n - X_m) + (Y_n - Y_m) + (Z_n - Z_m)}{\sqrt{(X_m - X_n)^2 + (Y_m - Y_n)^2 + (Z_m - Z_n)^2}} \tag{4}$$

5. **Line to Line Angle:** Angle between the line vectors has given us some extra features to recognize the activities. Angles (LL_A in Fig. 5b) have been extracted by applying the formula:

$$\cos\theta = \frac{L_k \cdot L_{k+p}}{|L_k| \times |L_{k+p}|} \quad (5)$$

where L_k and L_{k+p} are line vectors and $n = 1, 2, 3, \ldots$

6. **Line-to-Line Distance:** This part determines perpendicular distances between the line vectors.
7. **Joint-to-Plane Distance:** Three joints have created some planes, and the distance of those planes from different joints has been pulled out.

After extracting all the possible statistical and geometrical features, we have been left with over 4000 features, which can be categorized in 22 unique divisions (shown in Fig. 4).

4.3 *Feature Selection*

When developing a machine learning model, it is hardly ever the case that all of the variables in the dataset help generalize the model. In our scenario, from 11 sensors, we have extracted over 4000 features, including geometrical and statistical features. We have utilized the Python Sklearn library and filtered less important features using (1) mutual information gain and (2) ANOVA f-test. Note that some of the markers might be mislabeled in this dataset, so we have chosen over 700 essential features to ensure no loss of information while reducing the dimensionality of features.

4.4 *Model Selection and Evaluation*

In this study, we have explored several classifiers to classify the provided activities. Most of the classes have similar features overlapping, so we have selected popular algorithms for multi-class classification. As we have a fair amount of feature vectors, we need to be careful not to overfit our model (Table 2).

Table 2 Accuracy (in %) comparison chart of different models

Classifier	Train accuracy	Test accuracy
Support vector machine	93.2	53.7
Random forest	97.5	63.4
Extra trees	94.7	64.6

4.4.1 Support Vector Machine (SVM)

SVM is suitable for multi-class classification using the 'One vs. All' method which splits the multi-classes into multiple binary classifications and makes predictions based on the most confident model. As SVMs use regularization, they resist over-fitting even when the number of feature inputs is large. Regularization reduces the SVM's sensitivity to outliers and improves its overall generalization. In this case, we considered polynomial kernel with degree=3 and regularization parameter as 0.9.

4.4.2 Random Forest (RF)

Random forest splits the data based on certain decisions and tries to generalize the classification problem. This model utilizes bagging to construct trees. It sub-samples the input data with replacement. Random forest can handle large datasets with higher dimensionality and identify the most significant variables making it a powerful classification tool. In this work, the following parameters are considered: number of estimators = 300, criterion = 'entropy', maximum depth = 12, and maximum features = 0.9.

4.4.3 Extra Trees (ExT)

Extra trees is a type of ensemble learning which builds a set of decision trees from all of the given samples [20]. The decision rule is chosen randomly during tree construction. The benefit of ExT over RF is that the former split the trees based on random selection, which significantly reduces variance and computational cost. In this work, the following parameters are considered: number of estimators = 300, criterion = 'entropy', minimum samples split = 3, maximum depth = 10, maximum features = 0.9.

5 Result and Discussion

We have used fivefold cross-validation and leave-one-subject-out cross-validation for model evaluation (LOSOCV) [19]. As the activities overlap each other, LOSOCV gives more realistic results over fivefold cross-validation. Accuracy and F1-score have been used to evaluate the models. 70–20–10 split formation was used for the train–validate–test set. Extra trees classifier reduces variance with random splits of all observations, which has helped us tackle outliers. SVM has shown quick calculation regarding the output but has a comparatively low accuracy level, while random forest has a lengthy computational time with better generalization. Within all classifiers used in this project, extra tree classifier has cooked up the best possible outcome out of all classifiers that have been at our disposal. Extra tree classifier is the best suited

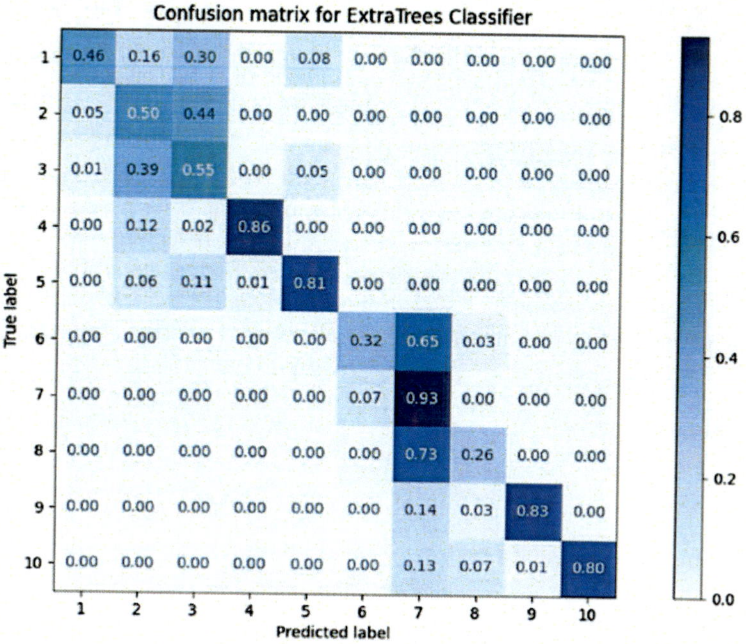

Fig. 6 Confusion matrix for extra tree classifier demonstrates how much the model has become confused while making predictions and classifying the activities

as it has managed to balance the bias and the variance of the data much better than other classifiers used for this project. So, at the end of the day, extra tree classifier puts us in a very convenient position (Fig. 6).

The confusion matrix reveals the problematic situation between activities 2 (normal (outward)) and 3 (forgot to put ingredients (inward)), and 6 (failed to put ingredients (outward)) and 8 (turn over bento box (outward)). We have plotted the various activities for better visualization. We have noticed that activities 2 and 3, as well as, 6 and 8 have significant resemblances. Therefore, they have signal overlapping in terms of distances and angles among various joint points. We need to decipher related activities and their corresponding relationships to find smarter features for better accuracy. Analysing the behaviour of the three classifiers, it emerges that extra tree demonstrated the best performance, allowing them to recognize more than 60% of the activities correctly.

6 Conclusion and Future Works

We are awed at the data harvesting procedure for this challenge. The attention to the details and sophisticated approach to extract data has mesmerized us. We did our level best to process the data and cohesively put together a model, train for maximum accuracy and receive meritorious output. We have explored different machine learning algorithms using multiple sets of features in order to classify the packaging activity with a short computational period. Please note that we were provided with only thirteen sensory data (some of them mislabeled) instead of all twenty-nine sensory data. So, we did our work based on the parts provided data and managed to get some crucial insights through it. We can infer that if we have the data of all of the twenty-nine sensors, the model accuracy would be enhanced even further. In addition to that, if twenty-nine sensory data were present, the dataset would have been large enough for us to explore deep learning-based models (e.g. recurrent neural network). We plan to study the data further by improving our method regarding this dataset in the future.

Acknowledgements This research has been partially assisted by ***Shadmin Sultana*** (University of Dhaka, Bangladesh) with some illustration works.

7 Appendix

Sensor modalities	Front head, left and right shoulder, left and right elbow, left and right wrist, right offset, v sacral.
Features used	Peak-to-peak distance, peak-to-peak time, upper peaks number, Lower peaks number, mean, RMS, maximum, minimum, variance, IQR, MAD, SMA, skewness, kurtosis, entropy, joint-to-joint Distance, joint-to-joint orientation, joint-to-plane distance, angles, joint-line distance, line-line distance, line-plane distance
Programming language	Python 3.9
Libraries	Numpy, Pandas, scipy, sklearn, matplotlib
Window size	2000
Post processing	N/A
Machine specification	RAM: 8 GB, CPU: Intel COREi5 @2.3 GHz, GPU: N/A
Training and testing time	SVM: Training time 10.56 s and Testing time 5.31 Random Forest: Training time 1060.11 s and Testing time 0.17 Extra Trees: Training time 103.49 s and Testing time 0.41

References

1. Mahmud, S., Tonmoy, M., Bhaumik, K.K., Rahman, A.K.M., Ashraful Amin, M., Shoyaib, M., Khan, M.A.H., Ali, A.A.: Human Activity Recognition from Wearable Sensor Data Using Self-attention. arXiv preprint arXiv:2003.09018 (2020)
2. Su, B., Wu, H., Sheng, M.: Human action recognition method based on hierarchical framework via Kinect skeleton data. In: 2017 International Conference on Machine Learning and Cybernetics (ICMLC), vol. 1. IEEE (2017)

3. Abir, F.F., Faisal, M.A.A., Shahid, O., Ahmed, M.U.: Contactless human activity analysis: an overview of different modalities. In: Ahad, M.A.R., Mahbub, U., Rahman, T. (eds.) Contactless Human Activity Analysis. Intelligent Systems Reference Library, vol. 200. Springer, Cham (2021)
4. De-La-Hoz-Franco, E., Ariza-Colpas, P., Quero, J.M., Espinilla, M.: Sensor-based datasets for human activity recognition—a systematic review of literature. IEEE Access **6**, 59192–59210 (2018)
5. Masum, A.K.M., Bahadur, E.H., Shan-A-Alahi, A., Chowdhury, M.A.U.Z., Uddin, M.R., Noman, A.A.: Human activity recognition using accelerometer, gyroscope and magnetometer sensors: deep neural network approaches. In: 2019 10th International Conference on Computing, Communication and Networking Technologies (ICCCNT), IEEE (2019)
6. Demrozi, F., Pravadelli, G., Bihorac, A., Rashidi, P.: Human activity recognition using inertial, physiological and environmental sensors: a comprehensive survey. IEEE Access (2020)
7. Miura, T., Kaiga, T., Shibata, T., Tajima, K., Tamamoto, H.: Low-dimensional feature vector extraction from motion capture data by phase plane analysis. J. Information Process. **25**, 884–887 (2017)
8. Hossain, T., Sarker, S., Rahman, S., Ahad, M.A.R.: Skeleton-based human action recognition on large-scale datasets. In: Vision, Sensing and Analytics: Integrative Approaches, Springer Nature Switzerland AG, pp. 125–146 (2021)
9. Sarker, S., Rahman, S., Hossain, T., Ahmed, S.F., Jamal, L., Ahad, M.A.R.: Skeleton-based activity recognition: preprocessing and approaches. In: Contactless Human Activity Analysis, Springer Nature Switzerland AG, pp. 43–82 (2021)
10. Cao, X., Kudo, W., Ito, C., Shuzo, M., Maeda, E.: Activity recognition using ST-GCN with 3D motion data. In: Adjunct Proceedings of the 2019 ACM International Joint Conference on Pervasive and Ubiquitous Computing and Proceedings of the 2019 ACM International Symposium on Wearable Computers (2019)
11. Lin, Z., Jiang, Z., Davis, L.S.: Recognizing actions by shape-motion prototype trees.. In: 2009 IEEE 12th International Conference on Computer Vision. IEEE (2009)
12. Su, B., Wu, H., Sheng, M., Shen, C.: Accurate hierarchical human actions recognition from kinect skeleton data. IEEE Access **7**, 52532–52541 (2019)
13. Zhang, S., Yang, Y., Xiao, J., Liu, X., Yang, Y., Xie, D., Zhuang, Y.: Fusing geometric features for skeleton-based action recognition using multilayer LSTM networks. IEEE Trans. Multimedia **20**(9), 2330–2343 (2018)
14. Xia, L., Chen, C.-C., Aggarwal, J.K.: View invariant human action recognition using histograms of 3d joints. In: 2012 IEEE Computer Society Conference on Computer Vision and Pattern Recognition Workshops. IEEE (2012)
15. Chaudhry, R., Ofli, F., Kurillo, G., Bajcsy, R., Vidal, R.: Bio-inspired dynamic 3d discriminative skeletal features for human action recognition. In Proceedings of the IEEE Conference on Computer Vision and Pattern Recognition Workshops (2013)
16. Tarek, M.H., Kadir, M.E., Mahbub, M., Akash, P.S., Ali, A.A., Shoyaib, M.: Mutual Information based feature selection for nurse care activity recognition. In: 2020 Joint 9th International Conference on Informatics, Electronics & Vision (ICIEV) and 2020 4th International Conference on Imaging, Vision & Pattern Recognition (icIVPR), pp. 1–6. IEEE (2020)
17. Alia, S.S., Adachi, K., Nahid, N., Kaneko, H., Lago, P., Inoue, S.: Bento Packaging Activity Recognition Challenge (2021). Available at: https://doi.org/10.21227/cwhs-t440
18. Siraj, M.S., Shahid, O., Ahad, M.A.R.: Cooking activity recognition with varying sampling rates using deep convolutional GRU framework. In: Ahad M.A.R., Lago P., Inoue S. (eds.) Human Activity Recognition Challenge. Smart Innovation, Systems and Technologies, vol. 199. Springer, Singapore (2021)
19. Kadir, M.E., Akash, P.S., Sharmin, S., Ali, A.A., Shoyaib, M.: Can a simple approach identify complex nurse care activity? In: Adjunct Proceedings of the 2019 ACM International Joint Conference on Pervasive and Ubiquitous Computing and Proceedings of the 2019 ACM International Symposium on Wearable Computers (2019)
20. Geurts, P., Ernst, D., Wehenkel, L.: Extremely randomized trees. Mach. Learn. **63**(1), 3–42 (2021)

Bento Packaging Activity Recognition Based on Statistical Features

Faizul Rakib Sayem, Md. Mamun Sheikh, and Md Atiqur Rahman Ahad

Abstract Due to the fast advancements of low-cost micro-embedded sensors and MoCap sensors, human action recognition has become an essential study topic and is garnering a lot of interest in different sectors. Recently, it is drawing a lot of attention in human-robot collaboration to assist human to preform regular tasks step-wise because it is difficult to obtain human labor at a lower wage to monitor industrial works. In this work, we have presented a straightforward machine learning paradigm to recognize ten different *Bento* (lunch-box) packaging activities in real-time world. Unlike other skeleton-based human activity recognition domain, it is a very challenging task due to the absence of lower-body marker information. Under these circumstances, we have provided an in-depth statistical analysis of different Bento packaging activities. After feature extraction process, we have used several machine algorithms and obtained best results in random forest classifier using hyperparameter tuning. We have achieved 64.9% validation accuracy using leave-one-out method.

1 Introduction

Human action recognition (HAR) in real-time applications is both an exciting and difficult problem because it differs from the diverse settings and behaviors of a person. It has become a popular research area with numerous applications in surveillance, health care monitoring, robot vision, fall detection, sports analysis, entertainment, autonomous driving, security, and smart homes, and so on [1, 2]. The research domain of HAR can be divided into two categories: vision-based or sensor-based techniques. The majority of the research focuses on the spatial and temporal aspects of an action

F. Rakib Sayem · Md. M. Sheikh
University of Dhaka, Dhaka, Bangladesh
e-mail: faizulrakib-2017214832@eee.du.ac.bd

Md. M. Sheikh
e-mail: mamunsheikhdueee52@gmail.com

M. A. R. Ahad (✉)
University of East London, London, UK
e-mail: atiqahad@du.ac.bd; atiqahad@yahoo.com

M. A. R. Ahad et al. (eds.), *Sensor- and Video-Based Activity and Behavior Computing*, Smart Innovation, Systems and Technologies 291,
https://doi.org/10.1007/978-981-19-0361-8_13

recognition video sequence recorded by RGB cameras. Illumination, varied angles of view, color videos reduce the overall performance significantly in vision-based HAR. Skeleton-based HAR has made remarkable progress because of the ease of environmental setups, faster execution speed, and low cost of Kinect sensors. In the skeleton-based HAR domain, research on aged people's daily activity monitoring [3] and physical rehabilitation exercise assessment of patients [4] has recently gained a lot of traction. It is very useful since it will track their regular activities, provide real-time feedback on their physical health status in daily basis, and supply physicians with current information regularly without costing transportation problem and huge health care cost burdens [5, 6].

Researchers have made remarkable progress that explored several models for automatic recognition and assessment of human actions in real-time applications. Machine learning (ML) techniques such as support vector machine [7], random forest [8], and KNN [9] have been used to tackle the HAR problem for a long time. In addition, Bayesian networks [10] and Markov models [11] have been used with promising results. Deep learning models have sparked a lot of interest recently, and they deliver excellent results in the HAR domain with their superior feature extraction abilities. Researchers in [12] provided 3D CNN model to classify human actions in the real-time surveillance videos. Zhu et al. [13] proposed a deep LSTM model to extract the concurrence features in HAR domain. Lee et al. [14] proposed a temporal sliding LSTM model for skeleton-based HAR. Chaudhry et al. [15] provided a 3D discriminative skeleton features to recognize human actions.

Very recently, HAR has gained a lot of interest for its use in tracking the actions of workers in many sectors. There have been some research progress of HAR domain in real-time applications for hospitals and nursing homes [16, 17]. Unlike conventional activities such as jogging, walking, running, standing, sitting [18], recognizing nursing services toward is a difficult and challenging process because traits of an activity rely on both patients and nurses, and so, there is a lot of intra-class diversity in nursing activities. Besides nursing activities, complex cooking activity recognition [19] was arranged in 2020. When it comes to cooking, for example, HAR is quite good for reminding a lonely old person of a missing step or ensuring that a nutritious diet is being maintained. This sort of industrial activity dataset collection is really difficult to come by. In SHL challenge [15], HAR has been employed to classify eight different locomotion and transportation activities.

This is a major issue for a variety of sectors that demand a large number of workers at a cheap wage. HAR has a significant influence on human-robot collaboration. For example, When cooking in a industry, the procedures and materials applied in the dish are entirely up to the user. However in packaging task, it is extremely usual to insert an in-gradient. If robots can be utilized to help people with these kind of small tasks, they might be a perfect solution to this issue. In this paper, we provide a simple machine learning framework to recognize Bento packaging activities. Our machine model is very efficient and can be trained with low computational cost.

The paper is organized as follow: In Sect. 2, we have provided a short description of this challenge dataset [17]. In Sect. 3, we represent our proposed workflow to solve this problem. The later Sect. 4 provides our results. The final Sect. 5 provides a summary of our work and some future works.

Fig. 1 Activity list of Bento packaging activity recognition

Activity No	Scenarios	Patterns
1	Normal	Inward
2		Outward
3	Forgot to put ingredients	Inward
4		Outward
5	Failed to put ingredients	Inward
6		Outward
7	Turn over bento-box	Inward
8		Outward
9	Fix/rearranging ingredients	Inward
10		Outward

2 Dataset Description

The dataset [20] for this Bento Packaging Activity Recognition Challenge comprises a high number of *NaN* values and solely contains skeletal joint 3D coordinates obtained by MoCap sensor. The train dataset contains ten different activities performed by three subjects. Each action contains five repetitions performed by each subject. The participants are instructed to do activities in five different scenarios such as normal, forgot to put ingredients, failed to put ingredients, turn over Bento box, and fix/rearranging ingredients. Length of each activity segment is about 50–70 s. The dataset is perfectly balanced which is very rare in other HAR domain. Skeleton joints coordinates were captured 100 Hz, and no preprocessing technique is applied to this data. The dataset contains no information about the lower-body joints. The dataset is difficult to work with since it contains just 13 joints from the upper-body parts and a high number of empty values. The test data consists of one subject, and the format is same as train dataset (Fig. 1).

3 Methodology

In general skeleton-based HAR, 3D coordinates of different markers in body are provided. Human behaviors can be described as time sequences of skeleton positions, according to our basic premise. Our main purpose of this work is to classify ten different Bento packaging activities in real-time applications. In this section, we will introduce our proposed approach to classify ten different Bento packaging activities. A simple block diagram of our proposed approach to solve this challenge is shown in Fig. 2. Our method consists of three different major steps: (1) data preprocessing, (2) feature extraction, and (3) model training.

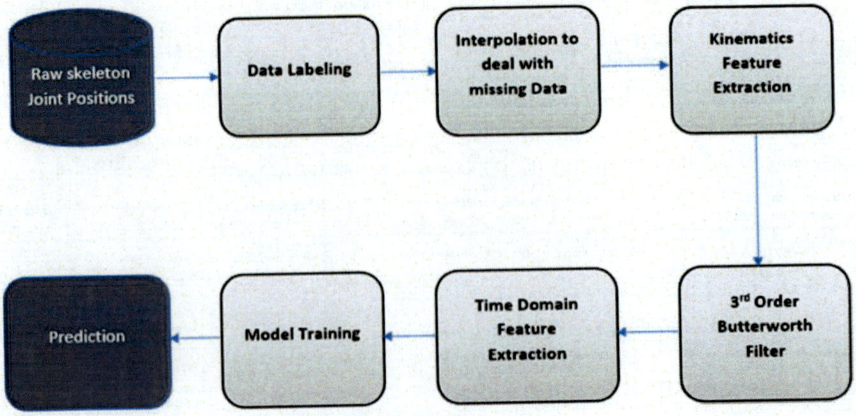

Fig. 2 Simple system flow diagram of the employed method

3.1 Data Preprocessing

The skeleton joint positions acquired by MoCap sensor are preprocessed via several steps. First, we collect raw skeleton joints positions and their corresponding action labels from different folders and merge them into a single dataframe. In most cases, the issue of missing data is overlooked while collecting data from MoCap sensors. In this challenge, almost every repetition of an action has a large number of missing values. To solve this problem, we employed the linear interpolation approach to fill the empty values considering real-time circumstances. We did not apply any segmentation method because the initial and last segments of an action frequently show different characteristics due to both technical errors and human mistakes.

3.2 Feature Extraction

Feature extraction is a dimensional reduction procedure that converts raw input data into a set of features that may be used to distinguish certain actions. In this challenge, the dataset was provided with only skeleton joint positions. This is a very challenging dataset because only 13 upper-body joint coordinates are available. We have extracted various joint angles, joint distance, and joint vectors. For angles, we have extracted both elbow and shoulder angles and their corresponding difference. For joint distances, we have extracted elbow-elbow, wrist-wrist, and both shoulder-wrist distances. We have extracted different joint vectors in all 3D coordinates. After extracting all the motion features, we have employed a third-order Butterworth low-pass filter to remove random noises and spikes of skeleton data. In total, we used 47 different spatial features including joint distances, joint angles, and joint vectors.

After that, we used several important time-domain features which are likely relevant to solve our classification problem. In general, we employed minimum, maximum, mean, and standard deviation, median absolute deviation, peak-to-peak range, mean-to-peak range, as in earlier HAR research. Besides, we have used some other time-domain features. These features are listed below along with their definitions and mathematical expressions:

25th Percentile: It is also described as the first quarter ($Q1$). The 25th percentile refers to a data value that is less than or equal to 25% of the sorted dataset.

$$Q1 = \left(\frac{25}{100}\right)n \tag{1}$$

Here, n is the total number of samples in a repetition.

75th Percentile: It is also known as the third quartile ($Q3$). The 75th percentile is the data value that is less than or equal to 75

$$Q3 = \left(\frac{75}{100}\right)n \tag{2}$$

Interquartile Range (IQR): It is the calculation of the statistical variation which denotes the difference between 75th and 25th percentiles.

$$\mathrm{IQR} = Q3 - Q1 \tag{3}$$

Skewness: Skewness calculates the asymmetry of a real-valued random variable's probability distribution around its mean. The skewness value can be any of the following: positive, zero, negative, or undefined.

$$\mathrm{Skewness} = \frac{n}{(n-1)(n-2)} \sum \frac{(Xi - \bar{X})^3}{\sigma^3} \tag{4}$$

After all spatial and time-domain feature extraction, we have found total 615 features. Then, we train our dataset with various machine learning algorithms such as random forest classifier (RFC), extra tree classifier (ETC), support vector machine (SVM), and K-nearest neighbors (KNN).

4 Result and Analysis

We have suggested a simple machine learning paradigm to solve the classification problem of Bento packaging activities. The overall performance of our suggested method employing multiple machine learning algorithms will be described in this section. We have used hyperparameter tuning to get the best results in validation data for random forest classifier. We have tuned the following paramters: maximum depth, number of estimators, minimum samples for split, and number of jobs. Among them, *maximum depth* is the most dominant parameter. It refers to the depth of each tree in the forest. If it is very high, then the model overfits the test data. Only tuning this parameter increases an average accuracy of 10% and reaches an average accuracy of 58%. However, by tuning all the mentioned hyperparameters, we have been able to increase the overall performance by 17%, and finally, our average accuracy reaches 64.9%.

The train dataset consists of total three subjects. For each subject, total repetitions for each activity is five, except for Activity 6 and Activity 9. For these two activities, we got six repetitions. We have used leave-one-out cross-validation strategy to test the robustness of our proposed method. Each time, we have trained our model with two subjects and validated our results on the activities of the other subject. In this manner, we have achieved three different accuracies using three different combinations of data. We have obtained the highest accuracy in RFC model, which is 64.9%. Using leave-one-out method, our results are shown in Figs. 3, 4, and 5, respectively. Random forest is an ensemble machine learning model, in which each tree in the forest produces a class prediction, and the class having the most votes becomes the prediction of the model. Besides, we have found 61.6%, 58%, and 57% in ETC, SVM, and KNN models, respectively. We have obtained a promising result on validation dataset.

Fig. 3 Confusion matrix while employing leave-one-out method for Subject 1

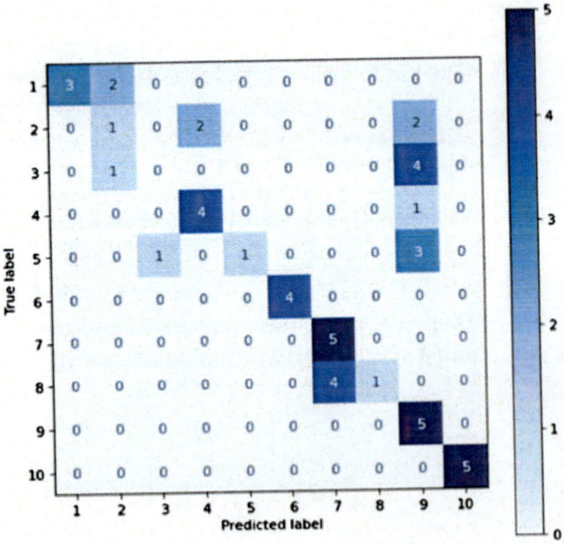

Fig. 4 Confusion matrix while employing leave-one-out method for Subject 2

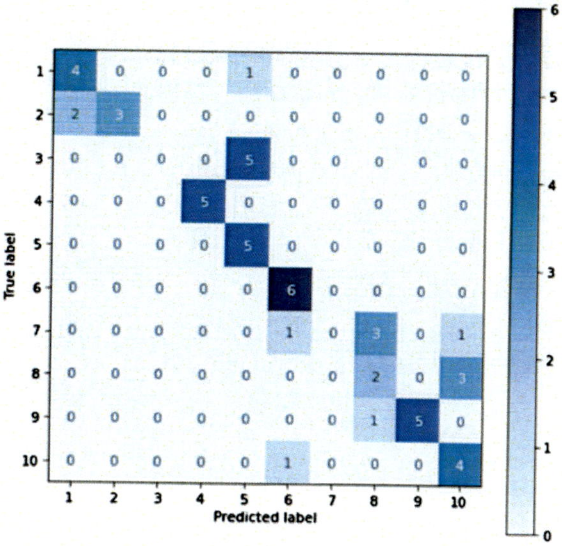

Fig. 5 Confusion matrix while employing leave-one-out method for Subject 3

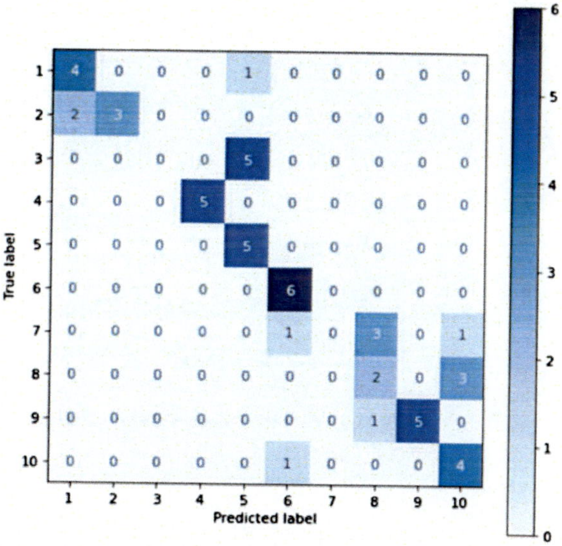

5 Conclusion

Skeleton-based HAR is drawing a lot of attraction in human-robot interaction in various industrial applications. However, research progress in this domain has not been flourished yet due the lack of publicly available challenging dataset. In this paper, we have provided a simple yet efficient machine learning framework to recognize complex Bento packaging activities. Our proposed method is very practical and can be trained costing less computational resources. Our experimental result illustrates that our proposed workflow can provide a decent accuracy. The primary difficulty we encountered when working on this difficult data was large missing data, which we solved using the linear interpolation approach. In the future, we will add some more complex features to improve the robustness of our model. In addition, we will explore several hybrid deep neural networks to improve overall performance for automatic recognizing of packaging activities. We are optimistic that our method will yield superior outcomes on the final test data as well.

The Appendix information of our dataset and methodology and computation resources are shown in Fig. 6.

Used sensor modalities	Skeletal 3D joints (MoCap Sensor)
Features used	Minimum, Maximum, Mean, Standard Deviation, Median Absolute Deviation, Peak-Peak Range, Mean-Peak Range, Percentile (25th and 75th), Interquartile Range, Skewness.
Programming language and libraries used	Language: Python. Libraries: panda, NumPy, Matplotlib, Sci-kit Learn, SciPy.
Window Settings and Post Processing	No windowing technique and post processing are applied.
Training and Testing time	Training time: approximately 1.5 second. Testing time: Less than 0.5 second.
Machine specification (RAM, CPU, GPU)	PC specification: RAM: 8 GB. CPU: AMD RYZEN 4000 @ 3 GHz. GPU: NVIDIA GEFORCE GTX 1650 Ti. Google Colab: Free web version with CPU: 2 Intel® Xenon® @2.30 GHz. RAM: 12 GB.

Fig. 6 Appendix information of our paper

Question Answer of the Reviewer

Reviewer 1

Answer: Thanks a lot for your valuable time and corrections. Our Answers are given below:

1. We have tried but failed to do so. We will correct it within 6th October.
2. The authors have found it also appropriate to use Fig. 1 instead of Table If you totally disagree, then we will change it.
3. We don't see free space in page 3. The free spaces before table and section are generated automatically.
4. We have corrected the naming of the heading.
5. We have corrected the punctuation problem in that Result and Analysis Sect. 6. We have changed the location of our image and now it does not interfere with references.
6. We have added Appendix Information in a table.

Reviewer 2

Answer: Thanks a lot for assessing our paper and providing good corrections. Our answers are given below:

1. We have corrected these language and punctuation errors.
2. We have added an appendix and it contains all the features used in our model.
3. Leave-one-out method means dropping a subject from train data and using it in validation data to test the performance of different models. I have added it clearly in Result and Analysis Section.
4. Cross Validation means leave-one-out method. We have now only used leave-one-out method in our paper to remove confusion.
5. We have now added results of hyperparameter tuning clearly in Result and Analysis Section.
6. We have added Appendix Information in a table.

References

1. Ahad, M.A.R.: Vision and sensor-based human activity recognition: challenges ahead. https://doi.org/10.4018/978-1-7998-2584-5.ch002 (2020)
2. Ahad, M.A.R., Antar, A.D., Shahid, O.: Proceedings of the IEEE/CVF Conference on Computer Vision and Pattern Recognition (CVPR) Workshops, pp. 1–11 (2019)
3. Abbate, S., Avvenuti, M., Corsini, P., Light, J., Vecchio, A.: Monitoring of human movements for fall detection and activities recognition in elderly care using wireless sensor network: a survey, wireless sensor networks: application—centric Design, Geoff V Merrett and Yen Kheng Tan, IntechOpen, https://doi.org/10.5772/13802 (2010)
4. Liao, Y., Vakanski, A., Xian, M., Paul, D., Baker, R.: A review of computational approaches for evaluation of rehabilitation exercises, Comput. Biol. Med. **119** (2020)
5. Ho, I.K., Goldschneider, K.R., Kashikar-Zuck, S., Kotagal, U., Tessman, C., Jones, B.: Healthcare utilization and indirect burden among families of pediatric patients with chronic pain. J. Musculoskeletal Pain **16**(3), 155–164 (2008)

6. Machlin, S.R., Chevan, J., Yu, W.W., Zodet, M.W.: Determinants of utilization and expenditures for episodes of ambulatory physical therapy among adults. Phys. Therapy **91**(7), 1018–1029 (2011)
7. Abidine, B.M., Fergani, L., Fergani, B., Oussalah., M.: The joint use of sequence features combination and modified weighted SVM for improving daily activity recognition. Pattern Anal. Appl. **21**(1), 119–138 (2018)
8. Hu, C., Chen, Y., Hu, L., Peng, X.: A novel random forests based class incremental learning method for activity recognition. Pattern Recognition **78**, 277–290 (2018)
9. Förster, K., Monteleone, S., Calatroni, A., Roggen, D., Troster, G.: Incremental kNN classifier exploiting correct-error teacher for activity recognition. In: Ninth International Conference on Machine Learning and Applications **2010**, 445–450 (2010)
10. Xiao, Q., Song, R.: Action recognition based on hierarchical dynamic Bayesian network. Multimed Tools Appl. **77**, 6955–6968 (2018)
11. Sok, P., Xiao, T., Azeze, Y., Jayaraman, A., Albert, M.V.: Activity recognition for incomplete spinal cord injury subjects using hidden Markov models. IEEE Senso. J. **18**(15), 6369–6374 (2018)
12. Ji, S., Xu, W., Yang, M., Yu, K.: 3D convolutional neural networks for human action recognition. IEEE Trans. Pattern Anal. Mach. Intell. **35**(1), 221–231 (2013)
13. Zhu, W., Lan, C., Xing, J., Zeng, W., Li, Y., Shen, L., Xie, X.: Co-occurrence feature learning for skeleton based action recognition using regularized deep LSTM networks. In: Proceedings of the AAAI Conference on Artificial Intelligence, vol. 30 no. 1 2016)
14. Lee, I., Kim, D., Kang, S., Lee, S.: Ensemble deep learning for skeleton-based action recognition using temporal sliding LSTM networks. IEEE Inter. Conf. Comput. Vis. (ICCV) **2017**, 1012–1020 (2017)
15. Wang, L., Gjoreskia, H., Murao, K., Okita, T., Roggen, D.: Summary of the sussex-huawei locomotion-transportation recognition challenge. In: Proceedings of the 2018 ACM International Joint Conference and 2018 International Symposium on Pervasive and Ubiquitous Computing and Wearable Computers (UbiComp'18), 1521–1530 (2018)
16. Lago, P., Alia, S.S., Takeda, S., Mairittha, T., Mairittha, N., Faiz, F., Nishimura, Y., Adachi, K., Okita, T., Charpillet, F., Inoue, S.: Nurse care activity recognition challenge: summary and results. UbiComp/ISWC'19 Adjunct, pp. 746–751 (2019)
17. Alia, S.S., Lago, P., Adachi, K., Hossain, T., Goto, H., Okita, T., Inoue, S.: Summary of the 2nd nurse care activity recognition challenge using lab and field data. In: Adjunct Proc. UbiComp-ISWC'20, pp. 378–383 (2020)
18. Pinilla, M., Medina, J., Nugent, C.: UCAmI Cup. Analyzing the UJA human activity recognition dataset of activities of daily living. Proceedings **2**, 19, 1267
19. Alia, S.S., et al.: Summary of the cooking activity recognition challenge. In: Ahad M.A.R., Lago P., Inoue S. (eds) Human activity recognition challenge. Smart innovation, systems and technologies, vol. 199. Springer (2021)
20. Alia, S.S., Adachi, K., Nahid, N., Kaneko, H., Lago, P., Inoue, S.: Bento packaging activity recognition challenge. IEEE Dataport. (2021). https://dx.doi.org/10.21227/cwhs-t440.s
21. Chaudhry, R., Ofli, F., Kurillo, G., Bajcsy, R., Vidal, R.: Bio-inspired dynamic 3D discriminative skeletal features for human action recognition. In: *IEEE Conference on Computer Vision and Pattern Recognition Workshops*, vol. 2013, pp. 471–478 (2013)
22. Ahad, M.A.R., Ahmed, M., Antar, A.D., Makihara, Y., Yagi, Y.: Action recognition using kinematics posture feature on 3D skeleton joint locations. Pattern Recogn. Lett. **145**, 216–224 (2021)
23. Adachi, K., Alia, S.S., Nahid, N., Kaneko, H., Lago, P., Inoue, S.: Summary of the bento Packaging activity recognition challenge. In: The 3rd International Conference on Activity and Behavior Computing (ABC2021) (2021)

Using K-Nearest Neighbours Feature Selection for Activity Recognition

Björn Friedrich, Tetchi Ange-Michel Orsot, and Andreas Hein

Abstract As Team *2A&B Core*, we contributed a K-nearest neighbour approach for classifying ten different activities for the Bento Packing Activity Recognition Challenge. We used hand-engineered features from motion capture data. Before classifying the data, we scaled it and applied a principal component analysis. We used the K-nearest neighbour classifier to find the best feature, and we found that the best feature was one that was related to a fixed position. Our approach achieved an accuracy of 38.78% on our validation subject and 42.00% on our test subject.

1 Introduction

The industry is using robots for a variety of tasks, because robots are faster and have more power than humans. Moreover, robots can work in hazardous environments and do tasks which are too dangerous for humans. This advantages are coming at the costs of some disadvantages like the need of structured environments and well-defined tasks and operations. Usually, humans and robots have distinct workspaces, because industrial robots can easily harm humans. To support humans at their work, robots and humans can work in a joint workspace, or the robot can work in a distinct workspace to prepare workpieces, materials, or further process the produce of a human. If the human makes a mistake, then the robot is not able to process the faulty workpiece. If the robot is able to detect a faulty workpiece, the robot can either sort it out or fix it. In both cases, the robot needs a mechanism to faulty workpieces. In cases where the workpiece is well-defined, deviations from the correct workpiece can be measured

B. Friedrich and T.A.-M. Orsot: Both authors contributed equally to this research.

B. Friedrich (✉) · A. Hein
Carl von Ossietzky University of Oldenburg, Ammerländer Heerstraße 114-118, 26129 Oldenburg, Germany
e-mail: bjoern.friedrich@uni-oldenburg.de

A. Hein
e-mail: andreas.hein@uni-oldenburg.de

M. A. R. Ahad et al. (eds.), *Sensor- and Video-Based Activity and Behavior Computing*, Smart Innovation, Systems and Technologies 291,
https://doi.org/10.1007/978-981-19-0361-8_14

by sensors, e.g. dimensions. However, there are several cases where the deviation can not be measured directly. In the later case, the system must detect the faulty workpiece in another way. One way is to observe the human and use activity recognition. The system can detect an activity that is not supposed to be executed or executed in a way that differs from the correct execution. Activities can be derived from motion, and motion can be accurately measured motion capture systems (MoCap). MoCaps are usually comprised of markers and cameras. The markers are attached to the human, and the cameras are tracking the motion of the markers. This research is part of the *Bento Packaging Activity Recognition Challenge* organised by *Sozo Lab* held as part of the *3rd International Conference on Activity and Behaviour Computing (ABC2021)* [1, 2]. The task is to classify ten different activities executed while packing Bento boxes at a conveyor belt in a laboratory. Four different participants executed ten activities five times, one participant was kept as test participant by the organisers. We used one participant for training, one for validation, and the last one as our internal test participant. Our approach uses hand-engineered features derived from trajectories. After computing the bag-of-words model of the trajectory features, we preprocessed the data by scaling and reducing the dimensions. All steps are done for each feature and participant separately. We were classifying each feature with a K-nearest neighbour classifier. We evaluated all possible combinations of classifiers, and the final ensemble was comprised of one classifier and achieved an accuracy of 38.78% on our validation participant and 42.00% on our internal test participant.

In the next section, we are giving a brief overview over activity recognition using MoCap data. In Sect. 3, we introduce the dataset and explain our feature engineering, preprocessing, and classification steps. In Sect. 4, we present our results and we discuss them in the following section. At last, we conclude our approach and mention some possible future work.

2 State of the Art

MoCap data has been used to classify activities in several domains. In [3], neural networks, random forests, and support vector machines were used to classify gym activities and karate techniques. The authors in [4] and [5] used temporal convolutional neural networks and histograms with density comparison to classify common human motion like walking. In the field of healthcare, a spatial-temporal graph convolutional network was designed to classify nurse care activities [6]. The research in [7] showed that MoCap data improves nurse care activity classification accuracy even though it is only used during the training of a classifier.

The mentioned approaches were used to classify motion where the whole body was involved. The task for the Bento packing challenge is slightly different because the subject's position is fixed, and the activity is mainly done using the upper body especially the arms.

3 Materials and Methods

3.1 Dataset

The dataset (151 csv files) is a set of ten activities repeated five times by three subjects. Each file contains the coordinates of 29 marker in a 3D coordinate system, the subject, and the activity. Each marker describes the movement of a part of the human body on the x, y, and z axes. This makes a total of 89 columns and several rows of frames for the execution of the activity. The following Table 1 provides details on the data for each activity.

3.2 Feature Engineering

In order to be able to create our features from these data, we produced some videos of these markers allowing to see the person in activity, to locate, and verify the position of the markers on the human body. After a deep analysis, we decided to focus on the markers on the arms and ignore the other markers on the body. Markers 4, 6, and 7 represent the right arm, and Markers 8, 9, and 10 represent the left arm. Markers

Table 1 Details of activity data

Activity	Index	Total frames	Average frames	Standard deviation	Total NaN
Normal (inward)	1	93,521	6235.00	688.08	80,778
Normal (outward)	2	92,218	6148.00	474.62	94,632
Forgot to put ingredients (inward)	3	93,128	6208.53	372.01	101,274
Forgot to put ingredients (outward)	4	93,894	6259.60	400.26	147,303
Failed to put ingredients (inward)	5	93,487	6232.46	378.10	154,074
Failed to put ingredients (outward)	6	98,929	6595.26	1175.86	43,815
Turn over Bento box (inward)	7	94,081	6272.06	892.97	39,900
Turn over Bento box (outward)	8	97,613	6507.53	918.40	44,088
Fix/rearranging ingredients (inward)	9	98,817	6176.06	1349.31	83,019
Fix/rearranging ingredients (outward)	10	94,947	6329.80	593.77	57,564

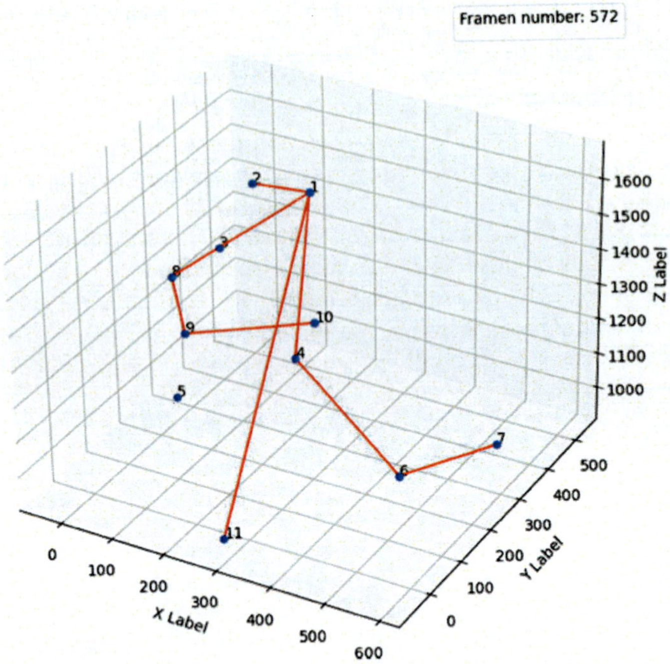

Fig. 1 Motion visualisation

10 and 7 are precisely the hands of the subject (Fig. 1). The videos proved that the coordinates of the work space did not change for all the activities. So, our idea was to define categories of movement allowing the learning and understanding of the activities. These movement categories for each hand marker are defined as follows and build the columns of features:

Let be the set $M = \{m_6, m_7, m_9, m_{10}\}$ of the markers of the hands of the subjects, let be X the set of the coordinates of the hands on the x-axis, let be Y the set of the coordinates of the hands on the y-axis, and let be Z the set of the coordinates of the hands on the z-axis, let be $n \in \mathbb{N}$ the set of the number of recorded frames.

- Motion category: *forward*, $\forall m \in M \wedge \forall y \in Y, y_{n-1} < y_n$,
- Motion category: *backward*, $\forall m \in M \wedge \forall y \in Y, y_{n-1} > y_n$,
- Motion category: *stop_on_y*, $\forall m \in M \wedge \forall y \in Y, y_{n-1} == y_n$,
- Motion category: *turn_left*, $\forall m \in M \wedge \forall x \in X, x_{n-1} > x_n$,
- Motion category: *turn_right*, $\forall m \in M \wedge \forall x \in X, x_{n-1} < x_n$,
- Motion category: *stop_on_x*, $\forall m \in M \wedge \forall x \in X, x_{n-1} == x_n$,
- Motion category: *downward*, $\forall m \in M \wedge \forall z \in Z, z_{n-1} > z_n$,
- Motion category: *upward*, $\forall m \in M \wedge \forall z \in Z, z_{n-1} < z_n$,
- Motion category: *stop_on_z*, $\forall m \in M \wedge \forall z \in Z, z_{n-1} == z_n$,

- Position category: *right*, $\forall m \in M$, $\forall$ angle in $[\angle(\overrightarrow{m_6, m_7}, \overrightarrow{OX}) | \angle(\overrightarrow{m_9, m_{10}}, \overrightarrow{OX})]$, $angle > 270°$ or $angle < 90°$,
- Position category: *left*, $\forall m \in M$, $\forall$ angle in $[\angle(\overrightarrow{m_6, m_7}, \overrightarrow{OX}) | \angle(\overrightarrow{m_9, m_{10}}, \overrightarrow{OX})]$, $angle < 270°$ or $angle > 90°$,
- Position category: *front*, $\forall m \in M$, $\forall$ angle in $[\angle(\overrightarrow{m_6, m_7}, \overrightarrow{OY}) | \angle(\overrightarrow{m_9, m_{10}}, \overrightarrow{OY})]$, $angle > 270°$ or $angle < 90°$,
- Position category: *behind*, $\forall m \in M$, $\forall$ angle in $[\angle(\overrightarrow{m_6, m_7}, \overrightarrow{OY}) | \angle(\overrightarrow{m_9, m_{10}}, \overrightarrow{OY})]$, $angle < 270°$ or $angle > 90°$,
- Position category: *top*, $\forall m \in M \wedge \forall z \in Z, z_n > 0$,
- Position category: *bottom*, $\forall m \in M \wedge \forall z \in Z, z_n < 0$,
- Position category: *same*, if both have the same motion.
- Position category: *different*, if both have the different motion.
- Position category: *over_table*, $\forall m \in M \wedge \forall y \in Y, y_n > 500$,
- Position category: *away_from_table*, i$\forall m \in M \wedge \forall y \in Y, y_n < 500$,

We have a total of 15 features. Each feature has been polished to compensate the trembling recorded movements of the subject, and the numbers were derived from the videos.

3.3 Bag-of-Words

The bag-of-words model is usually used in natural language processing. A bag-of-words feature can be considered as a histogram of words. The frequency of occurrence of words is counted and saved. This disregards all structure of the input and especially the length. We counted the occurrence of different trajectories for each of our features and saved them in a bag-of-words. We had six bag-of-words for each activity repetition.

3.4 Preprocessing

In the first step, we divided our data in training, validation, and test set. We used the data of Subject 1 for validation, the data of Subject 2 for training, and the data of Subject 3 for testing. We preprocessed our features by scaling them to [0, 1]. Afterwards, we used the principal component analysis (PCA) to reduce the feature dimensions. We kept 99% of the variance. We used separate scalers and PCAs for each participant.

3.5 *K*-Nearest Neighbour Feature Selection

We trained one KNN classifier for each feature and evaluated every possible combination of classifiers. The best performing combination was used as final model. The KNN algorithm classifies based on spatial distances and majority vote. In the training phase, all training samples and labels are stored. In classification phase, the distances of the new sample to all training samples are computed, and the maximum of the labels of the K-nearest training samples is assigned to the new sample. We used the Euclidean distance for our classifiers. We trained one KNN classifier for each feature and optimised the parameter K on the validation participant. The feature selection step revealed that the best combination was one classifier for the feature *over belt* only.

4 Results

The results of our final model are shown in Table 2. Table 3 shows the confusion matrix of the final model. The best feature on the training subject was *away from belt* and the worst *front*. The best feature on the validation subject was *over belt* and the worst *upward*. The test subject *over belt* outperformed all other features, and the least performance was on the feature *upward*.

The confusion matrix shows the best performance of our classifier on Activities 2, 5, and 6. The most false classifications occurred for Activities 7–10 without any correct classification. They were all classified as Activity 6.

5 Discussion

Our results show that it is difficult to engineer features that are subject independent. The best feature was the feature *over belt* which was computed by using a fixed position as reference. All subjects had to stick to the position because the task had to be performed there. Moreover, the second best feature was *away from belt* and that supports the assumption. The difference between the accuracy on the validation subject and the test subject was about 4%. So, we assume that the sensitivity to inter-subject variations was small, and the result on the challenge test set will be about 40% as well.

Table 2 Results of the KNN classifiers for each feature (accuracy in %)

Feature (word)	K	Training	Validation	Test
Away from belt	09	63.46	22.45	38.00
Backward	24	25.00	12.24	16.00
Behind	44	15.38	10.20	08.00
Different	20	23.08	18.37	12.00
Downward	14	42.31	10.20	08.00
Forward	23	32.69	20.41	04.00
Front	42	11.54	08.16	10.00
Left	44	13.46	12.24	08.00
Over belt[a]	11	57.69	38.78	42.00
Right	41	19.23	10.20	14.00
Same	44	13.46	14.29	10.00
Stop on x	01	13.46	10.20	12.00
Stop on y	03	17.31	12.24	10.00
Stop on z	19	15.38	12.24	10.00
Turn left	26	32.69	24.49	14.00
Turn right	23	46.15	18.37	12.00
Up	42	19.23	10.20	16.00
Upward	34	19.23	06.12	02.00

[a]The final model

Table 3 The confusion matrix of the final classifier on the test subject

	1	2	3	4	5	6	7	8	9	10
1	1	0	4	0	0	0	0	0	0	0
2	0	5	0	0	0	0	0	0	0	0
3	2	0	3	0	0	0	0	0	0	0
4	0	0	3	2	0	0	0	0	0	0
5	0	0	0	0	5	0	0	0	0	0
6	0	0	0	0	0	5	0	0	0	0
7	0	0	0	0	0	5	0	0	0	0
8	0	0	0	0	0	5	0	0	0	0
9	0	0	0	0	0	5	0	0	0	0
10	0	0	0	0	0	5	0	0	0	0

6 Conclusion and Future Work

We contributed an approach using KNN for classifying different activities using MoCap data as part of the *Bento Packaging Activity Recognition Challenge*. We reduced the set of markers and engineered several features by hand. We selected the best feature by applying KNN classifiers to each feature and evaluate each classifier combination. We found that only one feature (*over belt*) was used for the best result of 38.78% on our validation subject and 42.00% on our test subject. The feature did not work for Activities 7–10. All those were classified as Activity 6. The difference for both subjects was small, and we expect the challenge results being about 40% as well. There are two more promising next steps. The first one is to analyse the activities in more detail, engineer more features, and find a good combination of single classifiers. The second one is to build one-versus-all classifiers to find the best feature for each of the ten activities.

Acknowledgements The experiments were performed at the HPC cluster CARL, located at the University of Oldenburg (Germany), and funded by the DFG through its Major Research Instrumentation Programme (INST 184/157-1 FUGG) and the Ministry of Science and Culture (MWK) of the Lower Saxony State.

Appendix

Sensor modalities	MoCap markers
Marker left hand	8 9 10
Marker right hand	4 6 7
Features	Hand-engineered
Language and libraries	Python 3.6, Scikit-learn [8], NumPy [9], Pandas [10]
Window size and post-processing	No windows were used, no post-processing was applied
Training/testing time	3.1473 s/0.0027 s
Machine specifications	2x Intel Xeon E5-2650 12 × 2.2 GHz, 256 GB DDR4 RAM, no GPU

References

1. Adachi, K., Shamma Alia, S., Nahid, N., Kaneko, H., Lago, P., Inoue, S.: Summary of the bento packaging activity recognition challenge. In: The 3rd International Conference on Activity and Behavior Computing (ABC2021) (2021)
2. Shamma, A.S., Adachi, K., Nahid, N., Lago, P., Inoue, S.: Bento Packaging Activity Recognition Challenge. Haru Kaneko (2021)

3. Hachaj, T., Ogiela, M.R., Koptyra, K.: Human actions recognition from motion capture recordings using signal resampling and pattern recognition methods. Ann. Oper. Res. **265**(2), 223–239 (2018)
4. Paul Ijjina, E., Krishna Mohan, C.: Human action recognition based on motion capture information using fuzzy convolution neural networks. In: 2015 Eighth International Conference on Advances in Pattern Recognition (ICAPR), pp. 1–6 (2015)
5. Barnachon, M., Bouakaz, S., Boufama, B., Guillou, E.: Ongoing human action recognition with motion capture. Pattern Recogn. **47**, 238–247 (2014)
6. Cao, X., Kudo, W., Ito, C., Shuzo, M., Maeda, E.: Activity recognition using ST-GCN with 3D motion data. In: Adjunct Proceedings of the 2019 ACM International Joint Conference on Pervasive and Ubiquitous Computing and Proceedings of the 2019 ACM International Symposium on Wearable Computers, UbiComp/ISWC'19 Adjunct, pp. 689–692. Association for Computing Machinery, New York, NY, USA (2019)
7. Lago, P., Okita, T., Takeda, S., Inoue, S.: Improving sensor-based activity recognition using motion capture as additional information. In: Proceedings of the 2018 ACM International Joint Conference and 2018 International Symposium on Pervasive and Ubiquitous Computing and Wearable Computers, UbiComp'18, pp. 118–121. Association for Computing Machinery, New York, NY, USA (2018)
8. Pedregosa, F., Varoquaux, G., Gramfort, A., Michel, V., Thirion, B., Grisel, O., Blondel, M., Prettenhofer, P., Weiss, R., Dubourg, V., Vanderplas, J., Passos, A., Cournapeau, D., Brucher, M., Perrot, M., Duchesnay, E.: Scikit-learn: machine learning in Python. J. Mach. Learn. Res. **12**, 2825–2830 (2011)
9. Harris, C.R., Jarrod Millman, K., van der Walt, S.J., Gommers, R., Virtanen, P., Cournapeau, D., Wieser, E., Taylor, J., Berg, S., Smith, N.J., Kern, R., Picus, M., Hoyer, S., van Kerkwijk, M.H., Brett, M., Haldane, A., del Río, J.F., Wiebe, M., Peterson, P., Gérard-Marchant, P., Sheppard, K., Reddy, T., Weckesser, W., Abbasi, H., Gohlke, C., Oliphant, T.E.: Array programming with NumPy. Nature **585**(7825), 357–362 (2020)
10. McKinney, W.: Data structures for statistical computing in Python. In: van der Walt, S., Millman, J. (eds.) Proceedings of the 9th Python in Science Conference, pp. 56–61 (2010)

Bento Packaging Activity Recognition from Motion Capture Data

Jahir Ibna Rafiq, Shamaun Nabi, Al Amin, and Shahera Hossain

Abstract Human activity recognition (HAR) has been an important research field for more than a decade due to its versatile applications in different area. It has gained significant attention in the health care domain. Although it has similarity with other form of activity recognition, it offers a unique set of challenges. Body movements in a food preparation environment are considerably less than many other activities of interest in real world. In this paper, a comprehensive solution has been demonstrated for the Bento Box Packaging Challenge activity recognition. In this case, we present a well-planned approach to recognize activities during packaging tasks from motion capture data. We use dataset obtained from motion capture system where subjects have 13 markers on their upper-body area and by special use of cameras and body suit. We obtain around 50,000 sample for each of the activities. We reduce the data dimensionality and make the data suitable for the classification purpose by extracting reliable and efficient features. After feature extraction process, three different classifiers, e.g., random forest classifier, extra trees classifier, and gradient boosting classifier are compared to check the result. We conclude that this challenging dataset has been observed to work most efficiently for random forest classifier using hyperparameter tuning.

J. I. Rafiq (✉) · S. Nabi · A. Amin · S. Hossain
University of Asia Pacific, Dhaka, Bangladesh
e-mail: jahir@uap-bd.edu

S. Nabi
e-mail: 18201050@uap-bd.edu

A. Amin
e-mail: 18201063@uap-bd.edu

S. Hossain
e-mail: shaherahossain@uap-bd.edu

M. A. R. Ahad et al. (eds.), *Sensor- and Video-Based Activity and Behavior Computing*, Smart Innovation, Systems and Technologies 291,
https://doi.org/10.1007/978-981-19-0361-8_15

1 Introduction

According to recent research, the human activity recognition (HAR) system is capable of deciphering human motion or gestures in a situation by processing a series of sensor data [1, 2]. Nowadays, the identification of general human movement such as walk, cycle, or run, count steps can be readily recognized using many cheap commercial products, but domain-specific activity understanding from real field data is very challenging [3]. In this regard, differentiating activities without a human intervention is a challenge for researchers. By correctly identifying an occurrence, we can prevent accidents and save valuable lives as well as able to improve work efficiency [1]. Therefore, we have observed a great number of studies that focus solely on identification of the movement of a living being, particularly in the last decade. The scope of the work has since been expanding due to several factors. As the study is increasingly becoming more and more mature, we are encouraged to solve more and more problems using HAR. We need to work on challenges that are conventionally carried out by a human being. We need to design a system that evaluates like a normal human, then we need to implement and test it against real-world setting.

Nowadays, we use a good number of sensors in our smartphones and many household items such as watch, car, and vacuum cleaner. Likewise, we can embed an item with sensors, spoof the data that comes off the sensors, use feature of the data, and identify what activity is taken in a certain time. Machine learning has been widely used for the framework, algorithm, and classification of data [4]. Learning context and identifying an activity have been studied for long time although the amount of research has increased significantly since the availability of many low-cost micro-embedded sensors.

Wearable sensors can be extremely useful in providing accurate and reliable information on people's activities and behaviors, but it is not the only solution. We can use motion capture device to learn about the movement of a person in a given area. It is accepted as an alternative to embedding sensors. This is due to the fact that the activities are difficult to classify, and very similar sort of tasks are performed for completely different jobs. Motion capture (MoCap) data has produced outstanding results in the detection of some repetitive and critical activities [5]. Data from MoCap includes vital joint information, and these high-level dynamic markers make the data more robust and help to identify different features for activity detection [6]. Therefore, the "Bento Packaging Activity Recognition Challenge" has been set with motion capture data to identify very challenging activities during Bento (lunch-box) packaging time.

In this paper, we present a approach to distinguish Bento packaging activities using a simple machine learning framework. We compared three machine learning models' performances to select the best model to handle this data. The provided datasets itself are challenging, and they have only 13 upper-body joint coordinates data. In this research, we address this challenge to recognize Bento box packaging activity from MoCap data. The remaining part of the paper proceeds as follows. First, Sect. 2 begins by reviewing the related work. Section 3 explains our method where it includes dataset description, data prepossessing, feature extraction process from MoCap data as well as classification and model selection. Section 4 explains result analysis, and finally, in Sect. 5, we conclude with conclusion remarks.

2 Related Work

Researchers have extensively investigated and showed that human activity recognition is best achieved using inertial sensor data [7]. Automated identification of human actions has been proposed in the ubiquitous and wearable research community [8]. High-dimensional feature vectors are obtained through sensors, which are later used for identifying a particular activity and differentiate among activities [9]. Ahmed et al.[9] have suggested that combined feature selection strategy which organizes the filter and binding methodologies to determining the best features. Statistical feature-based representing methods have been used as a innovative approach to activity recognition.

Classification algorithm, such as artificial neural network (ANN), K-nearest neighbors (KNN), quadratic support vector machine (QSVM), are used to detect sudden change in movement in several studies where each classifier produces different result after they receive input data [10, 11]. Hence, classification plays an important part in studies. At the same time, better approach for regular activity recognition and critical activity recognition is crucial. Researchers are struggling to reveal better method for daily life day-to-day activity recognition. Real-life activity contains both micro- and macro-level activities [12] with a sequence which makes more complex to reveal the actual scenario. In this regard, micro-movement in an ordinary kitchen has not been fully explored in many of the works although a significant amount of work did consider activities of daily living (ADL) movements in the kitchen. Accelerometer collects data while a subject works in the kitchen with utensils that are equipped with sensors. Ensemble-based approach where sequence of accelerometer data has been utilized to detect an actor in a kitchen. Similarly, in [13], a smart kitchen that helps a cook during a cooking session is explored. Here, utensils are integrated with radio frequency identification (RFID), and accelerometers' data is used to detect a cook's step.

In [14], researchers have used body-worn multisensory device to detect six activities involving head and mouth. For classification, support vector machine, random forest, K-nearest neighbor, and convolutional neural network were used, which means both machine learning and deep learning approaches were applied successfully here. MoCap data has been used in various recent research as it is proving to be quite effective in recognizing a high-level activity. Unlike body-worn sensors, actors are marked at several places using marker in MoCap that in turn produces robust data and obtain features that are easy to classify in activity recognition. In [15], the researchers used the data from motion capture sensor to detect the activity at an early stage before any conventional classification was done. As a result, it effectively detected an ongoing action. MoCap data was used to produce histogram of activities and then Hausdorff distance was used to compute action poses. It produced impressive outcome even with large datasets. In [16], MoCap helped identify walking and running by producing spectrograms of micro-Doppler. The provided Bento Packaging Challenge dataset contains MoCap data with different joint positions. The dataset has ten critical activities during Bento packaging time with a very small differences among each class. In this research, we take the challenge to understand these activities from MoCap data with a simple machine learning framework.

3 Method

The following section describes the procedure for the collection of motion capture data for understanding different Bento box preparation activities. Afterward, we explain about data preprocessing and features extraction method from the raw data. Later on, the models used to classify different activities are explained.

3.1 Dataset

The Bento Packaging Activity Recognition Challenge [17] dataset encloses data collected from Motion capture system with 13 body markers. Motion capture data is gathered by capturing a subject's motions using markers and cameras while wearing a body suit. Markers' position in the body is like front, top and rear head, right and left shoulder, right offset, left and right elbow, left and right wrist, and V sacral. These are 13 body markers in the body as explained in Fig. 1. Using a different number of markers and various marker placements is a result in a different skeleton. Each marker depicts the movement of a human body component along the x, y, and z axes. The data has been collected from four subjects. Three subjects along with all activity labels have been used for training data, and remaining subject with unlabeled activity has been used for test data. Individual subjects are informed to put three types of food in the Bento box based on five different situations or actions like putting food inside Bento box without mistake, forgot to put ingredients, failed to put ingredients, turn over Bento box, and fixing/rearranging ingredients. The subjects performed these five different actions with five trials. Actions are done in two different patters like inward and outward directions. Each trail has been recorded for 50–70 s. The raw motion capture data was labeled based on the different activities. There were approximately 50,000 samples for each activity with a total number of 130,000 samples. Figure 2 depicts the total number of ten different activity records counted by Subjects 1, 2, and 3. The sample count of Activity 6 (failed to place ingredients inward) is higher for Subjects 1 and 2 than Subject 3.

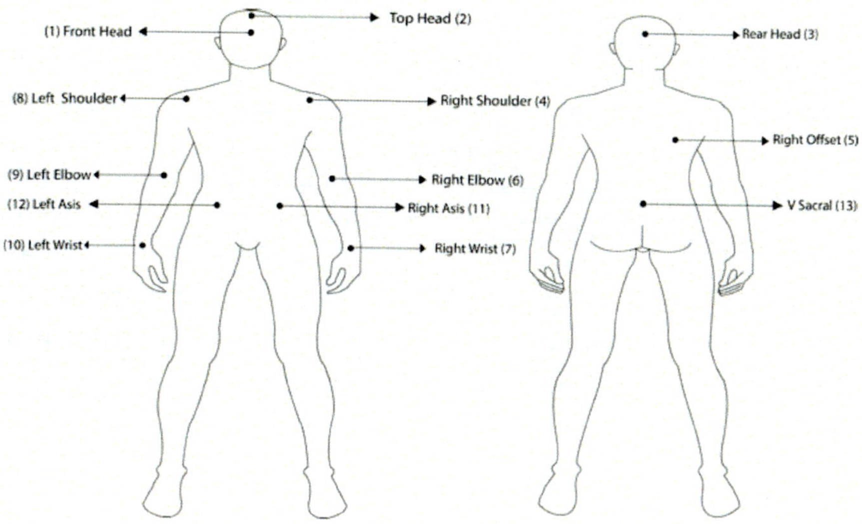

Fig. 1 Upper-body motion capture markers used for Bento packaging activity

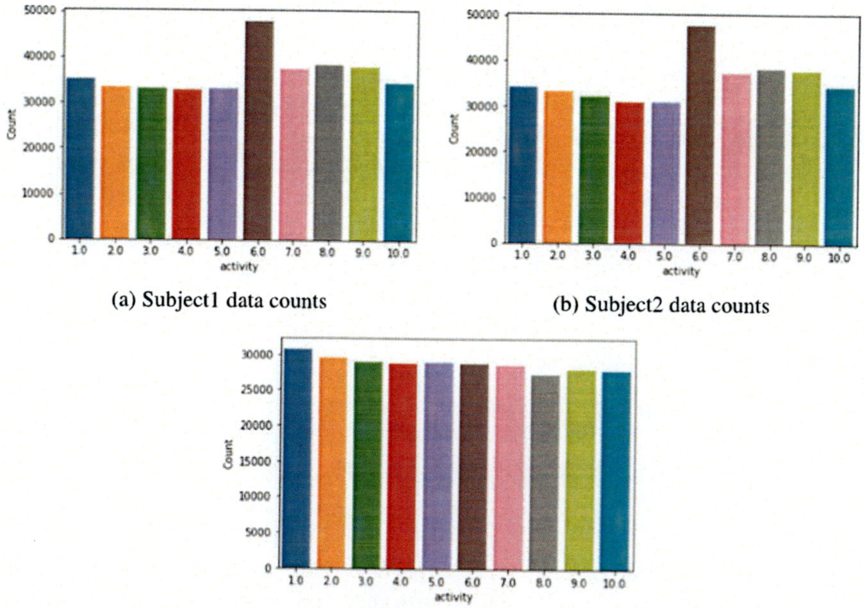

(a) Subject1 data counts

(b) Subject2 data counts

(c) Subject3 data counts

Fig. 2 Activity record count in Bento training dataset for three subjects

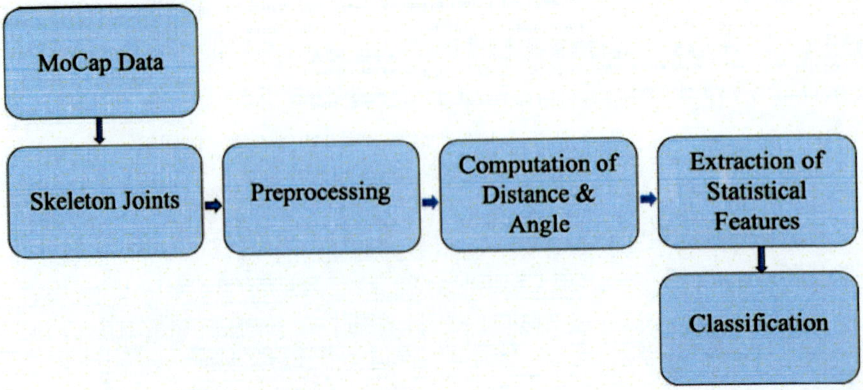

Fig. 3 Flow diagram of our method

3.2 Data Prepossessing

The basic flow diagram of the method is demonstrated in Fig. 3. During preprocessing, we simulated motion capture sensor data for a sampling rate 100 Hz. As a result, there were some missing values. We fill all missing values in the motion capture data with 0 as we assumed the missing values in the motion capture data means the subjects did not move. The joint positions and angles that are generated from 13 markers can result in vectors with hundreds of dimensions for every frame of the motion capture data. As a result, a massive volume of data must be displayed. Therefore, dimensionality reduction is an important step. We reduce the data dimensionality and make the data suitable for the classification purpose by extracting reliable and efficient features.

3.3 Feature Extraction

We initially used each MoCap sensor location to construct extracted sensor streams using the raw MoCap data. These streams included the distances and angles between some selected joints like hands, elbows, and shoulders, and the angles between different hand parts as shown in Fig. 1. We have extracted the elbow and shoulder angles, as well as the difference between them. The statistical feature we extract is listed in Table 1, which is minimum value (min), maximum value (max), diff (difference between maximum and minimum value), mean, standard deviation, skewness, kurtosis, and mean absolute deviation (MAD). Mean, median, and mean absolute deviation (MAD) values were checked to assess the dataset's central tendency. To check the data's variability, max, min, and standard deviation were calculated. We can assess the lack of symmetry in the data using skewness. It calculates the skewing

Table 1 Extracted time-domain features on the Bento packaging dataset

1. Mean
2. Min
3. Max
4. Difference
5. Standard deviation
6. Skewness
7. Kurtosis
8. Mean absolute deviation (MAD)

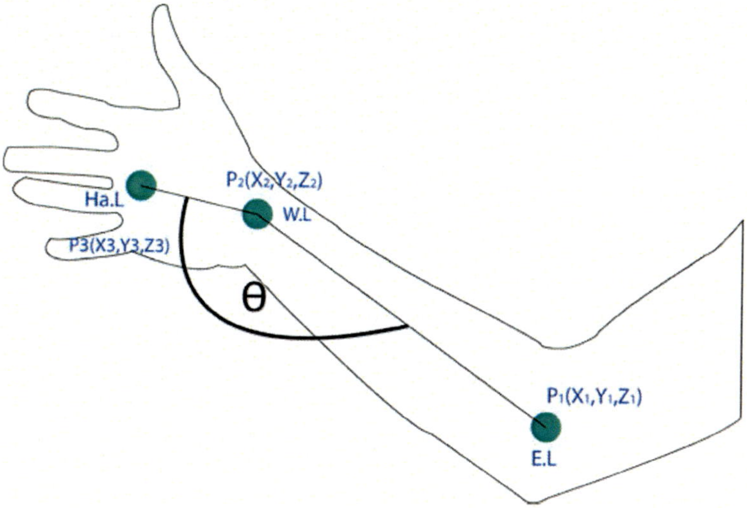

Fig. 4 Example of marker position in hand when we calculated angle and distance

rate, or irregularity, of a random variable's probability distribution around its mean value. The data distribution of flatness is measured by kurtosis [18, 19] (Fig. 4).

3.4 *Classification and Model Selection*

To detect the Bento activity, the process of detection is shown in Fig. 3. Initially, we select important joint position from data. After preprocessing the data, we measure the distance and angle between some selected joint position (specially from hands). Afterward, extract other time-domain features and split data for model training. Later on, we tested different classification model to evaluate the performance. To solve the problem of activity understanding, many different classification models have been used by researchers. There is no comprehensively approved approach for identifying a specific activity, and each classification model has its own set of pros and cons.

To compare the performance among classifiers, we explored random forest classifier, extra trees classifier, and gradient boosting classifier. To acquire the best results in validation data, we performed hyperparameter tuning like following way: random forest classifier (max_depth=1, n_estimators=500, min_samples_split=16, n_jobs=-1, random_state=1, extra trees classifier (n_estimators=500, criterion= “entropy”, verbose=1, n_jobs=3, max_depth=10, max_features=0.8, random_state=42), and gradient boosting classifier (n_estimators=100, max_features=300, learning_rate=0.2, max_depth=5). Moreover, after all, there have been trailed several models to train our data. In terms of this model training, we have assigned a splitting ratio of 0.7 whereby 70% of input data is separated as train set and used for training the model. The remaining 30% of the data is used as an internal test set to validate the model.

4 Result Analysis

The models’ classification accuracy on the previously separated test set is shown in the evaluation results in Table 2. We determined the model with the best performance based on the evaluation findings by comparing classification accuracies. The dataset has been observed to work most efficiently for random forest classifier. Other than this model, extra trees, and gradient boosting classifier have also been used. But, these models do not work as efficiently with the train and validation sets as random forest does. We have obtained highest accuracy in random forest classier which is 83%. On the other hand, extra trees classifiers obtained 63% and gradient boosting 31%. As we understand while handling this dataset, this is a very challenging dataset having only 13 upper-body joint coordinates. During classifiers comparison time, random forest performs best as it is a powerful classification tool since it can handle huge datasets with increased dimensionality and locate the most significant factors. The random forest classifier is made up of a set of basic decision tree classifiers that are generated at random based on the collected data in the training dataset. These decision trees learn on their own. Each class label is created in the test module based on the prediction levels of various classifiers. Random forests are the most inconsistency-tolerant classifier to handle this type of challenging dataset. The summary of the challenge is presented in [20].

Table 2 Classification results

Classifiers name	Accuracy
Random forest	83%
Extra trees	63%
Gradient boosting	31%

5 Conclusion

In this paper, we present a feasible way of recognizing ten different activities when packing a Bento box with food items. This is an important area of research as the demand for such automation will have positive impact on the catering industry as a whole. We have successfully recognized more than 80% of the activities using machine learning approach. Here, data is obtained from motion capture system, and no other sensors are used. Body markers are used to obtain data from the subjects at a conveyor belt in a laboratory. We have reduced the data dimensionality to keep the visualization better. Three classifiers showed different results as they have different approaches to data classifications. We did not use deep learning as the dataset was reasonably smaller than most deep learning applications would require. It is, overall, a quite challenging task to recognize the aforementioned tasks. This is mainly due to the fact that our dataset is relatively smaller. If we had a bigger dataset, possibly from multisensory devices, we would be able to extract better features, and recognition accuracy would increase significantly. Besides, in a full-body system, we usually have 29 markers. However, here we have only 13 markers, and we have only been given the top portion of the body. Hence, challenges are slightly different here and plenty of room for improvisation. On balance, this work will help shape more macro- and micro-level activity recognition work especially in the area where constraints are natural and help food industry.

6 Appendix

Used sensor modalities
Motion capture (MoCap)
Features Used
As described in Sect. 3.3 and summarized in Table 1
Programming Language and Libraries
Programming language: Python
Libraries: NumPy, Pandas, Matplotlib, Scikit-learn, Sci-Py

Machine Specification

- RAM: 8 GB
- Processor: 2.2 GHz Dual-core Intel Core i7
- GPU: N/A

Training and testing time
Training: 10.8 min
Testing: 3 min

References

1. Inoue, S., Lago, P., Hossain, T., Mairittha, T., Mairittha, N.: Integrating activity recognition and nursing care records: the system, deployment, and a verification study. Proc. ACM Interact. Mob. Wearable Ubiquitous Technol. **3**(3) (2019)
2. Saha, S.S., Rahman, S., Haque, Z.R.R., Hossain, T., Inoue, S., Ahad, M.A.R.; Position independent activity recognition using shallow neural architecture and empirical modeling. In: Adjunct Proceedings of the 2019 ACM International Joint Conference on Pervasive and Ubiquitous Computing and Proceedings of the 2019 ACM International Symposium on Wearable Computers, UbiComp/ISWC '19 Adjunct, pp. 808–813, New York, NY, USA. Association for Computing Machinery (2019)
3. Alia, S.S., Lago, P., Adachi, K., Hossain, T., Goto, H., Okita, T., Inoue., S.: Summary of the 2nd nurse care activity recognition challenge using lab and field data. In: Adjunct Proceedings of the 2020 ACM International Joint Conference on Pervasive and Ubiquitous Computing and Proceedings of the 2020 ACM International Symposium on Wearable Computers, UbiComp-ISWC '20, pp. 378–383, New York, NY, USA. Association for Computing Machinery (2020)
4. Hossain, T., Ahad, M.A.R., Tazin, T., Inoue, S.: Activity recognition by using lorawan sensor. In: Proceedings of the 2018 ACM International Joint Conference and 2018 International Symposium on Pervasive and Ubiquitous Computing and Wearable Computers, UbiComp '18, pp. 58–61, New York, NY, USA. Association for Computing Machinery (2018)
5. Cheema, M.S., Eweiwi, A., Bauckhage, C.:. Human activity recognition by separating style and content. Pattern Recogn. Lett. **50**, 130–138 (2014)
6. Aggarwal, J.K., Xia, L.: Human activity recognition from 3d data: a review. Pattern Recogn. Lett. **48**, 70–80 (2014)
7. Atallah, L., Yang, G.-Z.: Review: The use of pervasive sensing for behaviour profiling—a survey. Pervasive Mob. Comput. **5**(5), 447–464 (2009)
8. Guan, Y., Ploetz, T.: Ensembles of deep lstm learners for activity recognition using wearables. Proc. ACM Interactive Mobile Wearable Ubiquitous Technol. **1**, 03 (2017)
9. Ahmed, N., Rafiq, Islam.: Enhanced human activity recognition based on smartphone sensor data using hybrid feature selection model. Sensors **20**, 317 (2020)
10. Chelli, A., Pätzold, M.: A machine learning approach for fall detection and daily living activity recognition. IEEE Access **7**, 38670–38687 (2019)
11. Chelli, A., Pätzold, M.: A machine learning approach for fall detection based on the instantaneous doppler frequency. IEEE Access **7**, 166173–166189 (2019)
12. Alia, S., Lago, P., Takeda, S., Adachi, K., Benaissa, B., Ahad, M.A.R., Inoue, S.: Summary of the Cooking Activity Recognition Challenge, pp. 1–13 (2021)
13. Bonanni, L., Lee, C.-H., Selker, T.: Counterintelligence: Augmented Reality Kitchen (2005)
14. Hossain, T., Islam, M., Ahad, M.A.R., Inoue, S.: Human Activity Recognition Using Earable Device, pp. 81–84 (2019)
15. Barnachon, M., Bouakaz, S., Boufama, B., Guillou, E.: Ongoing human action recognition with motion capture. Pattern Recogn. **47**, 238–247 (2014)
16. Lin, y., le kernec, J.: Performance Analysis of Classification Algorithms for Activity Recognition Using Micro-doppler Feature, pp. 480–483 (2017)
17. Alia, S.S., Adachi, K., Nahid, N., Kaneko, H., Lago, P., Inoue, S.: Bento Packaging Activity Recognition Challenge (2021)
18. Bulling, A., Blanke, U., Schiele, B.: A tutorial on human activity recognition using body-worn inertial sensors. ACM Comput. Surv. **46**, 01 (2013)
19. Hossain, T., Ahad, M.A.R., Inoue, s.: A method for sensor-based activity recognition in missing data scenario. Sensors **20**, 3811 (2020)
20. Nahid, N., Kaneko, H., Lago, P., Adachi, K., Alia, S.S., Inoue, S.: Summary of the Bento Packaging Activity Recognition Challenge (2021)

Bento Packaging Activity Recognition with Convolutional LSTM Using Autocorrelation Function and Majority Vote

Atsuhiro Fujii, Kazuki Yoshida, Kiichi Shirai, and Kazuya Murao

Abstract This paper reports Bento Packaging Activity Recognition Challenge by team "RitsBen" held in the International Conference on Activity and Behavior Computing (ABC 2021). Our approach used an autocorrelation function in the preprocessing to isolate the data since the dataset was given with repetitive activity. We then use a model that implements convolutional layers and LSTM. The final decision is made by majority vote using sigmoid predictions output from all body parts. The loss is calculated using BCEWithLogitsLoss for each body part. The evaluation results showed that average accuracy of 0.123 was achieved among subjects 1, 2, and 3 in leave-one-subject-out manner. However, we did not achieve high accuracy as the possibility that the extraction of repetitive actions was not correct.

1 Introduction

This paper reports the solution of our team "RitsBen" to Bento Packaging Activity Recognition Challenge held at the International Conference on Activity and Behavior Computing (ABC2021). The goal of Bento Packaging Activity Recognition Challenge is to distinguish activities taking place during each segment based on the motion data collected with motion capture sensors while performing Bento-box packaging tasks [7]. Activity recognition is the process of automatically inferring what a user is doing based on sensor observations. Since activity recognition can enrich our lives by understanding the characteristics of human activity, there has been a lot of research on human activity recognition (HAR).

Lara et al. [8] surveyed the state of the art in HAR based on wearable sensors. Khan et al. [6] proposed an accelerometer-based HAR method. Bayat et al. [3] proposed a recognition system in which a new digital low-pass filter is designed. Anguita et al. [1] conducted a comparative study on HAR using inertial sensors in a smartphone. Attal et al. [2] presented a review of different classification techniques

A. Fujii · K. Yoshida · K. Shirai · K. Murao (✉)
Graduate School of Information Science and Engineering, Ritsumeikan University,
1-1-1 Nojihigashi, Kusatsu, Shiga 525-8577, Japan
e-mail: murao@cs.ritsumei.ac.jp

M. A. R. Ahad et al. (eds.), *Sensor- and Video-Based Activity and Behavior Computing*,
Smart Innovation, Systems and Technologies 291,
https://doi.org/10.1007/978-981-19-0361-8_16

in HAR based on wearable inertial sensors. In recent years, methods that use neural networks to improve the accuracy of activity recognition have also been actively researched. Yang et al. [11] proposed a systematic feature learning method based on deep convolutional neural networks (CNN) for HAR problem. Chen et al. [4] proposed a deep learning approach to HAR based on single accelerometer. Tsokov et al. [10] proposed an evolutionary-based approach for optimizing the architecture of one-dimensional CNNs for HAR. Dang et al. [5] introduced a classification of HAR methodologies and showed advantages and weaknesses for methods in each category.

In this paper, we construct a network with convolutional layers and LSTM layer to recognize the activities and detect repetition using the autocorrelation function. The outputs of the model are sigmoid values, the number of the outputs is as much as the number of sensors. The final output is a majority vote on those sigmoid values.

2 Challenge

In this challenge, each team competes in the recognition accuracy of activities related to Bento box packaging activities based on motion capture data. For more details, please refer to the article [9].

The data collected from four subjects (all males) who attached one motion capture system with 29 markers released by Motion Analysis Company.[1] The subjects packed three types of food according to the five different bento-box packaging scenarios. The subjects performed in two patterns of outward and inward, and five times each scenario. In total, 4 subjects × 5 scenarios × 2 patterns × 5 trials = 200 of data were collected. Training data contains data from three subjects (subjects 1, 2, 3) out of the four subjects and test data contains the data from the fourth subject (subject 4). Originally, the training dataset should be contained 150 trials for three subjects. However, activity 6 of subject 1 did not contain the fifth trial and the activity 6 and 9 of subject 2 contained the sixth trial. Therefore, the total number of training data was 151.

Table 1 shows a list of ten different activity names, movement direction patterns, and activity labels; there are five different activity types, and two movement direction patterns, for a total of 10 types (5 × 2 = 10). The segment is stored and divided by subject, activity label, and trials. For example, `[subject_1_activity_1_repeat_1]` contains the data of subject 1 having performed the first trial of activity whose label number is 1. Each file contains 89 types of data: 3-axis (X, Y, Z) data measured from each of 29 markers, subject number, and activity label. The measurement time for each file ranges from 50 to 70 s. Note that due to the complicated setup of the motion capture sensor, missing measurement data and incorrect activity labels may be included.

[1] https://motionanalysis.com.

Table 1 A list of ten different activity names, movement direction patterns, and activity labels

Activity name	Movement direction pattern	Activity label
Normal	Inward	1
	Outward	2
Forgot to put ingredients	Inward	3
	Outward	4
Failed to put ingredients	Inward	5
	Outward	6
Turn over bento-box	Inward	7
	Outward	8
Fix/rearranging ingredients	Inward	9
	Outward	10

Table 2 shows the number of recognized classes (ten classes in this challenge), the number of segments for each subject, the number of trials for each activity, and the maximum, mean, and minimum length of the segments.

Submissions from the participants will be evaluated by the accuracy of activity classification. The accuracy is given by $accuracy = \frac{P \cap G}{P \cup G}$; the number of correct labels predicted (logical product of prediction set P and groundtruth set G) divided by the number of total true and predicted labels (logical sum of P and G).

3 Method

This section describes the preprocessing to obtain the features from the raw data, the structure of the model, the loss function and the optimizer, the process of obtaining the activity labels from the predictions obtained by the one-hot vector, and implementation. Note that our method does not use motion capture data.

3.1 Preprocessing

Figure 1 shows the flow of preprocessing. The details of each process are described below.

- **Reading data process** reads raw data for each body part from a given dataset. The details of this dataset are described in Sect. 2.
- **Converting process** converts to velocity data from raw data. First, we interpolate the missing values in the raw data. The time when the missing data starts is t, the time when the missing data ends is $t + n$, the i-th missing time from the start time is $t + i$ $(0 \leq t \leq t + i \leq t + n \leq T)$, the raw data at t is $R(t)$, and the interpolated data at t is $I(t)$. $I(t + i)$ is calculated by $I(t + i) = R(t) + \frac{R(t+n)-R(t)}{n} \times i$. In

Table 2 Statistics of the dataset

Subject	Activity label	# of recognized classes	# of segments	# of trials	Length		
					Max	Mean	Min
1	1	10	49	5	5701	5311	5516
	2			5	6325	5120	5860
	3			5	6448	5956	6214
	4			5	6665	6257	6446
	5			5	6467	5955	6310
	6			4	5771	5427	5525
	7			5	5725	5323	5567
	8			5	6653	6307	6395
	9			5	6828	6252	6530
	10			5	6962	6269	6525
2	1	10	52	5	7660	6626	7037
	2			5	6788	6493	6667
	3			5	6827	6390	6610
	4			5	6933	6295	6564
	5			5	6690	6470	6608
	6			6	8441	7660	7996
	7			5	7719	7392	7511
	8			5	7870	7386	7667
	9			6	7434	1663	6343
	10			5	7420	6651	6343
3	1	10	50	5	6337	5972	6149
	2			5	6326	5724	5915
	3			5	5995	5582	5801
	4			5	5930	5596	5768
	5			5	5953	5523	5778
	6			5	6190	5402	5769
	7			5	6017	5408	5737
	8			5	5718	5223	5459
	9			5	5860	5357	5620
	10			5	5714	5351	5579
4	Unknown	Unknown	48	Unknown	5947	5024	5481

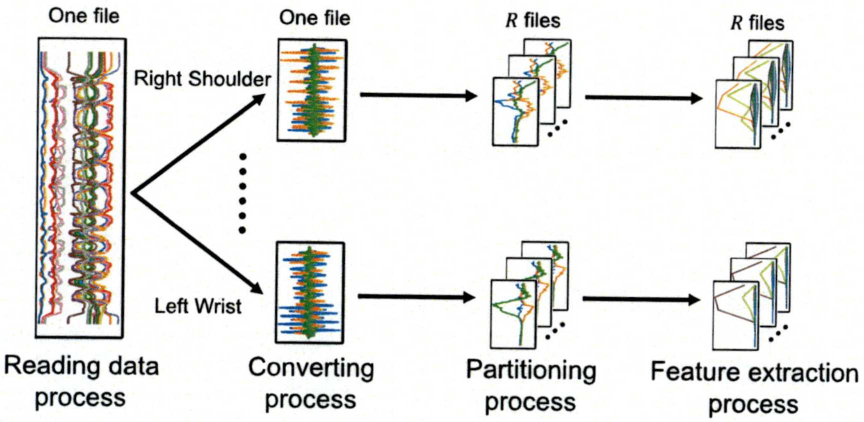

Fig. 1 Details of preprocessing. The first process is the raw data as it is provided. In the second process, the raw data is converted to velocity data. The partitioning process identifies and separates repetitive parts from the velocity data. The feature extraction process extracts 21-dimensional features from the separated velocity data

case of missing data at the beginning or end of a segment, the data that up to the time when the data was available at all markers was deleted and interpolated. The interpolated data was used to calculate the velocity data. The interpolated data at time j $(1 \leq j \leq T)$ is $I(j)$, and the velocity data is $V(j)$, which is calculated by $V(j) = \frac{I(j)-I(j-1)}{0.01}$. Since the dataset frequency in this challenge 100 Hz, the calculation was divided by 0.01.

- **Partitioning process** is the process of dividing the given data of approximately 60 s into data for one operation. The input is a single time-series velocity data, and the output is R time-series velocity data. R is the number of repetitive actions that were included. This time, we used the autocorrelation function. The autocorrelation function is the correlation between different points in a time series. When the time-series data has periodicity, the autocorrelation function also shows a peak at the same period. Therefore, by applying the autocorrelation function to the data set which was obtained by repeating the same operation, and finding the local maximum value, we aimed to extract the data of one operation of period T. We summed up all the sensor values in the data set to form a single synthetic wave and applied the autocorrelation function.
- **Feature extraction process** is to extract the characteristic data. Our method uses mean, variance, max, min, root mean square (RMS), interquartile range (IQR), and zero-crossing rate (ZCR) for the features. These features were extracted with a window size of 400 ms and an overlap of 50 ms. From these preprocessing, 7 features $\times$ 3 axes = 21 dimensions feature time series are obtained for one marker. We thought that upper body movements had a great influence on the activity. Therefore, we used only the data obtained from the markers attached to six parts of the upper body (Right Shoulder, Right Elbow, Right Wrist, Left Shoulder, Left Elbow, Left Wrist).

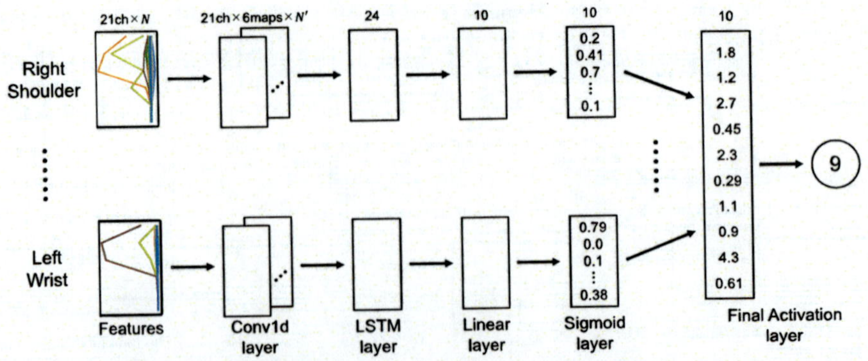

Fig. 2 Details of our model. The first layer is preprocessed 21-dimensional features. Conv1d layer is one-dimensional convolutional layer. This layer accepts 21-dimensional time-series features and maps each dimension to six (i.e., 21-dimensional features × 6 maps = 126-channel). The LSTM layer consists of 24 hidden layers, accepts 126-channel time-series data, and outputs 24-dimensional tensors. The linear layer transforms 24-dimensional tensors into 10-dimensional ones. After applying the sigmoid function in the sigmoid layer, the six predictions are merged to obtain the final prediction result

3.2 *Model*

The feature data created by the preprocessing is fed into our model. Figure 2 shows the structure of our model. The model consists of 1D convolutional layer, LSTM layer, Linear layer, and Sigmold layer. The models for six sensors are trained separately. The final activation layer determines one final prediction label from the six predictions. The details of each layer are described below.

- **Conv1d layer** has an input of 21 channels × sequence length N and an output of 21 channels × map size M × sequence length N'. N is the length of handcrafted time-series feature data, which is shorter than the raw data. N' is the length of time-series data after the one-dimensional convolution. This is equal to $N - K + 1$ (K is the kernel size). N and N' vary with the data because the dataset contains missing data. Kernel size K is set to 5. If N is 4, N' will be 0. Therefore, segments with N shorter than 5 are discarded and not fed into the model. Map size M is the number of filters and set to 6 × 21-dimensional features = 126. There are 6 filters for each channel, and the convolution is conducted for each channel.
- **LSTM layer** has an input of 126 channels × sequence length N' and an output of 24-dimensional tensors. This LSTM solves many to one task. We set the number of hidden layers to 24. The outputs obtained from the LSTM are not time-series data, but simply tensors.
- **Linear layer** has an input of 24-dimensional tensor and an output of ten-dimensional tensor which is the same as the number of activity classes.

- **Sigmoid layer** applies the sigmoid activation function to the ten-dimensional tensor. The output ten-dimensional tensor indicates the likelihood that the class is correct. This layer is not used in the training phase.

3.3 Loss Function and Optimizer

The model is trained by BCEWithLogitsLoss, which is a stable loss equipped with a Sigmoid function. Sigmoid function is usually used for classification when multiple labels are outputted. This challenge is a multi-class classification where one label is output from each file. Softmax function is usually used under this condition. However, the proposed method outputs the results for each model of body part and performs majority voting. We thought that it would be better to list all the classes that could be classified and then perform majority voting. We also tested training with CrossEntropyLoss, which is equiped with a Softmax function. Comparing the testing results, we found that the accuracy was higher when using BCEWithLogitsLoss, so we adopted it.

3.4 Final Prediction Classes Activation

Through the above process, the predictions for six sensors with ten labels of sigmoid values are obtained. Their labels are shown in Table 1. Six sensors are Right Shoulder, Right Elbow, Right Wrist, Left Shoulder, Left Elbow, and Left Wrist. Finally, our method integrates these predictions and outputs the final prediction. Specifically, the sigmoid values for each class are summed and the final prediction is made. If the total values are the same, the class that contains the largest value among each label is adopted.

For example, if the predicted values for activity 1 are [1.0, 0.0, 0.0, 0.0, 0.0, 0.0, 0.0, 0.0, 0.0, 0.0], [0.0, 0.5, 0.0, 0.0, 0.0, 0.0, 0.0, 0.0, 0.0, 0.0], [0.0, 0.5, 0.0, 0.0, 0.0, 0.0, 0.0, 0.0, 0.0, 0.0], [0.0, 0.0, 0.5, 0.0, 0.0, 0.0, 0.0, 0.0, 0.0, 0.0], [0.0, 0.0, 0.0, 0.0, 0.0, 0.0, 0.3, 0.0, 0.1, 0.0], [0.0, 0.0, 0.0, 0.0, 0.0, 0.0, 0.0, 0.0, 0.5, 0.0]. The summed sigmoid values are [1.0, 1.0, 0.5, 0.0, 0.0, 0.0, 0.3, 0.0, 0.6, 0.0], and the label with the largest value is adopted. However, in this case, the maximum value of 1 exists in label 1 and label 2, and therefore, we go back to the predicted values in each sensor. In the original prediction, the maximum value in label 1 is 1 and the maximum value in label 2 is 0.5, and therefore, we adopt label 1.

Table 3 Accuracy and loss for the six sensor positions at 5000 epochs by changing training and testing subjects

Training data	Test data	Sensor position	Accuracy	Loss
Subject 1, 2	Subject 3	Right Shoulder	0.135	0.238
		Right Elbow	0.137	0.266
		Right Wrist	0.127	0.272
		Left Shoulder	0.118	0.265
		Left Elbow	0.119	0.261
		Left Wrist	0.136	0.270
Subject 1, 3	Subject 2	Right Shoulder	0.136	0.250
		Right Elbow	0.121	0.290
		Right Wrist	0.133	0.284
		Left Shoulder	0.097	0.280
		Left Elbow	0.092	0.282
		Left Wrist	0.134	0.279
Subject 2, 3	Subject 1	Right Shoulder	0.142	0.236
		Right Elbow	0.130	0.276
		Right Wrist	0.115	0.282
		Left Shoulder	0.110	0.278
		Left Elbow	0.127	0.267
		Left Wrist	0.110	0.280

4 Evaluation

This section describes the evaluation experiments. We calculated the accuracy of the proposed model while changing the test subjects in leave-one-subject-out manner.

In partitioning process, repetitions were identified by calculating autocorrelation using `tsa.stattools.acf`[2] in `statsmodels` library. The model is developed in PyTorch. The loss function and optimizer were implemented using PyTorch libraries.[3,4]

In the training phase, all data of train subjects were used for training in one epoch, which was iterated 5000 epochs. Table 3 shows accuracy and loss for the six sensor positions at 5000 epochs by changing training and testing subjects. The loss was calculated using the ten-dimensional tensor output from the linear layer described in Sect. 3.2.

From these results, average accuracy of 0.123 was achieved among subjects 1, 2, and 3 in leave-one-subject-out manner. Even if we take into account the fact that there are 10 classes of labels, this accuracy is not high. The reason for the low accuracy

[2] https://www.statsmodels.org/stable/generated/statsmodels.tsa.stattools.acf.html.

[3] https://pytorch.org/docs/stable/generated/torch.nn.BCEWithLogitsLoss.html.

[4] https://pytorch.org/docs/stable/generated/torch.optim.Adam.html.

could be that some sensor data was missing or mislabeled. As described in Sect. 2, the training dataset may contain missing data and incorrect activity labels due to the complexity of the motion capture sensor setup. However, we did not take any action on the data with incorrect activity labels. Thus, there is a possibility that training was performed based on the wrong activity labels, and the accuracy was low. In addition, the proposed method uses the autocorrelation function in a preprocessing to extract the repetitive motion. However, it is possible that the data was not extracted correctly because the lengths of the waveforms after the partitioning process were significantly different. It is thought that the accuracy became low due to training on incorrectly extracted data.

Note that for the submitted result for the data of subject 4, our model was trained separately for the body parts with the data of subjects 1, 2, and 3, and the model at 5,000th epoch was used for testing the data of subject 4.

5 Conclusion

This paper reported the solution of our team "RitsBen" to Bento Packaging Activity Recognition Challenge. Our approach calculated the velocity data from the raw data at first. The repetitive motion data was separated from the velocity data by applying an autocorrelation function and extracted seven types of feature values including the mean value. Our approach model consists of 1D convolutional layer, LSTM layer, linear layer, and sigmold layer. The model was trained on the data of six parts attached to the upper body separately. The final activation layer, majority voting, was implemented to determine one final prediction label from the six predictions. BCEWithLogitsLoss was used as the loss function. The evaluation results showed that average accuracy of 0.123 was achieved among subjects 1, 2, and 3 in leave-one-subject-out manner. However, the high accuracy could not be achieved due to the fact that we did not deal with the case of incorrectly labeled actions and the possibility that the extraction of repetitive actions was not correct.

Appendix

See Table 4.

Table 4 Our resources

Used sensor modalities	Right Shoulder Right Elbow Right Wrist Left Shoulder Left Elbow Left Wrist
Features used	Mean Variance Max Min Root mean square Interquartile range Zero crossing rate
Programming language and libraries used	Python 3.8.8 statsmodels 0.12.2 PyTorch 1.9.0
Window size and post processing	Window size: 400 ms Overlap: 50 ms
Using resources in training and testing	CPU memory: 3043 MB GPU memory: 271 MB
Training and testing time	Training time (during 5000 epoch): 1112.233 s Testing time (at 5000 epoch): 5.577 s
Machine specification	OS: Windows 10 Pro CPU: Intel Core i9-10900K 3.70 GHz RAM: DDR4 128 GB GPU: NVIDIA GeForce RTX 3060 GDDR6 12 GB

References

1. Anguita, D., Ghio, A., Oneto, L., Parra, X., Reyes-Ortiz, J.L.: Human activity recognition on smartphones using a multiclass hardware-friendly support vector machine. In: International Workshop on Ambient Assisted Living, pp. 216–223. Springer, Berlin (2012)
2. Attal, F., Mohammed, S., Dedabrishvili, M., Chamroukhi, F., Oukhellou, L., Amirat, Y.: Physical human activity recognition using wearable sensors. Sensors 15(12), 31314–31338 (2015)
3. Bayat, A., Pomplun, M., Tran, D.A.: A study on human activity recognition using accelerometer data from smartphones. Procedia Computer Science 34, 450–457 (2014)
4. Chen, Y., Xue, Y.: A deep learning approach to human activity recognition based on single accelerometer. In: 2015 IEEE International Conference on Systems, Man, and Cybernetics, pp. 1488–1492. IEEE (2015)
5. Dang, L.M., Min, K., Wang, H., Piran, M.J., Lee, C.H., Moon, H.: Sensor-based and vision-based human activity recognition: a comprehensive survey. Pattern Recogn. **108**, 107561 (2020)

6. Khan, A.M., Lee, Y.K., Lee, S.Y., Kim, T.S.: A triaxial accelerometer-based physical-activity recognition via augmented-signal features and a hierarchical recognizer. IEEE transactions on information technology in biomedicine 14(5), 1166–1172 (2010)
7. Kohei, A., Sayeda, S.A., Nazmun, N., Haru, K., Paula, L., Sozo, I.: Summary of the bento packaging activity recognition challenge. In: The 3rd International Conference on Activity and Behavior Computing (2021)
8. Lara, O.D., Labrador, M.A.: A survey on human activity recognition using wearable sensors. IEEE communications surveys & tutorials 15(3), 1192–1209 (2012)
9. Sayeda, S.A., Kohei, A., Nazmun, N., Haru, K., Paula, L., Sozo, I.: Bento Packaging Activity Recognition Challenge (2021). https://doi.org/10.21227/cwhs-t440
10. Tsokov, S., Lazarova, M., Aleksieva-Petrova, A.: An evolutionary approach to the design of convolutional neural networks for human activity recognition. Indian Journal of Computer Science and Engineering 12(2), 499–517 (2021)
11. Yang, J., Nguyen, M.N., San, P.P., Li, X.L., Krishnaswamy, S.: Deep convolutional neural networks on multichannel time series for human activity recognition. In: Twenty-Fourth International Joint Conference on Artificial Intelligence (2015)

Summary of the *Bento Packaging Activity Recognition Challenge*

Kohei Adachi, Sayeda Shamma Alia, Nazmun Nahid, Haru Kaneko, Paula Lago, and Sozo Inoue

Abstract Human activity recognition (HAR) has a great impact on human-robot collaboration (HRC), especially in industrial works. However, it is difficult to find industrial activity data. With a goal of making the interactions between humans and robots more straightforward, we organized *Bento Packaging Activity Recognition Challenge* as a part of *The 3rd International Conference on Activity and Behavior Computing*. Here, the term *Bento* refers to a single-serving lunch box originated in Japan. We provided ten Bento packing activities data. The activities are performed by four subjects with a moving conveyor belt. In this work, we analyze and summarize the approaches of submission of the *challenge*. The challenge started on June 1st, 2021, and continued until August 25th, 2021. The participant teams used the given dataset to predict the ten activities, and they were evaluated using accuracy. The winning team used an ensemble model and achieved around 64% accuracy on testing data. To further improve the accuracy of the testing data, models particularly designed for small data with larger intra-class similarity could help.

K. Adachi (✉) · S. S. Alia · N. Nahid · H. Kaneko · S. Inoue
Kyushu Institute of Technology, Kitakyushu, Japan
e-mail: adachi@sozolab.jp

S. S. Alia
e-mail: alia@sozolab.jp

N. Nahid
e-mail: nazmun@sozolab.jp

H. Kaneko
e-mail: kaneko@sozolab.jp

S. Inoue
e-mail: sozo@brain.kyutech.ac.jp

P. Lago
Universidad Nacional Abierta y a Distancia, Bogotá, Colombia
e-mail: paula.lago@unad.edu.co

M. A. R. Ahad et al. (eds.), *Sensor- and Video-Based Activity and Behavior Computing*,
Smart Innovation, Systems and Technologies 291,
https://doi.org/10.1007/978-981-19-0361-8_17

1 Introduction

Human activity recognition (HAR) has been one of the most prevailing and persuasive research tospics in different fields for the past few decades [1]. The main idea is to comprehend individuals' regular activities by looking at bits of knowledge accumulated from people and their encompassing living environments based on sensor observations.

HAR has a great impact on human-robot collaboration (HRC) [2, 3]. With the betterment of lifestyle, it is getting harder to find human labor at a lower wage. This is a big problem for various industries where a big amount of workforce is required at a low wage. Robots can be a great solution for this problem if they can be used as an assistant for humans to do small tasks. To do so, the robot needs to first understand what the human is doing.

Though several datasets are available on cooking [4, 5] and daily living data [6], this type of industrial activity dataset is very hard to find. Cooking needs to follow a step-by-step workflow like food packing, which is another good place to implement human-robot collaboration, but there are a lot of differences between these two types. While cooking, the steps and ingredients used in the food solely depend on the user, but during packing a food, you need to put the items the company asked you to do. So, it is very common to forget to put an ingredient and forget to notice or sometimes when you notice the box is far away in the conveyor belt and if you hustle to put you might mess up the whole thing. Instances like this are very common in food-making companies, which create a lot of trouble. To help in this scenario, a robot hand can be a perfect assistant, but for that, it needs to know what the human is doing and if he/she has made any mistake and what type of mistake has been made. Also, recognizing these steps can be used for care quality assessment and for ensuring that safety protocols have been followed to avoid the human-robot collision. By keeping this in mind, Bento activity recognition data has been collected. Bento is a single-portion takeout or home-packed lunch box originated in Japan [7]. Here, subjects are asked to perform Bento box packaging tasks. This challenge aims at the recognition of the inside–outside activities and main activities taking place during Bento packing sessions. In this paper, we provide an overview of the submissions received in this *challenge* by the participant teams, analyzing their approaches, and share our observations from their activity identification processes.

2 Dataset Specification

The dataset is collected in an artificially created environment for Bento packaging, located in *Smart Life Care Unit* of the Kyushu Institute of Technology in Japan. Instructions on performing the activities were given to the subjects prior to the experiment. The subjects carried out five different activities. And, actions are done in two different patterns, inward and outward. The specifics about collected activities, format of the dataset, and experimental environment will be reported in this section.

Table 1 Activity name and associated label

Activity name	Label number
Normal (inward)	1
Normal (outward)	2
Forgot to put ingredients (inward)	3
Forgot to put ingredients (outward)	4
Failed to put ingredients (inward)	5
Failed to put ingredients (inward)	6
Turn over Bento box (inward)	7
Turn over Bento box (outward)	8
Fix/Rearranging ingredients (inward)	9
Fix/Rearranging ingredients (outward)	10

2.1 *Details of Activities*

The dataset of this *challenge* contains activities conducted in a scenario of Bento packing on a moving conveyor belt. Each of the subjects is instructed to put three types of food in the Bento box. There are five principal activities: normal, forgot to put ingredients, failed to put ingredients, turn over Bento box, and fix/rearranging ingredients. However, each of these five activities is executed in two different patterns: inward and outward. Therefore, in total, ten activity classes are in this dataset. Also, each activity was collected five times. Table 1 shows the activity names and label numbers in the training data. This same set is used also for the test data.

2.2 *Experimental Setting*

The whole experiment for collecting the dataset was conducted in *Smart Life Care Unit* of the Kyushu Institute of Technology in Japan. Four subjects (men) in their 20s and 30s participated during data collection, and there was no overlap between the subjects. A motion capture system from Motion Analysis Company [8] is used for this experiment. The data accumulated using this system has 29 body markers' information, even so we are opening only 13 body markers' data in this challenge. The places of the body are shown in Fig. 1. In the time of the experiment, we observed that the subjects were performing the activities mostly using upper-body parts. During our analysis on the dataset, we found conclusive evidence that there were no significant changes in accuracy when the removed 16 body markers were present. Hence, the data of the shown 13 markers is shared in this challenge.

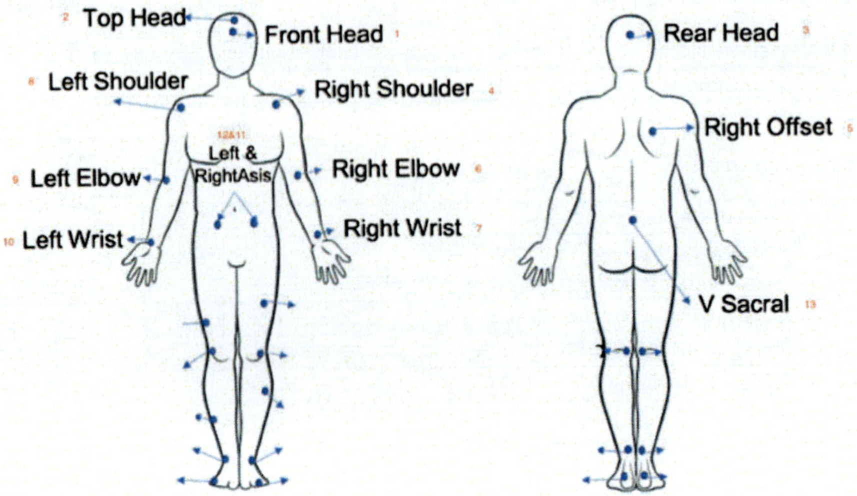

Fig. 1 Position of the markers

2.3 *Data Format*

The data has been separated into training data and test data. Training data contains data from three subjects, and test data contains the fourth subject's data. Each segment is assigned one activity which has approximately 50–70 s. The folder structure is shown in Fig. 2. Each activity's folder is nested within each subject's folder. Data from the 13 markers is in CSV files of each activity folder.

3 Challenge Tasks and Results

The goal of the Bento Packaging Activity Recognition Challenge is to distinguish activities taking place during each segment based on the motion data collected with motion capture sensors while performing Bento box packaging tasks. In the training dataset, we have provided data of three subjects along with all activity labels. In the test dataset, unlabeled data of the remaining subject has been given. Participants have to submit their predicted activity labels on the test dataset using their models.

Initially 22 unique teams registered and finally 9 teams submitted their prediction of the test data. However, among the submitted teams, two teams could not submit research papers containing details of their used formulas. Consequently following the rules of this challenge,[1] we had to disqualify that two teams. Therefore, we have seven final teams, and they are:

[1] https://abc-research.github.io/bento2021/rules/.

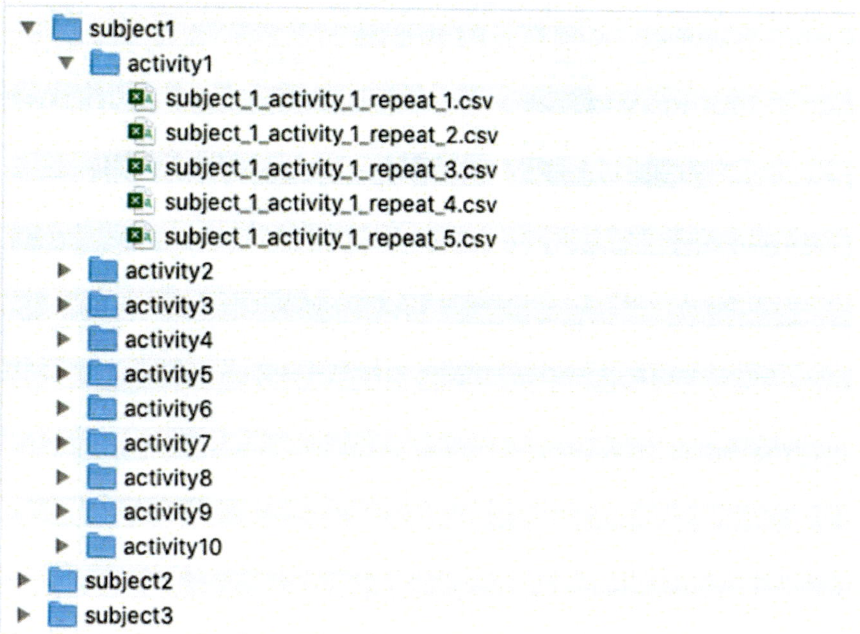

Fig. 2 Folder structure for the dataset

- Team Boson Kona [9]
- Hurukka [10]
- Horizon [11]
- Nirban [12]
- GreenRoad [13]
- 2A&B Core [14]
- RitsBen [15].

3.1 Evaluation Metric

To evaluate the submissions, we used accuracy as evaluation metric. The accuracy [16] is obtained using Eq. 1,

$$\text{Accuracy} = \frac{\text{TP} + \text{TN}}{\text{TP} + \text{FP} + \text{FN} + \text{TN}} \tag{1}$$

In the equation, the meanings of TP, TN, FP, and FN are stated below.

TP —True positive
TN —True negative

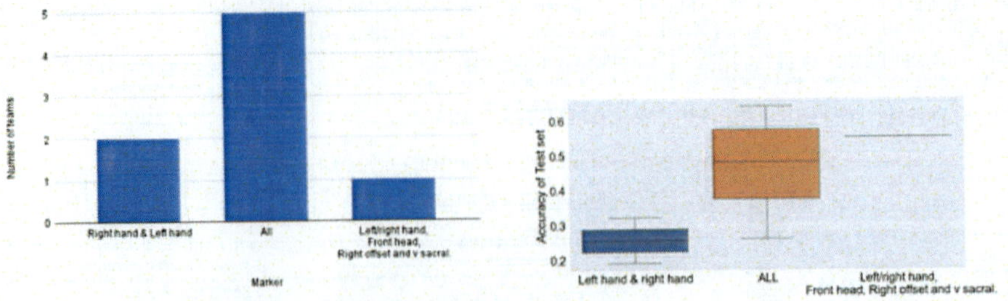

(a) (b)

Fig. 3 **a** Marker modalities used by teams and **b** Accuracy by different maker modalities

FP —False positive
FN —False negative.

3.2 Result

Usage of various combinations of traditional algorithms for classification, feature extraction by participants is observed in this challenge. Details of their used processes can be found in Table 3. As mentioned earlier, we provided data of 13 markers collected using motion capture system. Even so, the teams employed fusion of different markers and achieved several accuracies. Difference in the use of marker modalities is shown in Fig. 3. We can see in Fig. 3a that there are three types of teams,

- Used all the markers
- Used right and left hand
- Used left/right hand, front head, right offset, and V sacral.

In the analysis, it is perceived that the accuracy is higher when all makers are used (Fig. 3b).

Several algorithms are used by the participant teams. Just like previous challenges, in this one, we also observed use of random forest algorithm by different teams. Among the teams, five used machine learning (ML) algorithms, one used ensemble method, and one used deep learning (DL) algorithm (Fig. 4).

As for the implementation, all of the teams used Python. In the previous challenges [17, 18], wide employment of Python was also observed. In Fig. 5, the libraries which are used by multiple teams are shown in the figure.

The accuracy comparison of training and testing data is demonstrated in Fig. 6. Team Hurukka has almost same accuracy for training and testing. Team 2A&B and Team Boson Kona managed to achieve testing accuracy that is quite close with the training accuracy. However, in the most cases, training accuracy is higher than the testing accuracy. Team RitsBen was different in this case, because they had

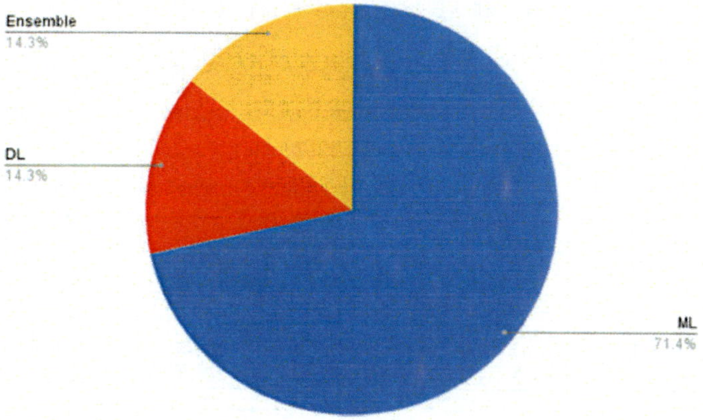

Fig. 4 ML and DL pipelines used by teams

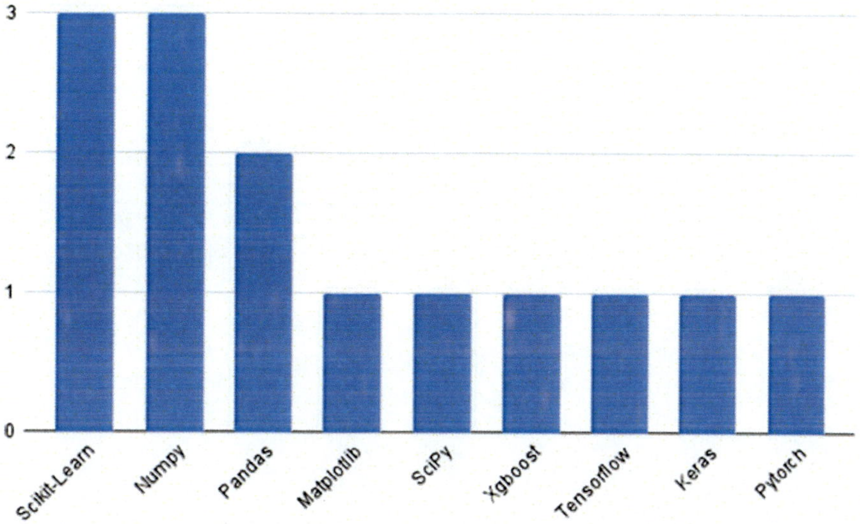

Fig. 5 Used libraries by teams

higher testing accuracy than in the training data. In spite of that, their training and testing accuracies were quite lower than the other teams. The team used LSTM for classification. According to the team, the reason can be mislabeling of several samples. However, according to our observations from different challenges organized by us, we can state that DL algorithms perform good when the amount of training data is large. In the case of limited training data and simple activities, ML algorithms perform far better. Another possible reason can be, using all of the markers gives better learning information. Team Horizon and GreenRoad attained very bizarre train-test accuracy combination despite having used same classifier (random forest) and markers. We assume that use of different feature set may have played a role here.

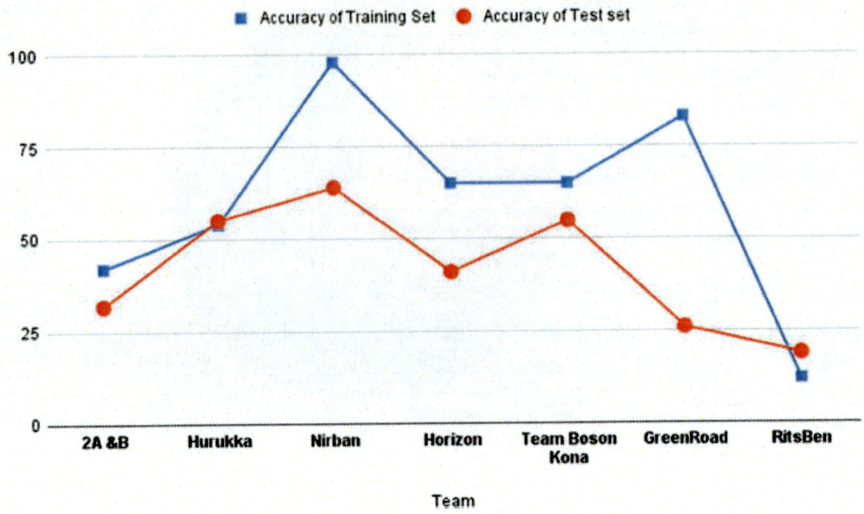

Fig. 6 Accuracy comparison of training and testing data

Table 2 F_1-score (%) of each activity by each team

Activity	2A&B Core	Hurukka	Nirban	Horizon	Boson Kona	GreenRoad	RitsBen
1	0.0	54.5	72.7	54.5	0.0	0.0	22.2
2	50.0	0.0	33.3	0.0	57.1	0.0	0.0
3	47.1	61.5	71.4	88.9	62.5	33.3	20.0
4	0.0	40.0	57.1	50.0	57.1	0.0	25.0
5	80.0	72.7	57.1	75.0	44.4	72.7	0.0
6	0.0	0.0	60.0	26.7	75.0	21.1	66.7
7	0.0	44.4	33.3	0.0	0.0	0.0	25.0
8	0.0	60.0	40.0	40.0	33.3	0.0	25.0
9	0.0	66.7	90.9	0.0	90.9	13.3	0.0
10	35.7	88.9	83.3	57.1	76.9	53.3	0.0
Average (macro-)	21.3	49.9	59.9	39.2	49.7	19.4	18.4

F_1-scores for each of the activity classes for all the teams are shown in Table 2. From the table, we can see that, Team 2A&B Core, GreenRoad, and Ritsben failed to identify many activity classes, thus leading to lower overall F_1-score. The other teams could identify most of the classes with comparatively better score. It is also observed that Activity class 5 (failed to put ingredients (inward)) has higher F_1-score compared to the other activities. However, Activity class 7 (turn over Bento box (inward)) has lower F_1-score in all teams.

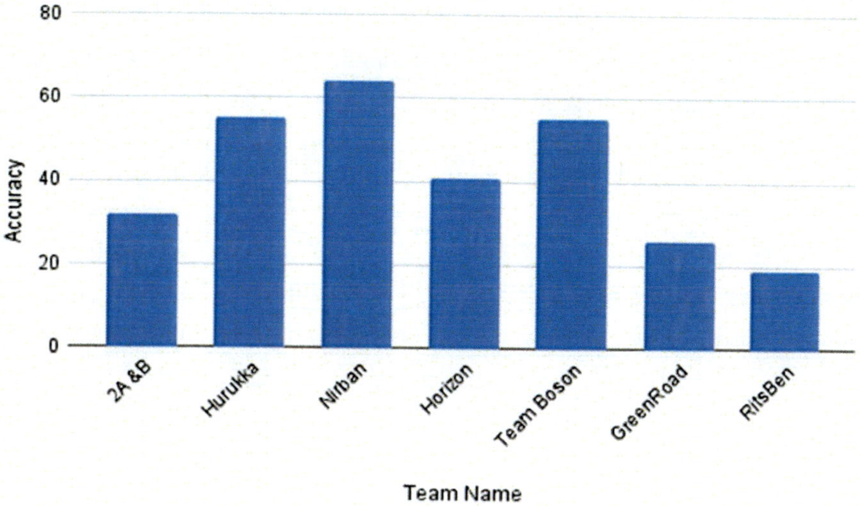

Fig. 7 Testing accuracy of each teams

Testing accuracy comparison for all the participant teams can be seen in Fig. 7. There we can see that Team Nirban achieved the highest accuracy among all the teams.

The confusion matrix on test data for the winning team is shown in Fig. 8. From the confusion matrix, misidentification of same type of activity between inward and outward can be found. So, in the future, for the betterment of testing accuracy, prediction model that works on small dataset should be developed. Also, more data collection in this scenario for each of the classes could help a lot to improve the overall accuracy. Furthermore, if the model identifies on intra-class similarity and focuses on differentiating these, it can result in an improved accuracy.

4 Conclusion

After summarizing the results of this challenge, we can say that all of the teams performed good, and the prediction accuracy varied between 19 and 64%. The winning team used an ensemble model and achieved high F_1-score for each of the activity compared to the other teams, which can be said to be the decisive factor. However, some teams had lower accuracy because of failure to identify all of the activity classes properly. So, it is important to recognize each activity rightly. In addition, cross-validation used by the participants is also important for evaluating the model. Because in this challenge, we provided test data of different subject than that was included in the training data. Therefore, the participant has to take into consideration to create a user-independent model. As a result, the participant who used leave-one-

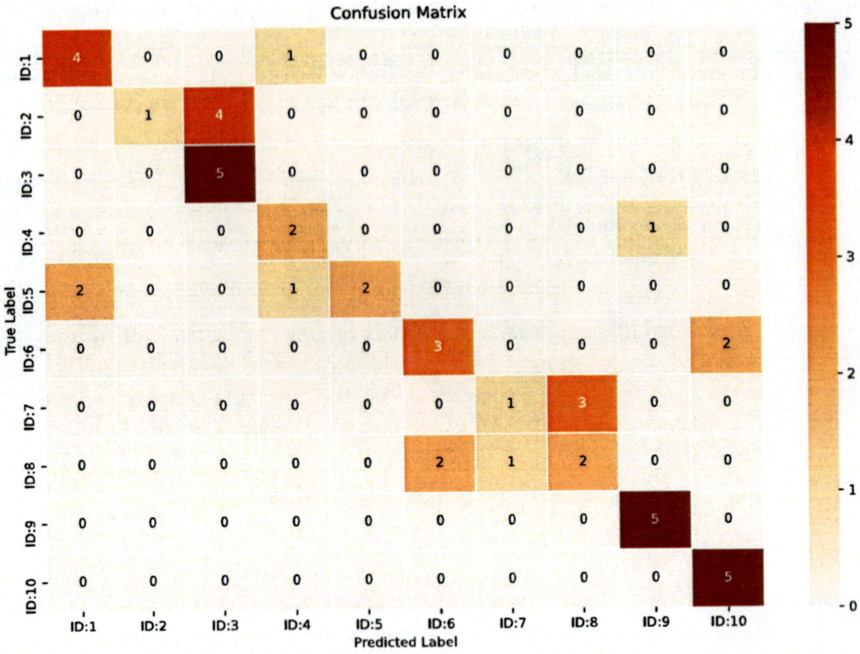

Fig. 8 Confusion matrix of the winning team

out cross-validation has a little accuracy divergence between training and testing data. This challenge aimed to recognize Bento packing sessions in anticipation of HAR for HRC. But, not only recognition accuracy but also subject usability and quick response are important viewpoints. To accelerate researching HAR for HRC, we want to collect data with collaborative robots using various sensors and share it with young researchers for more interesting results and observations.

Appendix

See Table 3.

Table 3 Details of each team

Team	Algorithm	Modalities	Programming language	Libraries	Classifier	Window size	Accuracy of training set	Accuracy of testing set	Training time	Testing time	RAM	CPU	GPU
2A&B [14]	ML	Left hand, Right hand	Python	Sklearn, NumPy, Pandas	KNN		42%	32%	3.1473 s	0.0027 s	25 GB	Xeon @2.2 GHz	NA
Hurukka [10]	ML	All	Python	Sklearn, NumPy, Pandas, Matplotlib	Extremely randomized trees	5 s	54%	55%	60 s	60 s	25 GB	Xeon @2.20 GHz	NA
Nirban [12]	Ensemble	All	Python	Pandas, NumPy, SciPy, Sklearn, XGBoost, TensorFlow, Keras	Ensemble		98%	64%	720 s	180 s	8 GB	i5 @2.50 GHz	NA
Horizon [11]	ML	All	Python	Sklearn, NumPy, Pandas, Matplotlib	Random forest	5 s	65%	41%	60 s	60 s	25 GB	Xeon @2.2 GHz	NA

(continued)

Table 3 (continued)

Team	Algorithm	Modalities	Programming language	Libraries	Classifier	Window size	Accuracy of training set	Accuracy of testing set	Training time	Testing time	RAM	CPU	GPU
Boson Kona [9]	ML	Front head, Right shoulder, Right elbow, Right wrist, Left shoulder, Left elbow, Left wrist, Right offset, V sacral.	Python	NumPy, Pandas, SciPy, Sklearn, Matplotlib	Extra tree	2000	65%	55%	103.49 s	0.41 s	8 GB	i5 @2.30 GHz	NA
GreenRoad [13]	ML	All	Python	NumPy, Pandas, Matplotlib, Scikit-learn, SciPy	Random forest		83%	26%	648 s	180 s	8 GB	i7 @2.20 GHz	NA
RitsBen [15]	DL	Right shoulder, Right elbow, Right wrist, Left shoulder, Left elbow, Left wrist,	Python	Statsmodels PyTorch	LSTM	0.4 s	12%	19%	1112 s	5.58 s	128 GB	i9 @3.70 GHz	RTX 3060

References

1. Liu, L., Peng, Y., Wang, S., Liu, M., Huang, Z.: Complex activity recognition using time series pattern dictionary learned from ubiquitous sensors. Inf. Sci. **340–341**, 41–57 (2016). https://doi.org/10.1016/j.ins.2016.01.020; https://sciencedirect.com/science/article/pii/S0020025516000311
2. Lee, S.U., Hofmann, A., Williams, B.: A model-based human activity recognition for human–robot collaboration. In: 2019 IEEE/RSJ International Conference on Intelligent Robots and Systems (IROS), pp. 736–743 (2019). https://doi.org/10.1109/IROS40897.2019.8967650
3. Roitberg, A., Perzylo, A., Somani, N., Giuliani, M., Rickert, M., Knoll, A.: Human activity recognition in the context of industrial human–robot interaction. In: Signal and Information Processing Association Annual Summit and Conference (APSIPA), Asia-Pacific, pp. 1–10 (2014). https://doi.org/10.1109/APSIPA.2014.7041588
4. Alia, S.S., Lago, P., Takeda, S., Adachi, K., Benaissa, B., Ahad, M.A.R., Inoue, S.: Summary of the cooking activity recognition challenge, pp. 1–13. Springer, Singapore (2021). https://doi.org/10.1007/978-981-15-8269-1_1
5. Damen, D., Doughty, H., Farinella, G.M., Fidler, S., Furnari, A., Kazakos, E., Moltisanti, D., Munro, J., Perrett, T., Price, W., Wray, M.: Scaling egocentric vision: the epic-kitchens dataset. In: European Conference on Computer Vision (ECCV) (2018)
6. Fabian Caba Heilbron Victor Escorcia, B.G., Niebles, J.C.: Activitynet: a large-scale video benchmark for human activity understanding. In: Proceedings of the IEEE Conference on Computer Vision and Pattern Recognition, pp. 961–970 (2015)
7. Wikipedia: Bento—Wikipedia, the free encyclopedia. http://en.wikipedia.org/w/index.php?title=Bento&oldid=1040941536 (2021). Online; Accessed 11 Oct 2021
8. Motion Capture Company. http://motionanalysis.com/movement-analysis/
9. Yeasin Arafat Pritom Md. Sohanur Rahman, H.R.R.M.A.K., Ahad, M.A.R.: Lunch-box preparation activity understanding from mocap data using handcrafted features. In: Bento Packaging Activity Recognition Challenge
10. Adrita Anwar Malisha Islam Tapotee, P.S., Ahad, M.A.R.: Identification of food packaging activity using mocap sensor data. In: Bento Packaging Activity Recognition Challenge
11. Faizul Sayem Md. Mamun Sheikh, M.A.R.A.: Bento packaging activity recognition based on statistical features. In: Bento Packaging Activity Recognition Challenge
12. Promit Basak, A.H.M., Nazmus Sakib, S.M.T.S.D.U.M.A.R.A.: Can ensemble of classifiers provide better recognition results in packaging activity? In: Bento Packaging Activity Recognition Challenge
13. Jahir Ibna Rafiq Shamaun Nabi, A.A., Hossain, S.: Bento packaging activity recognition from motion capture data. In: Bento Packaging Activity Recognition Challenge
14. Björn Friedrich Tetchi Ange-Michel Orsot, A.H.: Using k-nearest-neighbours feature selection for activity recognition. In: Bento Packaging Activity Recognition Challenge
15. Fujii, A., Yoshida, K., K.S.K.M.: Bento packaging activity recognition with convolutional lstm using autocorrelation function and majority vote. In: Bento Packaging Activity Recognition Challenge
16. Powers, D.: Evaluation: from precision, recall and f-factor to roc, informedness, markedness & correlation. Mach. Learn. Technol. **2** (2008)
17. Alia, S.S., Lago, P., Adachi, K., Tahera Hossain, Goto, H., Okita, T., Inoue, S.: Summary of the 2nd nurse care activity recognition challenge using lab and field data. In: UbiComp/ISWC'20 Adjunct: ACM International Joint Conference on Pervasive and Ubiquitous Computing and ACM International Symposium on Wearable Computers. ACM (2020)
18. Alia, S.S., Lago, P., Takeda, S., Adachi, K., Benaissa, B., Ahad, M.A.R., Inoue, S.: Summary of the cooking activity recognition challenge. In: Human Activity Recognition Challenge. Springer, Berlin (2020)

Author Index

M. A. R. Ahad et al. (eds.), *Sensor- and Video-Based Activity and Behavior Computing*, Smart Innovation, Systems and Technologies 291,
https://doi.org/10.1007/978-981-19-0361-8